# THE PSYCHOLOGY
# OF JEALOUSY AND ENVY

# THE PSYCHOLOGY
# OF JEALOUSY
# AND ENVY

Edited by

**Peter Salovey, PhD**
*Yale University*

THE GUILFORD PRESS
New York        London

© 1991 The Guilford Press
A Division of Guilford Publications, Inc.
72 Spring Street, New York, NY 10012

Printed in the United States of America

This book is printed on acid-free paper.

Last digit is print number:  9 8 7 6 5 4 3 2 1

**Library of Congress Cataloging-in-Publication Data**

The Psychology of jealousy and envy / edited by Peter Salovey.
    p.  cm.
    Includes bibliographical references and index.
    ISBN 0-89862-555-6
    1. Jealousy.  2. Envy.    I. Salovey, Peter.
  BF575.J4P79  1991
  152.4—dc20               90-23329
                               CIP

*For David L. Rosenhan and Judith Rodin, my mentors:*
*David sowed the seeds of my interest in jealousy and envy;*
*Judy cultivated and nourished what followed.*

# About the Contributors

**Robert G. Bringle** is an associate professor of psychology at Purdue University at Indianapolis. His research interests include interpersonal processes, evaluation of social and health problems, cognitive development, and the social psychology of aging. Correspondence can be addressed to: Department of Psychology, Indiana University–Purdue University at Indianapolis, 1125 East 38th Street, P.O. Box 647, KB54, Indianapolis, IN 46223.

**Jeff B. Bryson** completed his undergraduate work at the University of Texas at Austin and received a Ph.D. in social psychology from Purdue University. He is currently a professor of psychology at San Diego State University, where he is continuing his research on the personal, interpersonal, and cultural factors that influence reactions to jealousy-evoking situations. Correspondence can be addressed to: Department of Psychology, San Diego State University, San Diego, CA 92182-0350.

**Bram P. Buunk** is a professor of social psychology in the Department of Psychology at the University of Groningen, The Netherlands. His research interests are mainly in the area of close relationships, and include topics such as marital satisfaction, friendship, jealousy, alternative lifestyles, sex roles, and cross-cultural perspectives. Correspondence can be addressed to: Psychologisch Institut Heymans, Social and Organisational Psychology, University of Groningen, Grote Kruisstraat 2/1, 9712 TS Groningen, The Netherlands.

**Gordon Clanton** teaches sociology at San Diego State University. His 1977 book, *Jealousy* (with Lynn G. Smith), encouraged the social-scientific study of jealousy and contributed to the emergence of the study of emotions as a new specialty within sociology. Educated at the University of California–Berkeley in the late 1960s, Dr. Clanton also taught at Rutgers University. His research interests include the social psychology of emotions (especially love, jealousy, envy, and anger) and the dysfunctions of bureaucratic organizations. Correspondence can be addressed to: Department of Sociology, San Diego State University, San Diego, CA 92182.

**Gary L. Hansen** received his Ph.D. in sociology from Iowa State University in 1978. He is currently an associate extension professor in the Department of Sociology at the University of Kentucky. His research interests include the social-psychological aspects of emotions, the marital adjustment process, and rural families. Correspondence can be addressed to: Department of Sociology, University of Kentucky, 500 ASCS, Lexington, KY 40546-0215.

**Ralph B. Hupka** is a staff member of the Department of Psychology at California State University–Long Beach. He received his Ph.D. at the University of Massachusetts in 1969 in experimental psychology with a focus on classical conditioning. His current research interests are jealousy and the cross-cultural determinants of emotion. Correspondence can be addressed to: Department of Psychology, California State University–Long Beach, Long Beach, CA 90840-0901.

**David J. Kosins** is a licensed clinical psychologist in private practice in Seattle, Washington. Trained at the California School for Professional Psychology, San Diego, Dr. Kosins specializes in cognitive therapy for depression, treatment of anxiety and stress disorders, and group psychotherapy. Correspondence can be addressed to: P.O. Box 9014, Seattle, WA 98109.

**Eugene W. Mathes** received his doctorate in psychology, focusing on personality and social psychology, from Iowa State University in 1973. Since then, he has been a member of the Department of Psychology at Western Illinois University. His research interests include jealousy, romantic love, physical attractiveness, peak experiences, religion, values, and personality transformation. Correspondence can be addressed to: Department of Psychology, Western Illinois University, Waggoner Hall 100, Macomb, IL 61455.

**W. Gerrod Parrott** received his Ph.D. in psychology from the University of Pennsylvania in 1985 and is presently an assistant professor of psychology at Georgetown University. His scholarly interests center on the relation between emotion and cognition, and include research on cognitively complex social emotions and what they reveal about the self, the social world, and the nature of emotion. He also studies the effects of moods on memory, the self-regulation of mood, and the theory of cognition's role in emotion. Correspondence can be addressed to: Department of Psychology, Georgetown University, Washington, DC 20057.

**Alexander Rothman** is a doctoral candidate in social psychology at Yale University. His research interests include the implicit perception of social information and its influence on attitude formation and change. He is also concerned with intergroup behavior, especially the relationship between social identity and intergroup conflict. Correspondence can be addressed to: Department of Psychology, Yale University, Box 11A Yale Station, New Haven, CT 06520-7447.

**Peter Salovey** received his Ph.D. in clinical psychology from Yale University in 1986, where he is presently an associate professor contributing to both the social/personality and clinical psychology programs. His major research interest is the functions of human emotion, especially the ways in which emotions direct cognition, motivate social behavior, and color close relationships. Most recently, he has been concerned with complex emotions such as envy and jealousy, and the influence of emotions on perceptions of health and illness. Correspondence can be addressed to: Department of Psychology, Yale University, Box 11A Yale Station, New Haven, CT 06520-7447.

**Don J. Sharpsteen** received his doctorate in social psychology from the University of Denver and is currently an assistant professor of psychology at the University of Missouri at Rolla. His primary research interests are in the areas of emotions and close relationships, especially as they merge in the study of both jealousy and gossip. Correspondence can be addressed to: Department of Psychology, University of Missouri, Rolla, MO 65401-0249.

**Richard H. Smith** is an assistant professor in the Psychology Department at Boston University. He completed his doctoral work in social psychology at the University of North Carolina at Chapel Hill. After a postdoctoral fellowship in personality and social ecology at the University of Illinois at Urbana–Champaign, he took his present position at Boston University. Smith's research interests include social comparison processes, attribution theory, and social psychological factors affecting health. Correspondence can be addressed to: Department of Psychology, Boston University, 64 Cummington Street, Boston, MA 02215.

**Gregory L. White** is a social and clinical psychologist who received his B.A. at Stanford University and his Ph.D. at the University of California at Los Angeles. He currently directs the American Psychological Association-accredited clinical psychology internship program at Shasta Community Mental Health, Redding, California. His research and clinical interests include emotion, personality disorder, jealousy, stress and health, and the cultural psychology of contemporary masculinity. With Paul Mullen, he authored a volume on jealousy published in 1989 by Guilford Press. Correspondence can be addressed to: Shasta County Mental Health, 2630 Breslauer Way, Redding, CA 96049.

# Preface

Investigators interested in complex emotional states such as jealousy and envy quite commonly begin their chapters and articles with a brief lament: Why is it that major concerns such as these—concerns reflected upon by authors and playwrights, ruminated upon by philosophers, discussed on the couches of psychotherapists, and described on the glossy pages of the popular press—are virtually ignored by social scientists? I am delighted to feel no obligation to introduce this volume with a similar complaint. Although jealousy and envy have not received the thousands of person-years of research devoted to some other topics in psychology—from depression to causal attributions—it is now clear that scientists *are* interested in addressing these ubiquitous experiences. In the past few years, chapters on jealousy have been included in major anthologies of work on close relationships (Bringle & Buunk, 1986), as well as in the annual *Review of Personality and Social Psychology* (Bringle & Buunk, 1985; Salovey & Rodin, 1989). Integrative articles have appeared comparing various approaches to the measurement of jealousy or envy (Mathes, Roter, & Joerger, 1982; White, 1984). Moreover, a variety of books have been published recently as well—some directed toward clinicians (Bernhard, 1986), others aimed at educating the lay public about jealousy (Friday, 1985) or envy (Cohen, 1986), and still others offering new theoretical frameworks and taking stock of the entire research enterprise (White & Mullen, 1989).

After decades of banishment to popular magazines and advice columns, jealousy and envy, as complex interpersonal emotions, have certainly emerged as legitimate topics of scientific inquiry. This modern era of research was ushered in by a well-attended symposium at the 1977 convention of the American Psychological Association (APA), which included papers by Robert Bringle, Jeff Bryson, Ralph Hupka, and Gregory White, and a counterpoint by Gordon Clanton. In 1977, these individuals were essentially the only investigators committed to the scientific study of jealousy and envy, and their remarks were published in a special issue of a journal called *Alternative Lifestyles*. A symposium held 11 years later at the APA convention in 1988 provided an opportunity for several newer investigators in this field, Eugene Mathes, Gerrod (Jerry) Parrott, Richard Smith, and myself, to reflect on scientific progress in the area. Investigators from both the 1977 and the 1988 groups (Bringle, Buunk, Hupka, White, and myself) collaborated on a forward-looking symposium organized by Gregory White at the 1989 Iowa Conference on Personal Relationships. All of these investigators have contributed chapters to the present volume.

This volume represents the culmination of the recent interest in this field. The literature on envy and jealousy has grown to perhaps 100 empirical papers and several competing theoretical perspectives. It is now a viable field of inquiry among investigators of human emotions and among social scientists concerned with close personal relationships. The purpose of this volume is both to provide an exciting summary and synthesis of the research literature on jealousy and envy to date, and, primarily, to allow the major investigators in this field to state clearly their theoretical perspectives and particular contributions. The contributors have been asked to provide a coherent account of their work on jealousy and envy in the context of a specific jealousy/envy problem area (e.g., self-definition, marriage, culture). In this way, each chapter stands as an important integrative contribution, and we have avoided a series of chapters summarizing the same literature.

The volume is organized into three major sections. In the first section, jealousy and envy are discussed as emotions or as sets of beliefs that can best be described by examining individual personality processes. Part II focuses on the ways in which jealousy arises in the context of social interactions and close relationships. The broadest perspective is represented in the third section of the volume, covering family, societal, and cultural influences on the expression of envy and jealousy. Prior to each of these sections of the book, I have provided some introductory remarks in an attempt to acquaint the reader with the section's theme and highlight the major contribution of each chapter.

I would like to thank several people who helped make this volume possible. Most important is Seymour Weingarten, editor-in-chief at The Guilford Press, whose enthusiasm for the project never flagged. Our production editor at Guilford, Anna Brackett, has been enormously helpful as well. My research assistants during the past 2 years—Chloé Drake, Stephanie Fishkin, Sasha van der Sleesen and Michael Baron— have been an enormous help to me. The graduate students who collaborate on research with me at Yale University were instrumental in keeping the lab afloat while I attended to editing tasks. Finally, I would like to acknowledge the funding agencies that have supported my research during the past few years: the National Institute of Health Biomedical Research Support program (Grant No. BRSG S07 RR07015), the National Cancer Institute (Grant No. CA42101), the National Center for Health Statistics (Contract No. NCHS 200 88 7001), and the Presidential Young Investigator program of the National Science Foundation (Grant No. 9058020).

PETER SALOVEY
New Haven, Connecticut

## REFERENCES

Bernhard, K. F. (1986). *Jealousy: Its nature and treatment.* Springfield, IL: Charles C. Thomas.

Bringle, R. G., & Buunk, B. (1985). Jealousy and social behavior: A review of person, relationship, and situational determinants. In P. Shaver (Ed.), *Review of personality and social psychology* (Vol. 6, pp. 241–264). Beverly Hills, CA: Sage.

Bringle, R. G., & Buunk, B. (1986). Examining the causes and consequences of jealousy: Some recent findings and issues. In R. Gilmour & S. Duck (Eds.), *The emerging field of personal relationships* (pp. 225–239). Hillsdale, NJ: Erlbaum.

Cohen, B. (1986). *The Snow White syndrome: All about envy.* New York: Macmillan.

Friday, N. (1985). *Jealousy.* New York: Perigord Press.

Mathes, E. W., Roter, P. M., & Joerger, S. M. (1982). A convergent validity study of six jealousy scales. *Psychological Reports, 50,* 1143–1147.

Salovey, P., & Rodin, J. (1989). Envy and jealousy in close relationships. In C. Hendrick (Ed.), *Review of personality and social psychology* (Vol. 10, pp. 221–246). Beverly Hills, CA: Sage.

White, G. L. (1984). Comparison of four jealousy scales. *Journal of Research in Personality, 49,* 129–147.

White, G. L., & Mullen, P. E. (1989). *Jealousy: Theory, research, and clinical strategies.* New York: Guilford Press.

# Contents

xv

## PART II. THE EXPERIENCE OF JEALOUSY
## IN CLOSE RELATIONSHIPS

# PART I

# JEALOUS AND ENVIOUS THOUGHTS AND FEELINGS

At one level, jealousy and envy can be considered mental states of individuals resulting from the appraisal of certain provocative situations. Investigators considering envy and jealousy at this level are concerned primarily with the phenomenology of the emotional experience—what do envy and jealousy feel like?—and with the sets of beliefs that create vulnerability to these experiences. Part I of this volume contains four chapters that deal primarily with the thoughts and emotional reactions accompanying situations that provoke jealousy and envy.

In the first chapter, Gerrod Parrott describes such situations as "emotional episodes" that can be distinguished by distinct patterns of feelings. He integrates historical, philosophical, and literary analyses with first-person accounts of jealousy and envy that he has collected, in order to arrive at clear definitions of each. Parrott also provides very helpful distinctions as we consider jealousy and envy in the remainder of this volume. For example, he differentiates two types of jealousy, one based on suspected threats to relationships ("suspicious jealousy"), as compared to the emotional reaction experienced when the infidelities of one's partner are a foregone conclusion ("*fait accompli* jealousy").

In Chapter 2, Don Sharpsteen focuses particularly on jealousy, which he describes as an emotional blend containing primarily anger, sadness, and fear. He argues that jealousy may be most usefully viewed from a prototype perspective—in other words, that it is a category of emotional responding to which specific instances are more or less central. A prototype analysis has been quite successfully applied to a range of emotions and may be useful in the present context as well.

In the third chapter, Eugene Mathes uses Richard Lazarus's model of stress, coping, and emotional reactions to understand jealousy. In particular, he focuses on the importance of appraisals concerning one's loss of self-esteem and one's loss of the rewards provided by relationships as important cognitive triggers of jealous reactions. The situations in which jealousy is experienced are also determined by individuals' beliefs about morality, as well as by social expectations. Mathes presents results from several intriguing studies that he has conducted to underscore these points. One of these experiments involved asking people to describe the jealousy experienced by their pet cats and dogs; another study required that experimenters call students to ask whether they could date their boyfriends or girlfriends!

The final chapter in this section is a lovely analysis of envy by Richard Smith. Smith uses data from his own studies as well as analyses of literary works to pin down the hostile component of envious reactions. Smith argues that envy involves more than a discontent with one's own possessions or attributes; it also includes a hostility toward or resentment of those who have or appear to have advantages. Why is a sense of fairness and justice so important in envy? Smith provides some fascinating answers, based on his own research but also on intriguing descriptions of historical and literary figures.

## Chapter One

# The Emotional Experiences of Envy and Jealousy

W. GERROD PARROTT
*Georgetown University*

The principal task of this chapter is to present an account of the ways in which envy and jealousy are experienced. Both envy and jealousy can occur in several forms, which can be distinguished by the assessments and attentions of the person having the emotion. I contend that there is little that can be said in general about the experience of envy or jealousy. Envy and jealousy do not map as neatly onto the terms of emotion theory as do, say, sadness or fear; envy and jealousy exhibit greater variation in the conditions that elicit them and in the ways that people experience them. In order to speak clearly about these emotions, it is necessary to distinguish the important subtypes.

My analysis draws on a set of data being studied by Richard Smith and myself. We have collected several hundred detailed, first-person accounts of actual experiences of envy and jealousy, from subjects who were then asked to rate their experience on a number of scales. Analysis of these stories and of the data that accompany them has informed much of the account I present in this chapter, and I occasionally summarize the results of this research in support of my claims.

Underlying such an analysis of envy and jealousy are a number of conceptual issues concerning emotion, the relation between emotion and conscious experience, and the sources of emotional "feelings." These general issues need to be addressed prior to discussing envy and jealousy in particular.

## EMOTION AND EMOTIONAL EXPERIENCE

When people are asked to describe an actual experience of envy or jealousy, they usually provide a narrative of what I call an "emotional episode." An emotional episode includes the circumstances that lead up to an emotion or sequence of emotions, the emotions themselves, any attempts at self-regulation or coping that occur, subsequent events and actions, and the resolution or present status quo. In short, an emotional episode is the story of an emotional event, and it seems a natural unit of analysis for understanding human emotions. Most of the concepts in psychological theories of emotion are abstractions from the emotional episode: appraisals, "basic emotions," feelings, coping, display rules, effects of mood on cognition, cultural norms, and so on. These aspects may legitimately be studied in their own right, but to be properly understood, they must be returned to the context of the emotional episodes in which they occur (cf. Lazarus, Kanner, & Folkman, 1980; White, 1981).

Part of the difficulty in understanding envy and jealousy is in seeing how they map onto these narrower categories. Traditionally, the two are defined in terms that include the beliefs, motives, and emotional reactions of the emotional person, as well as the situations that evoke these responses (Parrott, 1988b). Envy may be said to occur when a person lacks what another has and either desires it or wishes that the other did not have it. It occurs when the superior qualities, achievements, or possessions of another are perceived as reflecting badly on the self. Envy is typically experienced as feelings of inferiority, longing, or ill will toward the envied person (Neu, 1980; Salovey & Rodin, 1984). Jealousy, on the other hand, may be said to occur when a person either fears losing or has already lost an important relationship with another person to a rival. Jealousy may be experienced in a number of ways, but typically these are thought to include fear of loss, anger over betrayal, and insecurity (Hupka, 1984; Mathes, Adams, & Davies, 1985). In analyzing envy and jealousy, I assume that the emotion people *experience* is determined by the cognitive appraisals that they make and by the aspects of those appraisals on which they focus their attention. This assumption is common to most cognitive approaches to emotion (for a review, see Smith & Ellsworth, 1985; for arguments concerning the consciousness of emotions and the role of attentional focus, see Ortony, Clore, & Collins, 1988).

Emotions, however, are not simply "feelings" or conscious experiences. Psychologists' conceptions of emotions include other elements in addition to experience, such as cognitive appraisals, social conventions, and physiological responses. These elements are conceptually distinct from conscious experience, even though they may in fact contribute to such experiences. Furthermore, as I discuss below, conscious experience is not always relevant to our use of emotion words, as when observers attribute envy or jealousy to others who do not believe themselves to be envious or jealous. Nevertheless, having certain experiences or "feelings" is often part of what is meant when a person is said to have a certain emotion, and it is sensible to speak of a person's having "feelings" of envy or jealousy. In this chapter I present a typology of these experiences.

Emotional experiences or "feelings" may result, in part, from changes in the body or from the activation of "primitive" or "noncognitive" areas of the brain, as some theorists have posited; however, it is important to note that emotional feelings can result from other sources as well. Feeling, as the term is used in speaking of emotion, may result from many high-level cognitive activities, such as having attention drawn to certain aspects of a situation, doubting, thinking hurriedly, and so forth (Parrott, 1988a). In addressing the experiences of envy and jealousy, I mean to include these aspects of experience, as well as those addressed by biologically oriented emotion theorists. I view emotional experience as inextricably bound up with such types of cognitive activity (Parrott, 1988a; Parrott & Sabini, 1989). This chapter concentrates on the perspective of people experiencing emotion: the manner in which they construe the situation, the aspects of the situation that they focus on, their evaluations of the situation, and their reactions to their own evaluations. These elements contribute to the emotional experience of envy and jealousy, just as limbic system activity or feedback from the body's periphery does (see also Frijda, 1986).

In focusing on emotional experience, I must distinguish those cases in which people are aware of being envious or jealous from those cases in which they are motivated by envy or jealousy yet do not know it. One important use of emotion words in everyday life is to explain a person's behavior (Peters, 1972). Both "envy" and "jealousy" can be used in this way: People may be said to be envious or jealous if their behavior is seen by others as being motivated by envy or jealousy. When envy or jealousy is meant in this way, no claim at all is made about the manner in which envious or jealous people are experiencing the situation—they may or may not realize that they are envious or jealous, and their feelings are irrelevant to the claim that envy or jealousy is the motive for their actions (Silver & Sabini, 1978b). In fact, it is easy to imagine situations in which an envious or jealous person is the *last* person to know that envy or jealousy motivates his or her actions.

In the case of envy, for example, one can imagine a woman who disparages the quick promotions given to her rival in the company as being obtained through obsequiousness, and is angry at this unfairness. This woman is *experiencing* anger. Suppose, however, that her friends see little evidence of the rival's obsequious behavior, and plenty of evidence of competence and hard work. They may interpret the woman's disparaging comments as being motivated by envy (Silver & Sabini, 1978a). So it would be fair to say that the woman is envious in this sense, but not in the sense of experiencing herself as being envious. The same can be true of jealousy. One can imagine situations (and recall numerous Hollywood plots) in which a man is made to realize his love for a woman by becoming sad or angry at the attention she gets from another man (sometimes a confederate of the woman) (see Neu, 1980). In at least some variations of this plot, there is a period in which the man is unaware that the source of his emotion is his love, and instead thinks that it is the woman's rudeness, ingratitude, poor taste, or some such thing. For both envy and jealousy, it seems quite correct to say that the person is envious or jealous *but does not know it.* I have more to say about this fact below, but for the moment I wish only to note the special case it creates for an account of the ways in which envy and jealousy are experienced.

These are the issues and assumptions that underlie my analysis of envy and jealousy. In the sections below I present a theory of the major types of envy and jealousy, after which I consider the distinctions between envy and jealousy.

## ENVY

Of the two emotions that are the subject of this chapter, envy is presently the less studied. This contrasts with the past, when envy was widely discussed as a perennial problem of human nature. For example, the well-known *Maxims* of La Rochefoucauld (1678/1959) include more on envy than on jealousy; a later, similar collection by British essayist William Hazlitt (1823/1932) contains numerous aphorisms about envy while neglecting jealousy almost entirely. In recent times, envy has been mentioned less often, and in fact the word "jealousy" has now come to be used frequently in its place, although the two emotions are quite distinct. The sociologist Helmut Schoeck (1966/1969) argued that the concept of envy has been actively repressed in the social sciences and in moral philosophy since the turn of the century, possibly because it is unpleasant to admit to. Yet Schoeck's thesis is that envy has an important role in all societies—that there are crimes of envy, politics based on envy, institutions designed to regulate envy, and powerful motives for avoiding being envied by others. Neglecting envy costs us a complete understanding of many interesting phenomena, so let us try to give envy its due.

At the heart of envy is social comparison, a common and powerful influence on the self-concept (Festinger, 1954; Heider, 1958). Much of our self-esteem comes from comparison with others (Morse & Gergen, 1970; Tesser & Campbell, 1980). When one's abilities, achievements, or possessions compare poorly with those of another, there is the potential for a decrease in one's self-esteem and public stature, and surely this is one route to envy (Heider, 1958; Silver & Sabini, 1978a; see also Salovey & Rothman, Chapter 12, this volume). Yet social comparison can lead to envy in other ways that have not been discussed as much. Social comparison can also stir up envy simply by heightening one's awareness of one's own deprivation, and it can promote envy by making salient the fact that one's own suffering is not shared by all.

Not all negative social comparisons lead to envy, however. Aristotle, in the *Nichomachean Ethics* and the *Rhetoric*, points out that envy is felt chiefly toward those who are our peers, for reasons having to do with notions of justice (Barnes, 1984). Spinoza (1677/1949, Part 3, Proposition 55) also noted this tendency, and attributed it to limits in what a person will desire. Contemporary research by Silver and Sabini (1978a) suggests that there are self-presentational reasons for this fact. People do not necessarily envy the Rockefellers' wealth, because the discrepancy does not reflect badly on them. It is only when the discrepancy between someone else's success and one's own failure serves to demonstrate or call attention to one's shortcomings that envy results.

Clearly, what Silver and Sabini demonstrated for public stature must be true for private self-esteem as well. A discrepancy between ourselves and dissimilar others does not suggest to us that we are inferior, whereas a discrepancy with persons who are comparable to ourselves in relevant respects provides strong evidence that our inferiority, not other factors, is the source of the discrepancy. This point was demonstrated experimentally in a study by Salovey and Rodin (1984), in which these factors were manipulated orthogonally in the laboratory. Undergraduates received either positive or negative feedback about a trait that was either

high or low in relevance to their self-concept, after which they anticipated interacting with another student who had performed well in an area
that was either related or not related to a subject's own aspirations. The
results suggested that symptoms of envy occurred in only one of the
eight conditions—the one in which students received negative feedback
about their abilities in a domain that was central to their self-concept, and
then faced interaction with a student who excelled in the same domain.
Other studies suggest that young children may experience envy with less
regard to the self-relevance of the aspects being compared. Bers and
Rodin (1984) found that envy was more associated with self-relevance of
comparison in children 10–11 years of age than in children 6–7 years of
age.

It is a fact of life that people are unequal. Certainly some inequalities
stem for injustice, but even in a just world some people would be born
with more beauty than others, some would receive more of a given talent
than others, some would fairly come to acquire more possessions than
others, and so forth. It is difficult to imagine that these differences among
peers could be made not to matter. When one contemplates how common
the situations promoting envy are, one appreciates envy's potential ubiq-
uity and influence.

Nevertheless nonsituational variables also influence the occurrence
of envy. The qualities that were once called "character" (and that social
scientists might today refer to as "personality variables") strongly influence whether a person succumbs to envy, even under the optimal conditions described above. Only if a person confronted with superiority is
predisposed to feel inferior and resentful, rather than inspired and motivated to improve—only if a person construes another's success as a
personal loss, rather than as a gain of a larger whole of which he or she is
a part—will envy be provoked by the circumstances outlined above. On
the whole, little is known about individual differences in susceptibility to
envy. Heider (1958) discussed some possibilities, including the ability to
make comparisons without inferring evaluations, the ability to join oneself with the other in a "we-group," and the ability to avoid the comparison of lots altogether. We (Smith, Parrott, & Diener, 1990) have constructed a scale designed to measure the propensity to become envious,
and have demonstrated that it successfully predicts envy both in the
laboratory and in everyday life. The scale has three factors: one that
assesses the frequency and intensity of envious experiences in the person's life; another that assesses feelings of inferiority; and a third that taps
resentment and perceptions of unfairness. The existence of these factors
suggests that the tendencies to feel inferior to others and to construe

one's shortcomings as due to unfairness predispose one to be envious. Further research on the characterological determinants of envy clearly remains to be done, however.

## Malicious and Nonmalicious Envy

Once the conditions for eliciting envy are met, the emotion can take several forms. I propose that at least six distinguishable emotions can be experienced as part of envy. This variety of envious experience can best be introduced by starting with a more general distinction, one between a sense of envy that is morally acceptable and one that is morally reprehensible. Since ancient times, authors have distinguished what I call "nonmalicious envy" from "malicious envy." The history of this distinction goes back to Aristotle, who distinguished envy from what he called "emulation." Modern authors continue to make similar distinctions. For example, Neu (1980) distinguishes "admiring envy" from "malicious envy"; Taylor (1988) distinguishes "admiring envy," "emulating envy," and "malicious envy"; and Rawls (1971) distinguishes "benign envy" and "emulative envy" from "envy proper." In inventing the term "nonmalicious envy" my aim is not to clutter the literature with additional terminology, but rather to reflect that Aristotle's emulation is not quite the same thing as modern conceptions of nonmalicious envy, and that such terms as "admiring envy" can be confusing. Aristotle distinguished emulation from envy by defining emulation as a longing, dissatisfaction, or angst

> caused by seeing the presence, in persons whose nature is like our own, of good things that are highly valued and are possible for ourselves to acquire; but it is felt not because others have these goods, but because we have not got them ourselves. It is therefore a good feeling felt by good persons, whereas [malicious] envy is a bad feeling felt by bad persons. Emulation makes us take steps to secure the good things in question, envy makes us take steps to stop our neighbour having them. (Barnes, 1984, p. 2212)

Aristotle's emphasis was that some forms of envy ("emulation") motivate people to improve themselves, whereas others motivate people to take good things away from others. When a modern writer such as Neu adopts such a distinction, much of Aristotle's meaning is retained, but the emphasis is altered to focus more on the roles of self-esteem and feelings of inferiority—notions that did not much concern Aristotle. An additional problem is that the term "admiring envy" is confusing, since admiration need not be present in it at all. For both these reasons, I think that "nonmalicious envy" is a preferable term for those varieties of envy that are, after all, distinguished primarily by their contrast with "malicious envy." Some authors do not consider nonmalicious envy to be envy at all. Aristotle did not, and neither do Schoeck (1966/1969), Rawls (1971), or Silver and Sabini (1978b); however, many authors do (e.g., Neu, 1980; Taylor, 1988). I follow this broader usage, in part because it is clear from my data that in everyday usage people mean the word "envy" to encompass both senses.

The focus of nonmalicious envy is "I wish I had what you have." It may be experienced in a variety of ways: as inferiority to the envied person, longing for what the other has, despair of ever having it, determination to improve oneself, or admiration of the envied person. The focus of malicious envy, on the other hand, is "I wish you did not have what you do" (Neu, 1980). Both varieties of envy are unpleasant, but only one seems worthy of envy's membership among the seven deadly sins: It is the malicious variety that earned envy that distinction. The focus of malicious envy is the removal or destruction of the envied object or quality. To the person suffering malicious envy, the marvelous car should be stolen or damaged, the virtuous person corrupted or killed, the beautiful face covered or disfigured. In malicious envy it is not necessary to desire what the other has—only to desire that it be taken away from the other. Nor is it necessary that the good fortune of the envied person be at the expense of the envier (consider envy of another's virtue). Malicious envy, however, may involve the delusion that the other is somehow the cause of one's inferiority, and thus of one's unhappiness (see Smith, Chapter 4, this volume). It thus may be experienced as anger or resentment over some alleged unfairness, and may be generalized to become hatred of the envied person. As Chesterfield said, "People hate those who make them feel their own inferiority" (Mahon, 1845, p. 9). It is this malicious form of envy that is considered a sin. For Aristotle, the evil of this envy was its desire to lessen the amount of goodness in the world, or, obversely, to experience joy at another's misfortune (an emotion for which there is no good word in English, but for which the Germans have a lovely word, *Schadenfreude*).

It should be apparent that there are strong similarities between malicious envy and anger. In fact, the distinction between the two rests primarily on whether the hostility is justified—a fact that illustrates the importance of including cognition and social standards in one's conception of emotion (see Fortenbaugh, 1975, for a discussion of Aristotle's position on this issue). If the superiority of the envied person results from what can reasonably be construed as unfair or unjustified actions (i.e., a transgression), then the anger it elicits may be considered to be justified, and may be called "righteous indignation" or "resentment" (the latter term was proposed by Rawls, 1971, to distinguish it from malicious envy). If, on the other hand, the superiority is not the result of injustice, then the anger is inappropriate and may be termed "malicious envy" (Silver & Sabini, 1978a).

The distinction between resentment and malicious envy is one that is made using the objective facts of the social world; in clear cases there will be agreement, whereas in ambiguous cases there will be debate (Sabini & Silver, 1982). At the moment an emotion occurs, however, a person may be wrong about whether anger is justified or not, and the distinction (mentioned above) between the explanatory and experiential meanings of emotion words may become relevant. In some cases judged by objective viewers as malicious envy, envious people may perceive themselves to be righteously indignant, not envious. They will be wrong in one sense, since the objective social facts will not support their claims of transgression or injustice; however, in such cases they will see themselves as justifiably angry or irritated, not as envious. In other cases of malicious envy, envious people may realize (to some extent, at least) that the anger felt toward the envied persons is unjustified. The perceptions of transgression that dominate their awareness and fuel their anger are not felt with total conviction, and are undermined to some extent by knowledge that their friends (or the judicial system) will not recognize their charges as valid. As much as one may *want* to believe that the person given the lead in the play is the pet of the drama coach, as much as one may *feel* that the newspaper reporter has been biased in giving so many more words to one's teammate, there may also be awareness of the self-protective function such thoughts can have and of the reasons to be skeptical about them. This awareness reduces the malevolence of the envy, or at least inhibits the envious person from acting on it. It may also bring on some guilt about unjustified ill will.

Awareness that anger is unjustified may also lead to a resentment that has as its object not the envied person, but rather the unfairness of life itself. One may feel angry at the fates for making some people beautiful without feeling angry at beautiful people for being beautiful; one may feel resentful of the fact that some children are born into families that have intact marriages or lots of money without blaming the children who come from such families. As William Hazlitt (1823/1932) observed, "Envy, among other ingredients, has a mixture of the love of justice in it. We are more angry at undeserved than at deserved good-fortune" (p. 169). Nietzsche (1880/1911) likewise noted the existence of what he called envy's "nobler sister":

In a condition of equality there arises indignation if A. is prosperous above and B. unfortunate beneath their deserts and equality. These . . . are emotions of nobler natures. They feel the want of justice and equity in things that are independent of the arbitrary choice of men—or, in other words, they desire the equality recognized by man to be recognized as well by Nature and chance. They are angry that men of equal merits should not have equal fortune. (p. 209)

## The Varieties of Envious Experience

Distinguishing malicious from nonmalicious envy illustrates how our concept of envy, in an important way, requires us to think in terms of emotional episodes, for in making this distinction we already are depicting envy as unfolding in time. Both malicious and nonmalicious envy start with social comparison—with the realization that there is someone who is superior to oneself in a respect that is of importance to oneself. From this point, a focus on oneself and one's shortcomings leads to some form of nonmalicious envy. At this point, one may also come to resent the unfairness of one's fate.

If, however, there is a focus on the envied person as a cause of one's shortcoming, the hostility and hatred of malicious envy will result. It is plausible in at least some cases to consider malicious envy to be the result of a defensive reappraisal of the circumstances, motivated by the desire to avoid feeling inferior. This possibility was advanced in the writings of Nietzsche (1887/1967), and can be seen in analyses ranging from José Ortega y Gasset's (1914/1961) discussion of failures in seeking truth ("Rancor emanates from a sense of inferiority," p. 35) to H. L. Mencken's (1922) essay on the antagonism of artists toward their critics ("Injustice is relatively easy to bear; it is justice that hurts," p. 101).

Such malicious envy may then be countered following consideration of the objective bases of one's interpretation, and feelings of guilt and shame may follow along with reappraisal of the situation. If malicious envy remains unchecked by any such objective reappraisal, the envious person will *experience* righteous resentment, not envy; this is the special case described above, which from an objective perspective may be called envy but from the subjective perspective of the emotional person will not be experienced as envy. Envy evolves over time; like many emotions, it does not hold still for the emotion theorist. Our concept of envy as an emotion refers to this set of objectively evaluated reactions—not to any single moment of experience, nor to any single sequence of experiences.

According to this analysis, we can distinguish at least six emotions that can be experienced as part of envy. This list is not meant to be

**TABLE 1.1. Emotional Experiences That Can Be Part of Envy**

| Emotional experience | Description |
|---|---|
| Longing | Longing for what another person has; frustrated desire |
| Inferiority | Sadness or distress over one's shortcomings or over inferiority to the envied person; anxiety over one's status; despair of ever obtaining what the envied person has |
| Agent-focused resentment | Resentment of a specific person or group; displeasure over their superiority; anger and hatred of those deemed responsible |
| Global resentment | Resentment of unfairness of circumstances or fate |
| Guilt | Guilt over ill will; belief that rancor is wrong; "enlightened malicious envy" |
| Admiration | Admiration; emulation |

exhaustive, but it does describe a substantial proportion of cases. Analysis of several hundred first-person accounts of envy confirms that emotional episodes of envy contain one or more of these six types of envious experiences.

First, envy usually includes an intense longing for what the other has. This longing is brought on by focusing on the desired object or quality, by being aware of how much it is desired, and by being frustrated in this desire both by lacking it and by knowing that another person has been able to possess it.

Second, when envious people focus on their own shortcomings relative to the envied persons, their thoughts include awareness of their inferiority and of the implications for their self-concept and their public stature. The "feelings of inferiority" resulting from such a cognitive focus include distress and sadness (due to the appraisal of shortcoming and inferiority) and anxiety (due to the prospect of undesirable future events and uncertainty about one's self). Interestingly, in the experiment by Salovey and Rodin (1984) described above, depression and anxiety were significantly greater in the envy condition than in other conditions.

When an envious person construes another's superiority as the result of a specific, objective unfairness, he or she may see the envied individual (or others) as guilty of a transgression that has caused this individual to be able to enjoy undeserved advantages that may rightfully belong to the envious person. Such a construing may well lead to anger or resentment over the transgression, and, quite possibly, to hatred of the envied person. I call this type of experience "agent-focused resentment," because it is a resentment of a specific unfairness for which a person or group of persons is perceived as responsible. Whether this type of experience can accurately be called "envy" depends on the correctness of the accusation from which it follows. If the resentful person is correct about the transgression that has occurred, then the person should not be considered envious, but rather righteously angry or justifiably resentful (Rawls, 1971). If, on the other hand, the accusation is unjustified, then this experience would be an example of "malicious envy."

When envious people focus on the unfairness of life itself, of the circumstances in which fate has placed them, then their experience is also one of anger and resentment. There is a difference in the object of the emotion, however, so this resentment is of a different type than agent-focused resentment—what I call "global resentment." Global resentment is experienced as anger about the unfairness of life itself—at the unfairness that mere luck can cause another person to possess qualities or objects that one desires for oneself. Global resentment is marked by an awareness that the envied person is not to blame for his or her superiority; that no one else is directly responsible either; and that if one were oneself blessed with this advantage, one would not be wrong to enjoy it as well.

A fifth way in which envy can be experienced follows from the knowledge that the ill will produced by agent-focused resentment is not warranted. In reaction to such resentment, the envious person may then feel guilty or shameful (cf. Mayer & Gaschke, 1988). This type of experience is characteristic of the moral struggle envious people may have with themselves. For guilt to occur, envious people must realize that their malicious thoughts are wrong or sinful. The occurrence of guilt often accompanies the beginning of attempts to inhibit malicious envy and to replace it with something more worthy of a good person. Agent-focused resentment that is accompanied by guilt about this ill will might be called "enlightened malicious envy." In contrast, malicious envy that is unaccompanied by guilt or other awareness of inappropriateness—that is, anger that is experienced as righteous anger but objectively deemed envy—might be called "unenlightened malicious envy."

A final form of envious experience is admiration, an appreciation of the envied person's good qualities. "Admiration is happy self-surrender; envy is unhappy self-assertion," wrote Kierkegaard (1849/1954, p. 217) in distinguishing the two. Although this type of experience does not fit the prototype (or definition) of envy, it does occur as part of episodes of envy. People whose envy has included feelings of inferiority and global resentment may experience admiration when they switch their attention from their own deficiencies and the unfairness of having them to the qualities of the person whose example has brought on these other experiences. Admiration is part of Aristotle's emulation—the reaction that Aristotle deemed the desirable one, the one that naturally occurs in the person of good character. Admiration may lead envious people to try to improve themselves, using the envied person as an example. So admiration has a place in a list of envious experiences.

Actual episodes of envy are hypothesized to consist of one or more of the above-described types of experiences. What experiences will occur will depend on how the situation is interpreted and what aspects of the situation are focused on. In principle, a particular episode of envy may consist of any combination of these six types of experience; in practice, certain combinations will prove more common than others, since certain of these experiences imply incompatible interpretations of the situation. For example, admiring and resenting the envied person would be expected to be relatively uncommon, while admiring and feeling inferior to the envied person would be expected to be relatively more common. These combinations can be examined empirically, either by having coders rate accounts of envy or by having subjects rate their own accounts. With either method, what I have consistently found is that inferiority and admiration tend to occur most frequently when agent-focused resentment is absent, and vice versa. Global resentment and longing seem to be consistent either with inferiority or with agent-focused resentment. Reports of intense guilt about ill will do occur, but are fairly uncommon.

These findings suggest that two basic determinants of the quality of an envious experience are whether one believes one has been unfairly treated and whether one believes that one's disadvantage is one's own fault. Our data suggest that when one's own qualities are seen as being responsible for one's poor showing by comparison with another, the most salient responses are those concerning feelings of inferiority as well as motivation to improve oneself. When unfair treatment is perceived, feelings of anger and resentment predominate.

## JEALOUSY

Jealousy is an emotion experienced when a person is threatened by the loss of an important relationship with another person (the "partner") to a "rival" (usually another person, but not necessarily so). A loss that does not involve the partner's starting up an analogous relationship with a rival does not produce jealousy. One does not become jealous when one's partner dies, or moves across the country; nor would one be said to be jealous if one were *rejected* by the partner without the partner's taking up a new relationship with anyone else (Mathes et al., 1985). The threat must involve the loss of the relationship *to a rival*, whether this loss is feared, is actual and present, or is a fact of the past. This latter point is often described, but rarely explained. Mathes et al. (1985) attribute the distinction between rejection and jealousy to "social custom." I argue below that there is more to the distinction than just this.

The commonest examples of jealousy involve romantic relationships, so it is important to realize that jealousy occurs in other types of relationships as well. Sibling jealousy is well known, and jealousy may also occur between friends, employees with the same boss, students of the same teacher, and so forth. The relationship need not involve love, and the rival need not even be a person: A man may be jealous of his wife's love of law school, a woman of her husband's new car (Tov-Ruach, 1980). What is always true is that jealousy involves a triangle of relations. One side of this triangle represents the relationship between two people, the jealous person and the partner; another side represents the relationship between the partner and the rival; the third side, the attitudes of the jealous person toward the rival.

Given the variety of relationships and rivals that can generate jealousy, it has proved to be something of a challenge to characterize just what threat they all have in common. It is not the loss of romantic love, since jealousy occurs in nonromantic relationships; it is not the loss of the public appearance of a relationship, since jealousy can occur if a partner is known to be attracted to another yet decides not to act on this attraction. One attractive characterization is that the threat of jealousy is the loss of another's attention—a hypothesis developed by Neu (1980) and especially Tov-Ruach (1980). Not just any loss of attention produces jealousy (one does not usually become jealous when the switchboard operator puts one on hold); it is a loss of what Tov-Ruach called "formative attention" that results in jealousy. Formative attention is attention that sustains part of one's self-concept. For example, if my regular chess partner begins playing chess with another player, I would not become jealous of the new partner unless my partner's regular company has been formative to me in some way. Perhaps his enjoyment of my play sustains my view of myself as an interesting, worthy opponent; perhaps some quality of my partner has helped me develop as a chess player; perhaps my partner's choosing me as his or her preferred opponent has allowed me to think that I have desirable qualities as an opponent that few others offer; perhaps my partner has a certain status among local chess players that has been conferred on me by merit of being his or her customary partner. It is because relationships with others can be formative in these ways that the threat of losing such a relationship can be so devastating to one's self.

One might say, then, that at the heart of jealousy is a *need to be needed*. This need exists because relationships with other persons create and confirm certain aspects of our selves. Certain aspects of the self are intrinsically interpersonal (Tov-Ruach, 1980). We think of ourselves as being fun to be with, sexually attractive, humorous, or worthy opponents. These concepts are meaningless when applied to a person who does not interact with others: There is no "fun to be with" without others to be fun with, no "sexually attractive" without someone to be attracted, no "humorous" without a laughing audience, no "worthy opponent" without another opponent. We need others not only to confirm these aspects of ourselves, but, in a real sense, to *create* these aspects of ourselves. A steady relationship involving these sorts of interactions is, among other things, a constant source of self-defintion. The threat of the loss of such a relationship is therefore the threat of a loss of self, not the loss of "property," as some have mistakenly claimed (e.g., Davis, 1936).

The fact that the prototypical cases of jealousy involve romantic love can be explained by the importance of the aspects of the self that are supported by this type of relationship in our culture. If one is jealous of one's chess opponent's interest in another player, the aspects of one's self that are threatened are not a central or substantial part of the self-concept (for most of us). On the other hand, if one is jealous of one's lover's interest in a romantic rival, the aspects of one's self that are threatened are both central and significant (for most of us). Interestingly, the most powerful jealousy of youth is sibling jealousy, and the relationship that appears threatened is the one that is most important—namely, that with one's parents. Surely one reason for the decline of sibling jealousy in adolescence and the ascent of romantic jealousy is the decline of parents and the ascent of romantic partners in sustaining the most important aspects of the self.

One approach to understanding the experience of jealousy is to define jealousy fairly narrowly, restricting it to a certain type of emotional experience. The advantage of this approach is that it will provide a fairly coherent category of emotional experience. The disadvantage is that in everyday parlance the word "jealousy" is used quite broadly, so a narrow definition will be useful as a technical term but will apply to only some of what is commonly called jealousy. Another approach is to define jealousy more broadly, which provides the advantage of including all usages of the term but also the disadvantage of conceptual looseness. The problem is that the situations that are said to cause jealousy tend to produce a variety of powerful emotions. If jealousy is defined broadly, as *all* of the emotions that tend to occur in these situations, then there will appear to be a bewildering variety of ways to experience jealousy. (I have found it convenient to define envy broadly in the preceding section only because the variety of experiences is tolerably small.) If jealousy is defined narrowly, then it will typically be only one of a variety of emotions that are experienced in the situations that produce jealousy. Below, I present one solution of each type. I find both to be useful—the narrower definition of jealousy because of its conceptual clarity; the broader one because of its usefulness in understanding the rich variety of experiences that occur during emotional episodes of jealousy.

## An Emotional Experience Characteristic of Jealousy

If jealousy were to be defined narrowly as a single type of emotional experience, I would propose that it be defined as a type of anxious insecurity following from the perception of threat to a relationship that provides formative attention. Perceiving such a threat makes a person feel insecure about the status of the relationship, and also about the aspects of the self sustained by the relationship. What distinguishes this anxiety from other anxieties is that it is at once a fear of losing a relationship and of losing one's self. If there is a unique experience corresponding to jealousy, whether romantic, sibling, or otherwise, it seems likely to be this feeling of fear and insecurity.

When jealousy is defined so narrowly, emotional episodes involving jealousy must often be said to include other emotional experiences as well. When the narrow definition is used, these experiences are best considered separate emotions that occur when the jealous person shifts the focus of attention to other aspects of the situation besides the threat of loss. On this account, jealous people are often also angry people, hurt people, depressed people, and even disgusted or happy people (Hupka, 1984), but when we speak of their being jealous we emphasize their fear of loss. The word "jealousy" is often meant in a broader sense, so the narrow definition is suggested primarily as a technical term that calls attention to an experience common to the many varieties of jealousy. An additional reason for considering this narrow sense to be central is that it is often the source of many of the other emotional responses that occur in jealous episodes.

## Suspicious Jealousy and Fait Accompli Jealousy

If the experience of jealousy were to be defined broadly, as a characteristic constellation of emotional experiences, then it would appear to take on a variety of forms. In order to make sense of this variety, several distinctions must be made between types of jealousy-inducing situations. The most important distinction concerns the nature of the threat to the relationship. Jealousy may occur when the threat is only suspected and its nature is unclear, or it may occur when the threat is unambiguously real and its effects on the relationship are known and achieved. When the threat is unclear or only suspected, we may call the resulting jealousy "suspicious jealousy," since the predominant reactions concern fears and uncertainties. When the threat to the relationship is unambiguous and damaging, we may term the resulting jealousy *"fait accompli* jealousy," since the threat is an accomplished fact, a thing that is known to be already done. In each of these situations jealousy may be experienced in a number of ways, but each situation is characterized by a different constellation of alternatives. This distinction is similar to one made by Hupka (1989 and Chapter 11, this volume), who has recently proposed that different experiences of jealousy follow from different levels of threat. Hupka distinguishes low, intermediate, and high levels of threat. His categories of low and intermediate threat correspond roughly to what I call suspicious jealousy; his category of high threat corresponds roughly to *fait accompli* jealousy. Hupka's emphasis on quantitative differences in level of threat differs from my emphasis on qualitative differences in the appraisals, motives, and concerns of people in these situations. Nevertheless, I consider his approach to be compatible with my own.

Suspicious jealousy occurs when a person believes that a partner may be transferring to a rival the type of attention that is formative in the relationship. The characteristic experience of this form of jealousy is that of anxiety and insecurity—the narrow sense of jealousy defined above. The importance of the relationship, the uncertainty concerning its status, and the jealous person's insecurity about the self create the anxiety, and this insecurity motivates the person to find out whether these fears are warranted. This motive, in turn, is responsible for a variety of cognitive symptoms that characterize the jealous person, including suspiciousness, inability to concentrate on other matters, ruminations and preoccupations, fantasies of the partner and rival enjoying a wonderful relationship, and an oversensitivity to slights or hints of dissatisfaction by the partner. These cognitive symptoms, I contend, are as much a part of the experience of suspicious jealousy as are the other aspects of anxiety (Parrott, 1988a). Other emotions may occur as well. It is not uncommon that the jealous person knows the rival, and focusing on that relationship may produce other emotional states; puzzlement, alarm, envy, anger, and hurt are commonly directed at the rival. I consider suspicious jealousy to be the prototype of jealousy. It accounts for the etymological relationship between "jealous" and "zealous," and it is most consistent with the usage of nonpsychologists (Hupka, 1989) and with historical usage. One of La Rochefoucauld's (1678/1959) *Maxims*, for example, is as follows: "Jealousy feeds on suspicion, and it turns into fury or it ends as soon as we pass from suspicion to certainty" (p. 41).

*Fait accompli* jealousy, on the other hand, is relatively free of anxiety concerning the status of the relationship—that much, at least, is usually clear. The characteristic experiences of this form of jealousy depend on the focus of attention. When the focus is on the loss of the relationship, the experience is one of sadness; when the focus is on the wrongdoing or betrayal of the partner or the rival, the experience is one of anger or hurt; when the focus is on one's inadequacy, the experience is one of depression and anxiety; when the focus is on the stress of coping with new social status, the experience is one of anxiety; and, let us not forget, when the focus is on the superiority of the rival, the experience can be one of envy (a point that has never been made more clearly than by Spinoza, 1677/1949, Part 3, Proposition 35). These are some of the common experiences found in our data, but they do not exhaust the possibilities by any means. Disgust, and even happiness or relief, can result from the proper focus of concern (Hupka, 1984).

One experience found in our data that is not much discussed in the literature is envy of the former partner. In *fait accompli* jealousy, people frequently see their former partners as being happy in their new relationships. They compare their own loneliness to the apparent happiness of their ex-partners; they compare the dependence and yearning they continue to feel for their ex-partners to the ex-partners' apparent lack of such need for them.

Under some conditions, it should be noted, suspicious jealousy can result in experiences similar to *fait accompli* jealousy. During episodes of suspicious jealousy, people vacillate between doubt and certainty that their suspicions are true. They usually feel unsure about what is true, but at some moments they believe their worst suspicions to be true, whereas at others they think these suspicions are most likely groundless and are the products of an overactive imagination. It stands to reason that when jealous people are feeling most certain that their relationships are actually threatened, their experience will most resemble that of *fait accompli* jealousy. Their beliefs may still have something of a provisional nature, because there may still be a lack of evidence, or because their partners may still insist that nothing has changed; but to the extent that the suspicions seem warranted, jealous people will tend to react to the likely loss of relationships in the ways that characterize *fait accompli* jealousy. The true distinction between these two forms of jealousy, then, is best described as a jealous person's subjective assessment of the threat, rather than the objective nature of the threat.

In our data, cases of suspicious jealousy are characterized by a greater salience of suspicion and distrust; by more fear, apprehension, anxiety, and worry; and by more intense feelings of being threatened and fearing loss. Cases of *fait accompli* jealousy, on the other hand, are characterized by more longing for what another has, and by more guilt about ill will toward others, both of which are symptoms of the envy that is often a component of this type of jealousy.

### Distinguishing Jealousy from Rejection

I can now address the question of how the experience of jealousy differs from that of rejection. First of all, note that the question is problematic only if jealousy is assumed to mean *fait accompli* jealousy (as was the case in the experiments by Mathes et al., 1985). Suspicious jealousy is clearly different from rejection, since in this common form of jealousy it is not clear that one has in fact been rejected. It is only with *fait accompli* jealousy that rejection and jealousy seem quite similar, since both involve loss of relationship rewards and loss of self-esteem (Mathes et al., 1985; White, 1981).

*Fait accompli* jealousy differs from rejection in a number of respects. First, as noted above, *fait accompli* jealousy may involve envy of the former partner. In contrast, when rejected, one may feel that one has failed to satisfy the partner and that one has lost a relationship that was desired; however, one's former partner is also without a relationship, may also be lonely, and may also be grieving and miserable (at least, one may hope that this is the case). A person who has been rejected finds some satisfaction in these facts, since the partner is usually perceived as the cause of his or her suffering. There appears to be a certain justice in the partner's also having to suffer as a result of having inflicted this suffering. With *fait accompli* jealousy, however, there is no such justice. The partner who inflicted all the suffering on the jealous person appears to be rewarded with more fun than ever. The partner appears to suffer no loneliness, no loss of affection, no loss of formative attention, no loss of the rewards of being in a relationship. The envy and resentment that this situation produces distinguish *fait accompli* jealousy from rejection.

A second difference is that jealousy may involve envy of the rival (Schmitt, 1988), whereas rejection does not. Thus, although rejection certainly can lower self-esteem, it does not present rejected people with rivals who appear superior in respects that are important to their self-concepts.

Finally, jealousy has greater potential for producing anger than rejection does. Although it is certainly possible for rejection to be accomplished in a manner that elicits anger, losing a relationship to a rival permits all of these insults and more, since the relationship with the rival may involve betrayal, and the public display of the new relationship may intensify the insult. Thus, the experience of jealousy can differ from that of rejection in a variety of ways, and these differences, plus the absence of rejection in suspicious jealousy, differentiate the two concepts.

### Jealousy of Relationships Past, Present, and Future

Independent of the distinction between suspicious and *fait accompli* jealousy is another distinction, based on the status of the relationship prior to the onset of jealousy-inducing threat. Our sampling of romantic jealousy reveals that although jealousy often occurs in the midst of an ongoing, committed relationship, it need not. Many instances of jealousy occur in response to threats to relationships that are only hoped for or are in an early, informal stage of development—for example, when a person to whom one is attracted but whom one has not yet approached seems receptive to the attentions of a rival. Other instances of jealousy occur long after a relationship is over—for example, when a former partner is spotted in a bar with a date. Three situations may be thus distinguished: relationships that are hoped for, those that are existing, and those that are already over.

When the relationship is merely hoped for, our data suggest that the most salient aspects of jealousy are likely to be wishfulness, longing for what another has, and embarrassment and guilt concerning the inappropriateness of more hostile jealous feelings that occur; notably nonsalient are suspicion, distrust, fear of loss, and upset over betrayal. When the relationship is existing, on the other hand, fear of loss, suspicion, and distrust are very much part of the experience, while longing and guilt are noticeably lacking. When the relationship is already over, longing returns as a salient feature, but guilt and embarrassment do not; feelings of betrayal, rejection, and suspicion prove to be as intense as they are when the relationship is ongoing.

Thus, jealousy occurs in a variety of situations, which differ in ways that significantly constrain the appraisals and concerns the jealous person is likely to have. Threats to relationships take on different significances when the threat is uncertain than when it is certain, as well as when the relationship is anticipated in the future than when it exists in the present or only in the past. Furthermore, even if these situations are considered one at a time, the experience of jealousy varies for the same reasons that the experience of envy does: The jealous person can focus on different aspects of the situation, and the focus can shift over time; the situation can be interpreted in different ways; and the person can cope with the situation in different ways.

## ARE ENVY AND JEALOUSY EXPERIENCED DIFFERENTLY?

In the analyses above, it has been taken for granted that the experiences of envy and jealousy are qualitatively distinct. There is considerable precedent for doing so. Philosophers, going back at least to Cicero's *Tusculan Disputations* (written in 45 B.C.), have argued that the two emotions are quite distinct. Recent arguments for their differentiation have been made by Sullivan (1953), Schoeck (1966/1969), Neu (1980), and Taylor (1988). These authors all agree on two things: (1) that envy and jealousy should be distinguished, and (2) that people frequently fail to do so. Let us consider each of these points in turn.

The arguments for distinguishing envy and jealousy are many. Envy occurs when another has what one lacks oneself, whereas jealousy is concerned with the loss of a relationship one has. Jealousy concerns relationships with other people, whereas envy extends to characteristics and possessions. In envy the rival's gain need not be at one's own expense; in jealousy one's own loss is someone else's gain. The most typical experiences of jealousy are fear of loss, suspicion, distrust, and anger; those of envy are inferiority, longing, and ill will. The hostility that accompanies envy is not socially sanctioned, whereas that accompanying jealousy often is, so the envious person's ill will may be accompanied by the belief that this hostility is unjustified and wrong.

Why these two emotions should be so readily conflated is best understood by considering some similarities between them. Both may involve hostility, although (as noted above) the betrayal of jealousy is frequently a legitimate transgression, whereas the resentment of envy is unsanctioned. Both also involve losses of self-esteem stemming from social comparison, although here too there are differences. As noted above, in envy the social comparison is made by the envious person, whereas in jealousy it is presumed to be made by the partner. Thus, in accounts of jealousy one often finds the jealous person wondering what in the world the partner sees in the rival; by contrast, the envious person *knows* what is superior about the rival. Nevertheless, the result is quite similar—a loss of self-esteem. Finally, jealousy and envy may frequently co-occur. Envy is frequently part of episodes of jealousy, and each of these emotions may lead to the other. The conditions that precipitate jealousy of one's partner may encourage comparisons with the rival, leading to envy. Furthermore, envy of a person may lead to thinking of that person as a rival for one's partner, and thus to the anxious insecurity of jealousy.

Given these similarities, one might wonder whether the average person makes distinctions between envy and jealousy. It seems increasingly common for the word "jealous" to mean *either* jealous or envious (Schoeck, 1966/1969). It would be permissible, for example, for a baseball player to say that he is jealous of his wife's attention to a handsome new rookie, and also for him to say that he is jealous of Nolan Ryan's fastball. The former situation fits the classic definition of jealousy, the latter that of envy, and yet the word "jealous" happily fits them both. Thus, people may not make much of a distinction between jealousy and envy.

In one study, my colleagues and I empirically investigated this possibility (Smith, Kim, & Parrott, 1988). Subjects were first asked to write a description of a situation in which they had felt either strong envy or strong jealousy; afterwards, they were asked to describe a situation in which they had felt whichever emotion they were not asked about initially. Raters then coded these descriptions for whether they best fit the traditional definition of envy or that of jealousy. When asked initially for envy, subjects by and large (93%) described envy, but when asked for jealousy they were less consistent, describing jealousy 75% of the time and envy the rest. Thus, the word "envy" seems to have a fairly fixed meaning, whereas the word "jealousy" seems to be capable of having a broader range of meanings. This interpretation received further support from the second set of descriptions subjects wrote. When subjects had initially written about jealousy, their subsequent accounts of "envy" mostly corresponded to the traditional definition (91%), just as with the first set of descriptions; however, when subjects initially wrote about envy, a large proportion of their subsequent accounts of "jealousy" (41%) were also about envy. This shows that the term "jealousy" did not necessarily *contrast* with the envy situations previously described, whereas "envy" did seem to imply a contrast with the jealousy situations previously described.

This study helps to clarify what ordinary people think about the sort of situations referred to by "envy" and "jealousy." Their conceptions matched those of scholars fairly well. The word "envy" evoked descriptions of situations in which one's personal qualities did not measure up to those of another; the word "jealousy" evoked some situations like this as well, but mostly descriptions of times when an actual or desired relationship (usually a romantic relationship) was threatened by another.

What about the affective experiences evoked in such situations? Do ordinary people share scholars' ideas about those as well? To find out, we gave subjects a list of affective states that have been theorized to be typical of envy and/or jealousy, and asked them to indicate for each whether it was more characteristic of envy or of jealousy. Subjects reliably rated most of these attributes as being more characteristic of one affect or the other. Envy was believed to be characterized by motivation to improve, longing, inferiority, and self-criticism. Judged as more characteristic of jealousy were suspicion, rejection, anger, hurt, fear of loss, desire to get even, and overall intensity. A number of basic affects such as anxiousness and sadness were among the several items that produced no reliable preference (Smith et al., 1988).

Thus, people do appear to distinguish between envy and jealousy, both in terms of the situations that produce them and in terms of the feelings that characterize them. There is a difference, though, between what subjects *say* they feel when envious or jealous and what they *actually* feel. There is one published paper investigating differences in actual experiences of envy and jealousy. Salovey and Rodin (1986) reported a series of three experiments in which they looked for different patterns of emotions or thought in the two; surprisingly, the most they ever found was that jealousy seemed much more intense than envy. Otherwise, envy and jealousy seemed to be experienced in basically the same way. The differences seemed more quantitative than qualitative.

Such a comparison presupposes, of course, that envy and jealousy can be addressed as coherent entities. The analyses I have provided above suggest that this is not entirely the case, and that one might be justified in asking "Which envy?" and "Which jealousy?" A global comparison of the experiences of envy and jealousy requires that certain assumptions be made about whether the types of envy and jealousy represented are typical of those experienced in real life, and whether it is informative to average across the various subtypes of envy and jealousy. Nevertheless, Salovey and Rodin's finding seems quite puzzling in light of the differences that have been postulated to exist.

There could be several explanations for this puzzling finding. One, suggested by Salovey and Rodin, is that "envy" and "jealousy" refer to different situations that both produce essentially the same sort of experience. Another possibility is that envy and jealousy co-occur much of the time, so empirical measures of one will be confounded by the presence of the other. Finally, it seems possible thtat the greater *intensity* of jealousy may serve to obscure differences in the *quality* of the two. Given that the typical case of jealousy seems to be so much more intense than the typical case of envy, comparing subjects' ratings of the two will show that jealousy swamps envy on most measures. But our notion of the *quality* of an affective experience is less closely related to the *absolute values* of the various affective components than it is to the *relative salience* of the components—the "affective profile" of the experience.

The accounts of envy and jealousy that I have collected represent a sample of real-life experiences. Subjects ($N = 149$) rated their experiences on scales designed to capture the differences between envy and jealousy (as well as their shared qualities). Examining these ratings of actual experiences of envy and jealousy clarifies these issues considerably (Parrott & Smith, 1990).

If one simply compares the ratings of envy and jealousy on these items, one finds a convincing replication of one of Salovey and Rodin's (1986) findings—namely, that jealousy produces more intense affective reactions than does envy. Of the 59 items, 32 were significantly greater for jealousy than for envy, while only 1 was significantly greater for envy (that item was "Others would disapprove if they knew what I was feeling").

In order to pursue the idea about relative salience, we equated the subjects' ratings for intensity by subtracting the mean of each subject's rating across all 59 items from each of his or her individual ratings. With these transformed ratings, one can again ask whether the envy and jealousy groups differ. If the same items are salient in both envy and jealousy, there should be no differences between the two groups on these transformed scores. On the other hand, any differences would suggest that there are qualitative differences between envy and jealousy that are not attributable to differences in intensity. What we found was strong evidence of the latter: qualitative differences. Overall, of the 59 items, 26 differed ($p < .10$); envy and jealousy were each greater in magnitude for 13 of these 26 (see Table 1.2). Feelings of inferiority, longing, resentment, and motivation to improve were more salient for envy than for jealousy. In addition, feelings of guilt about feeling ill will toward others and beliefs that one's feelings are unjustified were also more salient to the experience of envy. Jealousy, on the other hand, was characterized by a greater salience of distrust, fear of loss, self-doubt, and anxiety. So this analysis found some qualities to be more salient for envy than for jealousy, and others to be more salient for jealousy than for envy. To a remarkable extent, these differences correspond to those proposed by traditional definitions.

These results may offer a new insight or two as well. It is intriguing to note that three of the items, "inferior," "self-doubt," and "insecure,"

**TABLE 1.2. Questionnaire Items That Distinguish Envy and Jealousy (When Transformed to Equate for Intensity)**

| Envy | Jealousy |
|---|---|
| Feeling inferior | Afraid of a possible loss |
| Privately ashamed of myself | Threatened |
| Feeling unfairly treated by life | Rejected |
| Frustration | Worried |
| Bitter | Suspicious |
| Feeling wishful | Betrayed |
| Longing for what another has | Self-doubt |
| Others would disapprove if they knew what I was feeling | Lonely |
| | Uncertain |
| Embarrassing to admit to | Feeling degraded |
| Guilt over feeling ill will toward someone | Self-conscious |
| Feeling sinful | Insecure |
| At first denied to myself that I felt this emotion | Intense feeling |
| Motivated to improve myself | |

appear to have fairly similar meanings; however, the first was more salient for envy, whereas the latter two were more salient for jealousy. This finding suggests that a distinction might be made between different types of self-esteem, or between different routes to lowering self-esteem. "Inferior" implies that one evaluates oneself as comparing poorly with others, whereas "insecure" and "self-doubt" imply insecurities regarding getting along with others once they have judged one negatively. Thus, the data seem to confirm a point made above regarding the difference between envy and jealousy. In envy, one's own appraisal leads to dissatisfaction with oneself. In jealousy, the reflected appraisal of another leads to a lack of security and confidence.

## CONCLUSION

In what is perhaps the oldest recorded myth, the Egyptian myth of Osiris, both envy and jealousy figure as motives. In this myth, the god Osiris, tall, slender, and handsome, becomes king of Egypt. He marries his beautiful sister, and brings prosperity and civilization first to Egypt and then the rest of the world. However, Osiris has an ugly and evil younger brother named Seth, who hates him. Seth envies the attractiveness, power, and success of his older brother. Seth also has reason to be jealous of Osiris, since Seth's wife becomes so attracted to Osiris that she tricks him into sleeping with her and bears a child by him. Motivated by envy and jealousy, Seth sets a trap for Osiris and kills him (Griffiths, 1970). Envy and jealousy are as old as humanity, and apparently will remain. Their durable hold on us, and the problems they create for us, are what motivate us to try to understand them.

## ACKNOWLEDGMENTS

I am indebted to Richard H. Smith and Daniel N. Robinson for many pleasant discussions that helped develop my views on envy. I am grateful to both of them, and to Peter Salovey as well, for helpful comments on a draft of this chapter.

## REFERENCES

Barnes, J. (Ed.). (1984). *The complete works of Aristotle* (Vol. 2). Princeton, NJ: Princeton University Press.

Bers, S. A., & Rodin, J. (1984). Social-comparison jealousy: A developmental and motivational study. *Journal of Personality and Social Psychology, 47*, 766–779.

Davis, K. (1936). Jealousy and sexual property. *Social Forces, 14*, 395–405.

Festinger, L. (1954). A theory of social comparison processes. *Human Relations, 7*, 117–140.

Fortenbaugh, W. W. (1975). *Aristotle on emotion.* New York: Barnes & Noble.

Frijda, N. (1986). *The emotions.* New York: Cambridge University Press.

Griffiths, J. G. (1970). *Plutarch's de Iside et Osiride.* Cambridge, England: University of Wales Press.

Hazlitt, W. (1932). Characteristics: In the manner of Rochefoucault's Maxims. In P. P. Howe (Ed.), *The complete works of William Hazlitt* (Vol. 9, pp. 163–229). London: Dent. (Original work published 1823)

Heider, F. (1958). *The psychology of interpersonal relations.* New York: Wiley.

Hupka, R. B. (1984). Jealousy: Compound emotion or label for a particular situation? *Motivation and Emotion, 8*, 141–155.

Hupka, R. B. (1989, May). Components of the typical response to romantic jealousy situations. In G. L. White (Chair), *Themes for progress in jealousy research.* Symposium conducted at the Second Iowa Conference on Personal Relationships, Iowa City.

Kierkegaard, S. (1954). The sickness unto death. In W. Lowrie (Ed. and Trans.), *Fear and trembling and the sickness unto death* (pp. 131–262). Princeton, NJ: Princeton University Press. (Original work published 1849)

La Rochefoucauld, F. (1959). *Maxims* (L. Tancock, Trans.). Harmondsworth, England: Penguin. (Original work published 1678)
Lazarus, R. S., Kanner, A. D., & Folkman, S. (1980). Emotions: A cognitive-phenomenological analysis. In R. Plutchik & H. Kellerman (Eds.), *Emotion: Theory, research, and experience* (Vol. 1, pp. 189–217). New York: Academic Press.
Mahon, L. (Ed.). (1845). *The letters of Philip Dormer Stanhope, Earl of Chesterfield* (Vol. 2). London: S. & J. Bentley, Wilson, and Fley.
Mathes, E. W., Adams, H. E., & Davies, R. M. (1985). Jealousy: Loss of relationship rewards, loss of self-esteem, depression, anxiety, and anger. *Journal of Personality and Social Psychology, 48,* 1552–1561.
Mayer, J. D., & Gaschke, Y. N. (1988). The experience and meta-experience of mood. *Journal of Personality and Social Psychology, 55,* 102–111.
Mencken, H. L. (1922). *Prejudices: Third series.* New York: Knopf.
Morse, S. J., & Gergen, K. J. (1970). Social comparison, self-consistency, and the concept of self. *Journal of Personality and Social Psychology, 16,* 149–156.
Neu, J. (1980). Jealous thoughts. In A. O. Rorty (Ed.), *Explaining emotions* (pp. 425–463). Berkeley: University of California Press.
Nietzsche, F. (1911). The wanderer and his shadow (P. V. Cohn, Trans.). In O. Levy (Ed.), *The complete works of Friedrich Nietzsche: Vol. 7. Human all-too-human (Part II)* (pp. 179–366). London: George Allen & Unwin. (Original work published 1880)
Nietzsche, F. (1967). *On the genealogy of morals* (W. Kaufmann & R. J. Hollingdale, Trans.). New York: Vintage Books. (Original work published 1887)
Ortega y Gassett, J. (1961). *Meditations on Quixote* (E. Rugg & D. Marín, Trans.). New York: Norton. (Original work published 1914)
Ortony, A., Clore, G. L., & Collins, A. (1988). *The cognitive structure of emotions.* Cambridge, England: Cambridge University Press.
Parrott, W. G. (1988a). The role of cognition in emotional experience. In W. J. Baker, L. P. Mos, H. V. Rappard, & H. J. Stam (Eds.), *Recent trends in theoretical psychology* (pp. 327–337). New York: Springer-Verlag.
Parrott, W. G. (1988b, August). Understanding envy and jealousy. In W. G. Parrott (Chair), *Envy and jealousy: Experiencing and coping with negative social emotions.* Symposium conducted at the meeting of the American Psychological Association, Atlanta.
Parrott, W. G., & Sabini, J. (1989). On the "emotional" qualities of certain types of cognition: A reply to arguments for the independence of cognition and affect. *Cognitive Therapy and Research, 13,* 49–65.
Parrott, W. G., & Smith, R. H. (1990). *Distinguishing the experiences of envy and jealousy.* Manuscript submitted for publication.
Peters, R. S. (1972). The education of the emotions. In R. R. Dearden, P. H. Hirst, & R. S. Peters (Eds.), *Education and the development of reason* (pp. 466–483). London: Routledge & Kegan Paul.
Rawls, J. (1971). *A theory of justice.* Cambridge, MA: Harvard University Press.

Sabini, J., & Silver, M. (1982). *Moralities of everyday life.* New York: Oxford University Press.

Salovey, P., & Rodin, J. (1984). Some antecedents and consequences of social-comparison jealousy. *Journal of Personality and Social Psychology, 47,* 780–792.

Salovey, P., & Rodin, J. (1986). The differentiation of social-comparison jealousy and romantic jealousy. *Journal of Personality and Social Psychology, 50,* 1100–1112.

Schmitt, B. H. (1988). Social comparison in romantic jealousy. *Personality and Social Psychology Bulletin, 14,* 374–387.

Schoeck, H. (1969). *Envy: A theory of social behaviour* (M. Glenny & B. Ross, Trans.). Indianapolis, IN: Liberty Press. (Original work published 1966)

Silver, M., & Sabini, J. (1978a). The perception of envy. *Social Psychology, 41,* 105–117.

Silver, M., & Sabini, J. (1978b). The social construction of envy. *Journal for the Theory of Social Behaviour, 8,* 313–332.

Smith, C. A., & Ellsworth, P. C. (1985). Patterns of cognitive appraisal in emotion. *Journal of Personality and Social Psychology, 48,* 813–838.

Smith, R. H., Kim, S. H., & Parrott, W. G. (1988). Envy and jealousy: Semantic problems and experiential distinctions. *Personality and Social Psychology Bulletin, 14,* 401–409.

Smith, R. H., Parrott, W. G., & Diener, E. (1990). *The development and validation of a scale for measuring enviousness.* Unpublished manuscript.

Spinoza, B. (1949). *Ethics* (J. Gutman, Ed.). New York: Hafner. (Original work published 1677)

Sullivan, H. S. (1953). *The interpersonal theory of psychiatry.* New York: Norton.

Taylor, G. (1988). Envy and jealousy: Emotions and vices. *Midwest Studies in Philosophy, 13,* 233–249.

Tesser, A., & Campbell, J. (1980). Self-definition: The impact of the relative performance and similarity of others. *Social Psychology Quarterly, 43,* 341–347.

Tov-Ruach, L. (1980). Jealousy, attention, and loss. In A. O. Rorty (Ed.), *Explaining emotions* (pp. 465–488). Berkeley: University of California Press.

White, G. L. (1981). A model of romantic jealousy. *Motivation and Emotion, 5,* 295–310.

## Chapter Two

# The Organization of Jealousy Knowledge: Romantic Jealousy as a Blended Emotion

DON J. SHARPSTEEN
*University of Missouri—Rolla*

In this chapter, I propose that romantic jealousy is cognitively organized as a blended emotion. That is, people's mental abstractions (or prototypes) of jealousy, distilled from their experience with jealousy, share features with their prototypes of basic-level emotions such as anger, sadness, and fear. In this mental representation of jealousy episodes, the emotion-specific antecedents, responses, and self-control procedures associated with each of these basic-level emotions are interrelated (e.g., anger-like antecedents are linked to anger-like responses). The variables investigated by jealousy researchers often resemble the prototypic features of anger, sadness, and fear, and findings of some studies do suggest that emotion-specific appraisals generate emotion-specific responses. This cognitive organization has implications for social interaction, memory for jealousy experiences, and the approaches taken to studying and interpreting jealousy phenomena.

31

As with the study of emotions generally, the study of romantic jealousy has been fragmented; the antecedents, expressions, and consequences of jealousy have not yet been placed within a comprehensive emotion framework. However, recent research and theory in the field of emotion (Shaver, Schwartz, Kirson, & O'Connor, 1987) suggest that a prototype approach to understanding people's shared knowledge about jealousy would help to integrate research in the area. Shaver et al. explicitly assume that the emotion knowledge that people hold in common describes adequately, at least for everyday purposes, their common emotional experiences. That is, people's shared beliefs about emotional experiences reflect their similar experiences with emotions. A theory of romantic jealousy organized around people's shared knowledge of jealousy not only might provide a framework for existing research, but also might point researchers toward new avenues of study.

Shaver et al.'s (1987) approach to understanding emotion uses people's mental abstractions (viz., prototypes) of emotion events to describe the emotion process. A "prototype" is a set of organized features that characterizes the typical instance of a category of objects or events (Rosch, 1973, 1975). The prototype of a particular emotion (e.g., anger, fear) might include as its features the antecedents, responses, and self-control procedures most typically associated in the individual's mind with the emotion. To decide whether an event belongs in a particular emotion category, one can compare the feelings and behaviors associated with the event to the prototype for that emotion. If the features of the event resemble those of the prototype, and if they differ from those of other, related prototypes, then the event is considered an instantiation of the emotion. Shaver et al. found that people could reliably describe the antecedents, responses, and self-control procedures involved in a variety of emotional events. In addition, their subjects' use of emotion terms was found to form a three-tiered hierarchy. At the lowest level were the most concrete terms (subordinate-level emotion terms); at the highest level were the most abstract terms (superordinate-level emotion terms). Between subordinate- and superordinate-level terms were basic-level terms (viz., "joy," "love," "anger," "fear," "sadness"). Subordinate-level terms, such as "jealousy," were used to make finer distinctions between emotional experiences than those afforded by the higher-level terms. For example, "jealousy" was found to be a subcategory of "anger" in Shaver et al.'s subjects' implicit emotion hierarchy. This reflects the fact that most subjects sorted jealousy into emotion groupings containing anger-related terms.

Although jealousy's status as an emotion has been disputed by some researchers (e.g., Hupka, 1981; White, 1981c), its colloquial use as an emotion term (e.g., Friday, 1985) suggests the use of an emotion model, grounded in ordinary people's experience with emotion, in terms of which relevant research can be organized. That is, ordinary people use "jealousy" to label an emotion, and their understanding of the process of jealousy may be captured best by a model of emotion that parallels their use of the term. Because Shaver et al. (1987) have based their model on the common organization in people's descriptions of emotional experiences, their model may be most appropriate for the task.

## A COGNITIVE-MOTIVATIONAL MODEL OF EMOTION

Shaver et al. (1987) propose that ordinary people's mental representations of emotion concepts or categories are generic and script-like. In the individual's implicit model, emotion episodes begin with an appraisal of events in relation to motives or preferences. That is, one's motives and goals may be thwarted, advanced, or unaffected by the events being appraised. The outcome of that appraisal is the elicitation of emotional responses—action tendencies, expressions, subjective feelings, and physiological states—whose expression may ultimately be modified with the introduction of efforts at self-control. This model, based on perceivers' representations of emotional events, may be used as an organizational framework for talking about the events themselves.

Emotional responses reflect a person's appraisal of events vis-à-vis that person's motives, goals, or preferences. Emotion events are described by both concrete and cognitive antecedents (i.e., the elements physically or objectively present in a situation, perceptions of those elements, and assessments of their impact on motives and goals), responses and response tendencies, and efforts at self-control. Through experience with different categories of emotion events (e.g., anger, love, fear), people develop prototypes for those events. Through repeated exposure to jealousy (via television, movies, books, personal experience, etc.), and possibly, as Clanton and Smith (1986) suggest, through such events as the symbolic loss of the mother and sibling rivalry, people may distill jealousy's essential components (its antecedents, responses, and self-control procedures) and organize their understanding of those experiences into a jealousy prototype. Current theory and research on jealousy suggest that people's jealousy experiences, and thus their jealousy prototypes, have much in common with their prototypes for several basic-level emotions—in particular, anger, sadness, and fear.

## PREVIOUS CONCEPTUALIZATIONS
## OF ROMANTIC JEALOUSY

Several researchers (e.g., Bringle & Buunk, 1985; Constantine, 1976; White, 1981c) have proposed models of the romantic jealousy process that are similar to Shaver et al.'s description of emotion prototypes. These models share an emphasis on perceptions and interpretations in determining whether an individual considers himself or herself jealous, and on the links between these cognitive elements of the jealousy process and jealousy behaviors. Furthermore, each is consistent with Shaver et al.'s explication of the emotion process and emotion prototypes.

Based on clinical observation, Constantine (1976) described the jealousy process in terms similar to those used by cognitively oriented emotion theorists. In this model, "jealousy begins with perceptions, leading to interpretations, which generate feelings that may or may not be expressed behaviorally" (p. 385). An individual's feelings of security and interdependence in a relationship act as threshold mechanisms, determining whether a situation is interpreted as threatening the existence of the relationship. The threat of loss produces anxiety; actual loss produces emotional pain. These primary emotional responses may be followed by internalizing reactions such as grief, despair, and guilt, or by externalizing reactions such as anger, rage, and hate. At this point, jealousy behavior may emerge, unless the feelings dissipate or the situation changes. Obviously, this model maps onto the one described by Shaver et al. (1987), although the prototype approach will permit more specificity in describing the relations among elements of the jealousy process.

Other theorists, claiming that jealousy is not itself an emotion (Hupka, 1981; White, 1981c), have focused on the labeling of emotion as jealousy. According to Hupka (1981), emotional reactions are defined as jealous reactions by the situations in which they occur. For example, there are particular social contexts that would lead one to define anger as jealousy rather than as anger alone. These situations are defined by culture, although responses are determined by the situation's implications for an individual's well-being (i.e., by an appraisal of the situation vis-à-vis motives, goals, and preferences). Furthermore, the range of possible responses is culturally determined. Individuals' knowledge of the situations that call for jealousy and appropriate responses would be stored in their jealousy prototypes.

Similarly, White (1981c) has suggested that jealousy be viewed as a label given to a "complex of interrelated emotional, cognitive, and behavioral processes" that follows from a romantic threat (p. 295). White (1981c; White & Mullen, 1989) has used Lazarus's work on the coping process (Lazarus, 1966, 1968; Lazarus, Averill, & Opton, 1970; Lazarus & Launier, 1979) to describe how the emotional, cognitive, and behavioral components of jealousy may be interrelated. He describes jealousy events in terms of five broad sets of processes and variables. First, "primary appraisal variables" affect perceptions of (1) the potential for attraction between one's partner and a rival, and (2) the likelihood of the threat to the relationship from real or potential rivals. For example, one's sense of security in the relationship may attenuate the threat from a potential rival. "Secondary appraisal variables," such as comparing oneself to the rival or looking for alternatives to the present relationship, are assessments of coping strategies that might reduce threat. Following the perception of a threat, the jealous person experiences "emotional reactions" such as anger, depression, guilt, and anxiety. Then "coping behaviors" are enacted in order to reduce the threat to one's self-esteem or to the relationship. Finally, the "outcomes" from this process modify the influences of primary appraisal variables and provide information regarding the efficacy of various coping strategies. (A more extended discussion of jealousy from the standpoint of Lazarus's emotions theory can be found in Mathes, Chapter 3, this volume.)

This model is clearly similar to Shaver et al.'s (1987) model of emotion, although a prototype approach may help to define the links among specific appraisals, responses, and coping strategies. People's jealousy prototypes represent their knowledge of these elements and their interrelations. White (1980) himself has found that people report using ploys to induce jealousy in their partners. This suggests that they have jealousy prototypes permitting them to anticipate jealous reactions to the antecedents they create; in other words, they have knowledge of relations between at least some jealousy antecedents and responses.

As Bringle and Buunk (1985) point out, the characteristic affective, cognitive, and behavioral responses of jealousy have yet to be determined. Moreover, they ask whether the nature of the threat, the affective responses, and coping strategies are interrelated. A prototype approach to studying jealousy, geared toward the idea that jealousy is a blended emotion, may shed light on these issues.

## ROMANTIC JEALOUSY AS A BLENDED EMOTION

Shaver et al. (1987) and others (e.g., Arnold, 1960; Plutchik, 1980) suggest that some subordinate-level emotions, such as romantic jealousy, may be blended emotions. According to Arnold (1960), a blended emotion is "a compound of many emotions, all directed toward the same object, but aroused by various and often conflicting aspects of the object or situation" (p. 197). Several ways of conceptualizing jealousy as a blended emotion are consistent with Arnold's definition. First, jealousy affect may be a unique and recognizable blend of basic-level emotions, such as anger, sadness, and fear. That is, the jealous person may experience these emotions simultaneously. We (Sharpsteen & Schmalz, 1988) recently found that within subjects' actual jealousy episodes, the intensity of anger-, sadness-, and fear-like emotions each predicted variability in jealousy intensity over and above that predicted by the others. This might mean that the affect of jealousy is a singular blend of anger, sadness, and fear.

This finding could also result from reappraisals of the changing jealousy situation—another way to conceptualize romantic jealousy as a blended emotion. Several emotions may appear over the course of a jealousy episode as the jealous person reappraises the situation with respect to his or her partner, rival, or relationship. When Hupka (1984) asked his subjects to focus on different aspects of several jealousy scenarios (e.g., the onus of succeeding on one's own after losing the partner, or the manner in which the relationship was ended), he found that the different appraisals called for in the scenarios produced different attributions of primary emotions to the story's jealous character. For example, focusing on the partner's sharing of secrets with the romantic rival produced attributions of anger to the jealous person; focusing on the prospect of making it on one's own after depending on the partner produced attributions of fear. Of course, this might also mean that some jealousy episodes involve only anger, whereas others involve only sadness, fear, or other emotions (and the cognitions, affect, and behaviors associated with them), depending on the outcome of the individual's appraisal.

If romantic jealousy episodes involve several basic-level emotions (whether simultaneously, in succession, or across episodes), then people's jealousy prototypes are likely to have features in common with their prototypes for these basic-level emotions. That is, jealousy may be cognitively organized as a blended emotion. Many researchers emphasize jealousy's relations to anger, sadness, and fear (Mathes, Adams, & Davies, 1985; Pfeiffer & Wong, 1989). The prototypic features of jealousy should include some of the features of these emotions.

The variables measured and manipulated by jealousy researchers do resemble many of the prototypic features of anger, sadness, and fear. They can also be categorized as antecedents, responses, and self-control procedures, as Shaver et al. (1987) did with the features of the basic-level emotion prototypes delineated by their subjects.

## Antecedents

The antecedents of emotions are the elements physically or objectively present in a situation, along with the perceptions, interpretations, and appraisals of them. It is clear that a virtually infinite number of situations may produce romantic jealousy, but only one intervening interpretation seems to be required: that there is a rival for one's partner. In fact, loss of one's partner to a rival has been found to result in greater anticipated jealousy (and anger) than loss as a result of rejection, destiny, or fate (Mathes et al., 1985). That interpretation could be precipitated by the ostensible rival's behavior alone, the partner's behavior alone, or their joint behavior. In any case, the interpretation of that behavior is likely to be influenced by attributional processes. Berscheid (1983) suggests that jealousy requires an attribution of responsibility to the rival and partner following an interruption of one's own plans or activities. Also, White (1981a) has found that attributions of partners' motives differentially predicted perceived threat to the relationship and romantic jealousy.

Having decided that there is a rival, the individual assesses the implications of the rivalry with respect to his or her motives, goals, and preferences. The outcome of that assessment, or appraisal, is the elicitation of affect, behavior, and cognition associated with a particular emotion—most likely negative emotions, such as anger-, sadness-, or fear-like ones (e.g., Bush, Bush, & Jennings, 1988; Mathes et al., 1985; Pfeiffer & Wong, 1989).

As reported by White (1981c), a number of researchers (Benedictson, 1977; Hupka & Bachelor, 1979; Rosmarin, Chambless, & LaPointe, 1979; Rusch & Hupka, 1977) have identified primary appraisal variables related to romantic jealousy. In cognitive–motivational terms, these variables measure the relationship between one's motives, goals, and preferences and the event being appraised. White (1981b) discusses two primary appraisal variables that are assumed to influence a partner's attraction to a real or potential rival: the perception that one is inadequate to meet the needs and expectations of the partner, and the perception that one is more involved in the relationship than is one's partner. White derives these variables from Thibaut and Kelley's (1959) notions of "comparison level" (CL) and "comparison level for alternatives" (CLalt). CL represents what a person expects to receive from the relationship, whereas CLalt is the lowest level of outcomes acceptable in light of the available alternatives. Each partner is assumed to have estimates of the other partner's CL and CLalt, by which each infers the other's satisfaction and involvement with the relationship. One's own adequacy as a partner is a function of the other partner's CL, whereas

CLalt determines which partner is more involved in the relationship. That is, the one who has more or better alternatives should be less involved and more likely to leave the relationship.

White (1981b) has produced evidence to support the idea that comparison levels influence the likelihood of one's being chronically (frequently and intensely) jealous within a relationship. In what he described as a causal model, jealousy was found to be marginally related to relative involvement (a judgment based on an estimate of the partner's CLalt), which in turn was predicted by physical attractiveness as compared to one's partner, the partner's availability of opposite-sex friends, and the perception that the partner considers oneself more involved in the relationship. Perceived inadequacy (a judgment reflecting one's estimate of the partner's CL) was found to be moderately correlated with jealousy scores and was itself related to low self-esteem, the belief that one's partner is attracted to another, and the perception that the partner is dissatisfied with the relationship.

White (1981b) suggests that jealousy results when romantic rivalry (or the possibility of romantic rivalry) threatens a person's self-esteem or the quality or existence of the relationship. The antecedents of fear (threat of social rejection, possibility of loss or failure; see Figure 2.1) seem most similar to this sort of appraisal. In fact, we (Sharpsteen & Schmalz, 1988) asked subjects to rate the intensity of a variety of emotions that might occur during their typical jealousy episodes, and found that subjects' ratings of fear-like emotions (fear, distrust) accounted for variability in chronic jealousy scores better than ratings of emotions from other basic-level domains.

But lacking a sense of equity or adequacy may sometimes be less salient than the perception that the motive to maintain these things has been obstructed by the partner or rival. Berscheid (1983) suggests that the relationship between the partner and rival interferes with the jealous person's plans and activities. An implication of Berscheid's analysis is that the jealous person (though not necessarily the *chronically* jealous person) appraises the situation as frustrating or obstructing his or her motives and goals. Judgments of relative involvement and inadequacy (based on estimates of the partner's CL and CLalt) may also represent judgments about the likelihood of achieving one's goals. Threats to self-esteem or the relationship may be seen as interruptions of the psychological goals of maintaining feelings of security. Several prototypic antecedents of anger are related to the obstruction of goals: loss of power, violation of expectation, interruption of goal-directed activity, and possibly judgment of illegitimacy (see Figure 2.2). Jealousy, a branch of

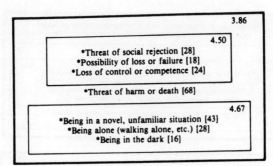
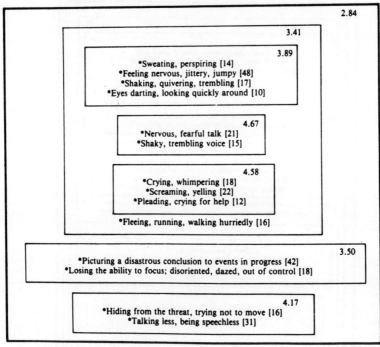

**FIGURE 2.1.** The prototype of fear. Antecedents are listed in the uppermost heavily outlined box, responses in the middle heavily outlined box, and self-control features in the lower box. The number in the upper right-hand corner of each box represents, on a 5-point scale, the average functional similarity rating of features in that box (higher numbers represent greater similarity). The numbers in brackets indicate the percentage of 120 subjects mentioning that feature. From "Emotion Knowledge: Further Explorations of a Prototype Approach" by P. Shaver, J. Schwartz, D. Kirson, & C. O'Connor, 1987, *Journal of Personality and Social Psychology, 52,* p. 1076. Copyright 1987 by the American Psychological Association. Reprinted by permission.

•Predisposition to anger, either because of previous similar or related
experiences or because of stress, overload, fatigue, etc. [18]

2.97

4.04

4.44

•Reversal or sudden loss of power, status, or respect; insult [43]
•Violation of an expectation; things not working out as planned [54]
•Frustration or interruption of a goal-directed activity [33]
•Real or threatened physical or psychological pain [57]

•Judgment that the situation is illegitimate, wrong, unfair,
contrary to what ought to be [78]

2.92

3.50

3.75

4.44

•Obscenities, cursing [30]
•Verbally attacking the cause of anger [69]
•Loud voice, yelling, screaming, shouting [59]
•Complaining, bitching, talking about how lousy things are [18]

4.04

4.83

•Hands or fists clenched [22]
•Aggressive, threatening movements or gestures [21]

4.33

•Attacking something other than the cause of anger
(e.g., pounding on something, throwing things) [35]
•Physically attacking the cause of anger [26]
•Incoherent, out-of-control, highly emotional behavior [18]
•Imagining attacking or hurting the cause of anger [31]

3.87

4.08

•Heavy walk, stomping [11]
•Tightness or rigidity in body; tight, rigid movements [17]
•Nonverbally communicating disapproval to the cause of anger
(e.g., slamming doors, walking out) [25]

4.25

•Frowning, not smiling, mean or unpleasant expression [18]
•Gritting teeth, showing teeth, breathing through teeth [13]
•Red, flushed face [33]

3.50

•Crying [17]
•Feelings of nervous tension, anxiety, discomfort [17]

4.00

•Brooding; withdrawing from social contact [14]

4.50

•Narrowing of attention to exclude all but the anger situation;
not being able to think of anything else [16]
•Thinking "I'm right, everyone else is wrong" [38]

4.00

•Suppressing the anger; trying not to show or express it [20]
•Redefining the situation or trying to view it in such a way
that anger is no longer appropriate [11]

40

anger in Shaver et al.'s (1987) implicit emotion hierarchy, may be distinguished from basic anger in part by the relationship of the individual to the person perceived to be the cause of his or her emotion. That is, jealousy, rather than anger alone, results when a motive is obstructed by one's romantic partner and a romantic rival. Salovey and Rodin (1986) have found anger, in tandem with jealousy, to be a common response to this set of emotional antecedents.

The prototypic antecedents of sadness seem less closely related to the theoretical antecedents described in the jealousy literature than do the antecedents of anger and fear. Undesirable outcomes, loss of the relationship, rejection, and discovering one's powerlessness (see Figure 2.3) may be most salient to the jealous person when his or her jealous feelings are nearing resolution. Most research and theory focus implicitly on initial reactions to jealousy-provoking situations. But because people do engage in sadness-like behaviors and coping responses when jealous (as discussed in the following sections), it seems likely that they also make sadness-like appraisals. Certainly, a person who feels inadequate and overinvolved when confronted with a romantic rival may at times focus on his or her powerlessness, especially if loss of the relationship appears inevitable (e.g., when loss is part of the person's jealousy prototype).

At least some of the prototypic antecedents of anger, sadness, and fear are similar to one another. For example, discovering one's powerlessness (sadness), loss of control (fear), and reversal or loss of power (anger) are seemingly similar antecedents from different emotion domains. This may appear daunting in light of the thesis that emotion-specific appraisals generate emotion-specific responses. But "antecedent" is a more inclusive term than "appraisal." It is how these antecedents are appraised, with respect to motives, goals, and preferences, that governs the affective, behavioral, and cognitive responses to the situation.

---

**FIGURE 2.2.** The prototype of anger. Antecedents are listed in the uppermost heavily outlined box, responses in the middle heavily outlined box, and self-control features in the lower box. The number in the upper right-hand corner of each box represents, on a 5-point scale, the average functional similarity rating of features in that box (higher numbers represent greater similarity). The numbers in brackets indicate the percentage of 120 subjects mentioning that feature. From "Emotion Knowledge: Further Explorations of a Prototype Approach" by P. Shaver, J. Schwartz, D. Kirson, & C. O'Connor, 1987, *Journal of Personality and Social Psychology, 52,* p. 1078. Copyright 1987 by the American Psychological Association. Reprinted by permission.

3.43

4.22

4.40

*An undesirable outcome; getting what was not wanted;
a negative surprise [40]
*Death of a loved one [58]
*Loss of a valued relationship; separation [57]
*Rejection, exclusion, disapproval [19]
*Not getting what was wanted, wished for, striven for, etc. [15]
*Reality falling short of expectations; things being
worse than anticipated [26]

*Discovering that one is powerless, helpless, impotent [15]

*Empathy with someone who is sad, hurt, etc. [26]

2.93

3.50

4.42

*Sitting or lying around; being inactive, lethargic, listless [41]
*Tired, rundown, low in energy [21]
*Slow, shuffling movements [16]
*Slumped, drooping posture [20]

4.50

*Withdrawing from social contact [50]
*Talking little or not at all [46]

3.71

4.33

*Low, quiet, slow, monotonous voice [21]
*Saying sad things [27]

4.33

*Frowning, not smiling [17]
*Crying, tears, whimpering [77]

4.67

*Irritable, touchy, grouchy [21]
*Moping, brooding, being moody [17]

3.92

4.33

*Negative outlook; thinking only about the negative side of things [38]
*Giving up; no longer trying to improve or control the situation [31]

*Blaming, criticizing oneself [18]

*Talking to someone about the sad feelings or events [20]

4.83

*Taking action, becoming active (either to improve the situation or to
alter one's feelings) [26]
*Suppressing the negative feelings; looking on the positive or bright
side; trying to act happy [20]

42

## Responses and Response Tendencies

A wide range of feelings, behaviors, and cognitions may follow the appraisal of a jealousy situation (Bringle & Buunk, 1985; Clanton & Smith, 1986; Pfeiffer & Wong, 1989; White, 1981b), although Buunk and Bringle (1987), Constantine (1976), and Pfeiffer and Wong (1989) suggest that these may sometimes be conditioned responses not requiring cognitive appraisal. In cases where cognitive appraisal does occur, responses that are typical of a particular basic-level emotion domain should be linked reliably to appraisals from the same domain. That is, to the extent that the characteristic antecedents, responses, and coping strategies associated with different basic-level emotions are distinct, response tendencies (and efforts at self-control) should reflect the basic-level antecedents from which a particular episode of jealousy arises. A fear antecedent that occurs in the context of a romantic relationship should evoke some fear-like responses. Anger antecedents should produce anger responses. As mentioned earlier, Hupka (1984) found that at least some jealousy antecedents reliably produced attributions of certain emotions to a jealous protagonist. Of course, this may not always happen: Emotion categories are fuzzy sets (Fehr & Russell, 1984), and some responses may be idiosyncratic, not typical of any emotion domain, or related to more than one domain. Nevertheless, to the extent that the links between antecedents and responses are reliable, an understanding of these links may be useful to jealousy researchers (and jealous people).

Jealousy responses can be categorized as behavioral, affective, and cognitive (Pfeiffer & Wong, 1989; White, 1981b). The behavioral concomitants of jealousy have not been considered as widely as the others, partly because behaviors vary tremendously from person to person, so much so that Constantine (1976) described jealousy behavior as "a unique personal statement" (p. 390). Shettel-Neuber, Bryson, and Young (1978) found that men were more likely than women to be angry

---

**FIGURE 2.3.** The prototype of sadness. Antecedents are listed in the uppermost heavily outlined box, responses in the middle heavily outlined box, and self-control features in the lower box. The number in the upper right-hand corner of each box represents, on a 5-point scale, the average functional similarity rating of features in that box (higher numbers represent greater similarity). The numbers in brackets indicate the percentage of 120 subjects mentioning that feature. From "Emotion Knowledge: Further Explorations of a Prototype Approach" by P. Shaver, J. Schwartz, D. Kirson, & C. O'Connor, 1987, *Journal of Personality and Social Psychology*, 52, p. 1077. Copyright 1987 by the American Psychological Association. Reprinted by permission.

at themselves, to get drunk or high, to verbally threaten the interlopers, and to feel flattered. Women were more likely to cry when alone, to make themselves more attractive to their partners, and to make the partners think they did not care. According to Bryson (1976, 1977), men's behavior appears to be aimed at maintaining self-esteem, whereas women's is aimed at maintaining their relationships.

These behavioral responses to jealousy seem to be those that would follow from anger, sadness, and fear antecedents. Some of these behaviors fit the prototypes of these basic-level emotions, as found by Shaver et al. (1987). Verbally attacking the cause of one's anger is a prototypical anger response. Blaming and criticizing oneself, taking action to improve the situation (e.g., trying to make oneself more attractive), and taking action to alter one's feelings (e.g., getting drunk or high) are elements of the sadness prototype. Acting unafraid (e.g., making the partner think that one is indifferent) is a prototypical fear response. Most of these and other behavioral responses to jealousy (e.g., Buunk, 1981, 1982a, 1982b) can be construed as coping behaviors, which are considered more fully later.

Perhaps because behaviors vary widely, most researchers focus on the affective responses to jealousy. Many of the emotional concomitants of jealousy can be considered anger-, sadness-, and fear-like emotions. Bush et al. (1988), for example, provided their subjects with a list of emotion and affect terms with which they were to evaluate their feelings both before and after imagining a jealousy-provoking scene. Feelings of possessiveness, shame, anger, disgust, and contempt increased following this manipulation, whereas feelings of joy decreased. In addition, feelings of surprise, distress, and fear were rated as more intense in highly threatening scenes than in low- or no-threat scenes.

Salovey and Rodin (1986) asked subjects to rate how angry, sad, embarrassed, and jealous or envious they would be in each of 53 situations. They found that unfair romantic situations produced more anger and sadness than other romantic or social comparison (envy) situations. This result is consistent with the findings of Shaver et al. (1987) that unfair or undeserved situations are prototypic of anger and sadness experiences.

Relevant to the proposal that jealousy is represented in people's prototypes as a blended emotion, 62% of the variability in ratings of situations as romantic jealousy versus social comparison jealousy (i.e., envy) could be accounted for by affect ratings. That is, jealousy and envy situations could be predicted by the affect each elicited, suggesting that people may be able to distinguish one from the other on the basis of the affective responses typically associated with each (Smith, Kim, & Parrott, 1988; see also Parrott, Chapter 1, this volume). Thus the responses cued by jealousy situations appear to be distinct from those of at least one related prototype.

The cognitions that have been studied as jealousy responses can generally be considered reappraisals of the jealousy situation. For example, one's ideas about the partner's motives or reasons for leaving the relationship (Mathes et al., 1985; White, 1981a), as well as paranoid worries and suspicions (Pfeiffer & Wong, 1989), may influence ongoing responses to a jealousy situation. White (1981a) found that the perception of dissatisfaction as the partner's motive predicted anger as the response to the jealousy situation. In addition, men said that they responded with anger when they perceived sex as their partners' motive, and women responded with anger when they perceived rivals' attractiveness (rivals' superior looks or personality) as their partners' motive.

How the partner is perceived to have left the relationship may also influence an individual's responses to the loss. Mathes et al. (1985) found type of loss (fate, destiny, rejection, rival) to affect subjects' anticipated loss of self-esteem. Of particular interest here, loss of a partner to a rival (an apparently prototypic jealousy antecedent) produced a significantly greater expected loss of self-esteem than loss resulting from fate or destiny, and about the same loss of self-esteem as loss resulting from rejection without a rival. Furthermore, loss of self-esteem was found to precipitate anger.

The appraisals generated by the motives and manner of a partner's behavior were not directly assessed in these studies, but because anger apparently was produced, subjects may have made anger-like appraisals. Dissatisfaction, sex, and rival attractiveness could all be construed as insults to the jealous partner, a prototypic anger antecedent. Similarly, the loss of self-esteem, as opposed to relatively static low self-esteem (which might produce fear-like appraisals), could be appraised as a reversal or loss of status.

Many of the responses that follow from jealousy can be considered coping behaviors. Like other responses, coping behaviors may vary as antecedents change, reflecting the basic-level emotion prototypes to which they are most similar.

## Coping and Efforts at Self-Control

Jealousy is a protective reaction aimed at coping with a perceived threat (Clanton, 1981) or interruptions in activities with one's partner. Buunk and Bringle (1987) define coping strategies as "cognitive and behavioral responses that are goal-directed attempts to change or influence the self, the partner, the relationship, or the situation" (p. 138).

Emphasizing the positive side of jealousy, Constantine (1976) suggests that it may be a warning signal to both partners that some aspects of their relationship need to be clarified or renegotiated. Jealousy may draw attention to differences in each partner's expectations and assumptions about the relationship. Thus jealousy is an opportunity to clarify personal differences. Presumably, jealousy behaviors will be directed toward accomplishing this.

Constantine's optimism notwithstanding, there seems to be a predominance in the literature of analyses explicating less constructive means of coping with jealousy. Whitehurst (1971) proposed that jealousy behaviors could be classified as isolational (e.g., withdrawal, refusal to fight or negotiate), antagonistic (e.g., attempts at revenge), redefinitional (e.g., externalizing problems through intellectualization and rationalization), or resolutional (e.g., joint problem solving, realistic negotiation). Even among the apparently less desirable coping behaviors, Whitehurst speculates that some may be more functional than others; for example, antagonistic behaviors may be preferable to isolational ones because the former involve contact with the partner.

From among partners in sexually open marriages, Buunk (1981) asked those who had said they were less jealous in their relationships now than in the past to rate the applicability of 16 potential causes of their reduced jealousy. A factor analysis of these data produced evidence of four broad attributed causes of reductions in jealousy. The first of these factors, Independence, involved increased security about one's good qualities and increased self-confidence. Over half of those who said that they had become less jealous over the course of their relationships indicated that Independence was the cause of the reduction in jealous feelings. Half of the respondents said that they attributed the reduction to a factor Buunk termed Accepting Jealousy, which included learning to express their feelings of jealousy. The importance of fostering a more secure relationship was reflected in the Trust and Communication factors. These four perceived causes for reduction of jealousy were, however, only weakly related to respondents' expectations of how jealous they would become in future jealousy-provoking situations.

Hatfield and Walster (1986), using Schachter's model, proposed two means of controlling jealousy. First, they suggested that societies encourage people to label their jealous feelings differently. In some cultures, a person will interpret a mate's extradyadic relationships as "sexual curiosity" or pride that others value the partner, rather than as dismay at the partner's poor taste or as an interruption of the pair's activities.

A second approach would be to reduce arousal. For example, a society could teach that self-worth is not dependent on one's partner (thus reducing threat, a prototypic fear antecedent, or powerlessness, a prototypic sadness antecedent) or on controlling someone (lack of control may co-occur with loss of power, a prototypic anger antecedent). In fact, Buunk (1982b) has found that emotional dependence is not related to jealousy among persons with extramarital sexual experience. Buunk suggests that such a person distinguishes between the partner's ability to provide emotional support and the partner's desire for his or her own satisfaction.

Like jealous responses in general, the coping behaviors and efforts at self-control presented in the studies cited resemble responses and self-control procedures from the anger, sadness, and fear prototypes (Shaver et al., 1987). For example, reactive retribution, confrontation (Bryson, 1976, 1977), and antagonism (Whitehurst, 1971) are aspects of the anger prototype. Hiding one's feelings from others, as in impression management (Bryson, 1976, 1977) or feigning indifference (Shettel-Neuber et al., 1978), are prototypic fear behaviors. Acceptance and soliciting trust or communication (Buunk, 1981, 1982a; Buunk & Bringle, 1987), redefinition (Whitehurst, 1971), and seeking social support (Bryson, 1976, 1977) fit with the behaviors and self-control procedures of the sadness prototype. Again, these conclusions are tentative; the self-control features of the anger, sadness, and fear prototypes (Shaver et al., 1987) at least partly overlap. Furthermore, the differential effectiveness of these strategies in reducing anger, sadness, fear, and jealousy has yet to be empirically shown.

## CONCLUSIONS

The main thesis of this chapter is that romantic jealousy is cognitively organized as a blended emotion. This organization reflects the fact that a variety of emotions, primarily anger-, sadness-, and fear-like ones, are typically involved within or across jealousy episodes. Furthermore, emotion-specific appraisals are theorized to generate emotion-specific affect, behaviors, and cognitions that take the form of responses and efforts at at self-control. These emotion-specific relations become a part of one's jealousy knowledge, and are therefore incorporated into one's jealousy prototype.

What are some of the implications of this cognitive organization? First, the knowledge represented in people's jealousy prototypes can help them to understand their own and others' jealousy behavior. For example, the jealous person's attributions about his or her partner's jealousy-provoking behavior—attributions based in part on information in the jealousy prototype—would almost certainly be a part of dialogue aimed at resolving the jealousy.

Second, the jealousy prototype is likely to influence people's perception and recollection of jealousy events, as when information that is prototypic is used to fill in for information that is not available (Schank & Abelson, 1977). Similarly, jealousy prototypes may be used to anticipate people's reactions to jealousy-provoking situations. For example, the methods used to induce jealousy in one's partner (White, 1980) probably reflect knowledge of the relations between antecedents and responses held in one's jealousy prototype.

In short, a jealousy prototype helps people to make sense of jealousy situations. This would be true, too, of the situations presented by researchers. Many studies implicitly tap jealousy prototypes by asking subjects to evaluate jealousy-provoking situations for which no one appropriate appraisal or emotional response is apparent (e.g., Bush et al., 1988; Salovey & Rodin, 1988). When given only a terse description of a jealousy situation, subjects may need to call on their jealousy prototypes (their ideas about the typical jealousy experience) in order to answer researchers' questions. Subjects may give what is, in their own minds, the most likely appropriate response, but not necessarily the response they would anticipate making if given enough information to appraise the situation. For example, situations that seem to engender anger, sadness, and fear may prompt only one of those responses when an appraisal is available or can be generated from information in the situation that is presented (Hupka, 1984). Thus, in the absence of knowledge about people's appraisals of a situation, caution should be used in drawing conclusions about the capacity of a given situation to elicit specific jealousy responses. In other words, it may not be properties of the situation alone that guide subjects' responses, but their ideas about any jealousy situation.

Shaver et al. (1987) aggregated data across subjects' accounts of actual and typical emotion episodes in order to determine the common elements within several categories of emotion events (anger, sadness, fear, joy, love). A variant of this approach was also used successfully by Fehr (1988) in her prototype analysis of the concepts of love and commitment. The same strategy could be used to delineate an idealized jealousy prototype, one that presumably would be a blend of predominantly anger-, sadness-, and fear-like features. That is, the common elements of people's jealousy experiences could be used as a model of their jealousy prototypes. That model could then be used as the basis for research investigating the links among jealousy's antecedents, responses, and self-control procedures, as well as the relations among the affective, behavioral, and cognitive facets of jealousy experiences.

## REFERENCES

Arnold, M. B. (1960). *Emotion and personality.* New York: Columbia University Press.

Benedictson, C. (1977). *The development of a scale for the assessment of jealousy.* Paper presented at the meeting of the Southeastern Psychological Association.

Berscheid, F. (1983). Emotion. In H. Kelley, E. Berscheid, A. Christenson, J. H. Harvey, T. Huston, G. Levinger, E. McClintock, L. Peplau, & D. Peterson (Eds.), *Close relationships* (pp. 110–168). San Francisco: W. H. Freeman.

Bringle, R., & Buunk, B. (1985). Jealousy and social behavior: A review of person, relationship, and situational determinants. In P. Shaver (Ed.), *Review of personality and social psychology: Vol. 6, Self, situations, and social behavior* (pp. 241–264). Beverly Hills, CA: Sage.

Bryson, J. (1976). *The nature of sexual jealousy: An exploratory study.* Paper presented at the meeting of the American Psychological Association, Washington, DC.

Bryson, J. (1977). *Situational determinants of the expression of jealousy.* Paper presented at the meeting of the American Psychological Association, San Francisco.

Bush, C. R., Bush, J. P., & Jennings, J. (1988). Effects of jealousy threats on relationship perceptions and emotions. *Journal of Social and Personal Relationships, 5,* 285–303.

Buunk, B. (1981). Jealousy in sexually open marriages. *Alternative Lifestyles, 4,* 357–372.

Buunk, B. (1982a). Strategies of jealousy: Styles of coping with extramarital involvement of the spouse. *Family Relations, 31,* 13–18.

Buunk, B. (1982b). Anticipated sexual jealousy: Its relationship to self-esteem, dependency, and reciprocity. *Personality and Social Psychology Bulletin, 8,* 310–316.

Buunk, B., & Bringle, R. (1987). Jealousy in love relationships. In D. Perlman & S. Duck (Eds.), *Intimate relationships: Development, dynamics, and deterioration* (pp. 123–148). Beverly Hills, CA: Sage.

Clanton, G. (1981). Frontiers of jealousy research. *Alternative Lifestyles, 4,* 259–273.

Clanton, G., & Smith, L. (Eds.). (1986). *Jealousy.* Lanham, MD: University Press of America.

Constantine, L. (1976). Jealousy: From theory to intervention. In D. Olson (Ed.), *Treating relationships* (pp. 383–398). Lake Mills, IA: Graphic.

Fehr, B. (1988). Prototype analysis of the concepts of love and commitment. *Journal of Personality and Social Psychology, 55,* 557–579.

Fehr, B., & Russell, J. A. (1984). Concept of emotion viewed from a prototype perspective. *Journal of Experimental Psychology: General, 113,* 464–486.

Friday, N. (1985). *Jealousy.* New York: Perigord Press.

Hatfield, E., & Walster, G. (1986). The social psychology of jealousy. In

G. Clanton & L. Smith (Eds.), *Jealousy*. Lanham, MD: University Press of America.

Hupka, R. B. (1981). Cultural determinants of jealousy. *Alternative Lifestyles, 4*, 310–356.

Hupka, R. B. (1984). Jealousy: Compound emotion or label for a particular situation? *Motivation and Emotion, 8*, 141–155.

Hupka, R. B., & Bachelor, B. (1979). *Validation of a scale to measure romantic jealousy*. Paper presented at the meeting of the Western Psychological Association, San Diego.

Lazarus, R. (1966). *Psychological stress and the coping process*. New York: McGraw-Hill.

Lazarus, R. (1968). Emotions and adaptation: Conceptual and empirical relations. In W. Arnold (Ed.), *Nebraska Symposium on Motivation* (pp. 175–266). Lincoln: University of Nebraska Press.

Lazarus, R., Averill, J., & Opton, E. (1970). Toward a cognitive theory of emotion. In M. Arnold (Ed.), *Feelings and emotions* (pp. 207–232). New York: Academic Press.

Lazarus, R., & Launier, R. (1979). Stress-related transactions between person and environment. In L. Pervin & M. Lewis (Eds.), *Perspectives in interactional psychology*. New York: Plenum.

Mathes, E., Adams, H., & Davies, R. (1985). Jealousy: Loss of relationship rewards, loss of self-esteem, depression, anxiety, and anger. *Journal of Personality and Social Psychology, 48*, 1552–1561.

Pfeiffer, S. M., & Wong, P. T. P. (1989). Multidimensional jealousy. *Journal of Social and Personal Relationships, 6*, 181–196.

Plutchik, R. (1980). *Emotion: A psychoevolutionary synthesis*. New York: Harper & Row.

Rosch, E. (1973). On the internal structure of perceptual and semantic categories. In T. Moore (Ed.), *Cognitive development and the acquisition of language*. New York: Academic Press.

Rosch, E. (1975). Cognitive representations of semantic categories. *Journal of Experimental Psychology: General, 104*, 192–233.

Rosmarin, D., Chambless, D., & LaPointe, K. (1979). *The survey of interpersonal reactions: An inventory for the measurement of jealousy*. Unpublished manuscript, University of Georgia.

Rusch, P., & Hupka, R. (1977). *Development and validation of a scale to measure romantic jealousy*. Paper presented at the meeting of the Western Psychological Association, Seattle.

Salovey, P., & Rodin, J. (1986). The differentiation of social-comparison jealousy and romantic jealousy. *Journal of Personality and Social Psychology, 50*, 1100–1112.

Salovey, P., & Rodin, J. (1988). Coping with envy and jealousy. *Journal of Social and Clinical Psychology, 7*, 15–33.

Schank, R., & Abelson, R. (1977). *Scripts, plans, goals, and understanding*. Hillsdale, NJ: Erlbaum.

Sharpsteen, D. J., & Schmalz, C. M. (1988). *Romantic jealousy as a blended emotion.* Paper presented at the meeting of the Colorado Psychological Association, Fort Collins.

Shaver, P., Schwartz, J., Kirson, D., & O'Connor, C. (1987). Emotion knowledge: Further explorations of a prototype approach. *Journal of Personality and Social Psychology, 52,* 1061–1086.

Shettel-Neuber, J., Bryson, J., & Young, L. (1978). Physical attractiveness of the "other person" and jealousy. *Personality and Social Psychology Bulletin, 4,* 612–615.

Smith, R. H., Kim, S. H., & Parrott, W. G. (1988). Envy and jealousy: Semantic problems and experiental distinctions. *Personality and Social Psychology Bulletin, 14,* 401–409.

Thibaut, J., & Kelley, H. (1959). *The social psychology of groups.* New York: Wiley.

White, G. (1980). Inducing jealousy: A power perspective. *Personality and Social Psychology Bulletin, 6,* 222–227.

White, G. (1981a). Jealousy and partner's perceived motives for attraction to a rival. *Social Psychology Quarterly, 44,* 24–30.

White, G. (1981b). Relative involvement, inadequacy, and jealousy: A test of a causal model. *Alternative Lifestyles, 4,* 291–309.

White, G. (1981c). A model of romantic jealousy. *Motivation and Emotion, 5,* 295–310.

White, G., & Mullen, P. E. (1989). *Jealousy: Theory, research, and clinical strategies.* New York: Guilford Press.

Whitehurst, R. (1971). Violence potential in extramarital sexual responses. *Journal of Marriage and the Family, 33,* 683–691.

## Chapter Three

# A Cognitive Theory of Jealousy

EUGENE W. MATHES
*Western Illinois University*

The theoretical framework that I have found most useful for organizing my research on romantic jealousy is Richard Lazarus's cognitive–phenomenological theory of emotions (Lazarus, 1966; Lazarus & Averill, 1972; Lazarus, Kanner, & Folkman, 1980). I am not the first researcher to apply Lazarus's theory to jealousy: Both White (1981b) and Hupka (1981) have done so before me, and I am especially indebted to White for his theorizing concerning primary appraisal and jealousy. In what follows, I plan to describe Lazarus's cognitive–phenomenological theory of emotion, and then use it to organize the presentation of my jealousy research.

## LAZARUS'S COGNITIVE-PHENOMENOLOGICAL THEORY OF EMOTION

Lazarus conceives of the individual as "an evaluating organism, searching the environment for cues about what is needed or desired, and evaluating each input as to its relevance and significance" (Lazarus & Averill, 1972, p. 242). Three kinds of appraisals take place: "primary appraisal," "secondary appraisal," and "reappraisal." Primary appraisal involves evaluating an event for its significance to the individual's well-being. Three evaluations are possible. The event may be evaluated as irrelevant, benign/positive, or stressful. Irrelevant events have no effect on the individual's well-being, whereas benign/positive events enhance the individual's well-being. Stressful events involve harm or loss (an injury has already taken place); threat (an injury is anticipated); or challenge (although injury may occur, there is also the possibility of positive gain, mastery, or growth). Secondary appraisal involves an evaluation of the possible alternative courses of action for dealing with the event, especially if the event is a stressful one. The extent to which an individual is threatened depends upon the individual's estimation of how effective he or she will be in dealing with the stressor. Reappraisal involves a changed evaluation of the situation because of a change in the situation (possibly brought about as a result of coping efforts) or further reflection on the original evidence.

The various cognitive appraisals lead to coping activities, which may involve either direct actions designed to change the external situation or intrapsychic coping processes (e.g., the use of defense mechanisms). If the primary appraisal of the event is that it is irrelevant, little or no emotion follows. If the primary appraisal is that the event is positive/benign, positive emotions follow. If the primary appraisal is that the event is stressful, negative emotions follow. Secondary appraisal and reappraisal dampen or amplify these emotions, depending upon whether these appraisals suggest that the individual can or cannot adequately cope with the event (secondary appraisal) or has or has not adequately coped with the event (reappraisal).

## PRIMARY APPRAISAL

When Lazarus's theory is applied to jealousy (see Figure 3.1), the stimulus event that leads to the various cognitive appraisals is a situation in which a person, P, has a romantic relationship with his or her beloved, B. A rival, R, then intrudes with the intention of establishing a romantic relationship with B, thus creating the possibility that P might lose B. Initially, P's claim to B is greater than that of R. Often this claim is a matter of precedence (P established a romantic relationship with B before R did). However, the claim may be legal in nature (even though R knew B before P knew B, B is married to P). If P and R have equal claim to B, the situation is not a jealousy situation but one of competition. If R has greater claim to B than P has to B, we have a situation of romantic envy

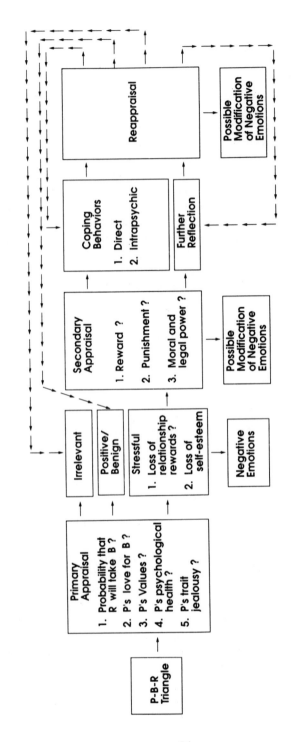

**FIGURE 3.1.** An application of Lazarus's cognitive–phenomenological theory of emotion to jealousy.

so far as P is concerned: P wants what R already has, B. My differentiation of romantic jealousy from romantic envy is based on research carried out by Smith, Kim, and Parrott (1988; see also Parrott, Chapter 1, this volume). Not everyone, however, would differentiate between romantic jealousy and envy (Bers & Rodin, 1984; Salovey & Rodin, 1986).

## Loss of Relationship Rewards and Self-Esteem

When faced with the P-B-R triangle, P initially engages in primary appraisal. P asks himself or herself whether this situation is irrelevant, positive/benign, or stressful with respect to his or her well-being. P's answer to this question is that it is stressful if (1) R is likely to take (or has already taken) B away from P and (2) P loves or otherwise wants to retain B for himself or herself. White (1981b) suggests that the unwilling loss of B to R is stressful to P for two reasons. The loss of B to R means a loss of relationship rewards and a loss of self-esteem. "Loss of relationship rewards" refers to the fact that P will no longer have B to dance with, talk to, sleep with, and so on. "Loss of self-esteem" refers to the fact that, at least in the eyes of B, P is inferior to R.

To test White's hypothesis that the loss of B to R means the loss of relationship rewards and self-esteem, Heather Adams, Ruth Davies, and I (Mathes, Adams, & Davies, 1985) compared the effects of the loss of B to R (the "rival" condition) with the effects of a no-loss control condition and of several other ways of losing B. The other ways included loss of B due to fate (the "fate" condition—e.g., B is killed in an automobile accident); loss of B due to B's destiny (the "lover's destiny" condition—e.g., B takes a job elsewhere), and loss of B due to B's rejection of P (the "rejection" condition—e.g., B tells P that B does not love P any more and ends the relationship). College student subjects were presented with four examples of the no-loss condition and each of the four types of loss, and after each example were asked about loss of relationship rewards and of self-esteem. To assess the loss of relationship rewards, subjects were asked: "If this happened to you, would you feel lonely?" To assess the loss of self-esteem, subjects were asked: "If this happened to you, would your self-esteem suffer?" Responses were made on 7-point scales ranging from "No, definitely" (1) to "Yes, definitely" (7).

It was hypothesized that the loss of relationship rewards and self-esteem would be low in the no-loss control condition. Loss of relationship rewards would be high in all of the other conditions, since they would all involve the end of the relationship. Loss of self-esteem would be low in the fate condition, moderate in the lover's destiny condition, and high in the rejection and rival conditions. These predictions were supported. Significant main effects for condition were found for both dependent variables—loss of relationship rewards and loss of self-esteem. As can be seen in Figure 3.2, loss of relationship rewards was minimal in the no-loss condition and high in the other conditions. Loss of self-esteem was minimal in the no-loss condition, slight in the fate condition, moderate in the lover's destiny condition, and high in the rejection and rival conditions. Therefore, losing B to R hurts because it means not only a loss of relationship rewards, but also a loss of self-esteem.

## The Probability That R Will Take B

P's next step in the primary appraisal process is to determine the extent to which (1) R is likely to take (or has already taken) B away from P, and (2) P loves or otherwise wants to retain B for himself or herself. To accomplish this, P will examine a number of aspects of the P-B-R triangle, one of which is the probability that R will succeed in taking B from P. If R has not succeeded and probably will not succeed in establishing a romantic relationship with B, P will appraise R's presence as irrelevant and devote no more time or attention to the situation. For example, if P were married to a kindergarten teacher, and one of B's students had a crush on her, P would probably construe the little rival's presence as irrelevant to P's well-being. On the other hand, if R has already succeeded or there is a high probability that R will succeed in establishing a romantic relationship with B and thus take B from P, P will evaluate the P-B-R triangle as highly stressful. One factor that will probably contribute to R's chances of success and P's stress is R's social desirability. If R has many socially desirable characteristics (is bright, physically attractive, rich, etc.), R has a greater chance of winning B than if R has few socially desirable characteristics. Evidence supporting this hypothesis comes from a study by Shettel-Neuber, Bryson, and Young (1978), in which they suggest that subjects were more threatened by a physically attractive rival than to a physically unattractive rival. On the other hand, Buunk (1982) found that his Dutch subjects stated that they would prefer that their spouses have sexual intercourse with a physically attractive and liked (by the subjects) R than with an unattractive and unliked R. Buunk suggests that his subjects chose a socially desirable R to preserve their own self-esteem. Research designed to determine when P works in terms of threat (prefers a socially undesirable R) and when P works in terms of self-esteem (prefers a socially desirable R) would seem to be in order.

A couple of studies have found that the most devastating event that can happen to P is sexual intercourse between R and B. Salovey and Rodin (1986) had subjects rate 53 different situations for jealousy/envy

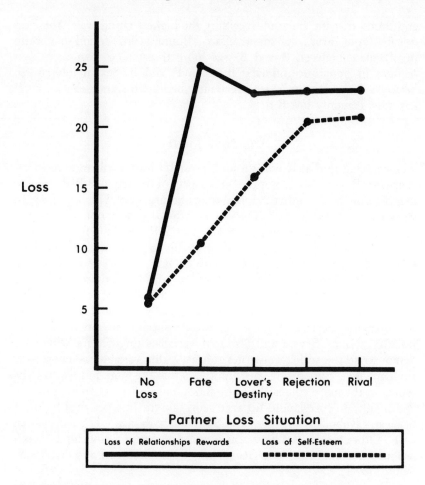

**FIGURE 3.2.** Loss of relationship rewards and loss of self-esteem as a function of type of partner loss. From "Jealousy: Loss of Relationship Rewards, Loss of Self-esteem, Depression, Anxiety, and Anger" by E. W. Mathes, H. E. Adams, & R. M. Davies, 1985, *Journal of Personality and Social Psychology, 42*, p. 1555. Copyright 1985 by the American Psychological Association. Adapted by permission.

and found that the situation receiving the highest rating was "You find out that your lover is having an affair." Buunk (1982) found that erotic involvement between R and B was more threatening than very high degrees of nonerotic intimacy between R and B. Sexual intercourse between R and B may be so threatening because it signals the worst: P has most certainly lost B to R.

### P's Love for B

The probability that R will succeed in establishing a romantic relationship with B, however, is not the only aspect of the actual P-B-R triangle that determines P's primary appraisal of the situation. The nature of P's romantic relationship with B is also a factor. If P does not want B, R's presence is not evaluated as stressful. In fact, if P is looking for some way to get rid of B, R's presence will probably be evaluated as positive/benign. However, if P is in love with B, R's presence is evaluated as stressful. Furthermore, the more in love P is with B, the more threatening R's presence is. The first jealousy study I carried out is relevant to this point (Mathes & Severa, 1981). Having just constructed the Interpersonal Jealousy Scale, a 28-item, relationship-specific measure of romantic jealousy, Nancy Severa and I sought variables to correlate with it to demonstrate the scale's construct validity. One variable we chose was romantic love. Supporting the hypothesis that the more in love an individual is, the more vulnerable he or she is to jealousy, we found positive and significant correlations between scores on the Interpersonal Jealousy Scale and Rubin's Romantic Love Scale for both men (.47) and women (.41). Other researchers have also found a positive relationship between jealousy and romantic love (Rosmarin, Chambless, & LaPointe, 1979; White, 1984).

Dependence functions in much the same way as romantic love. The more dependent P is on B (possibly because P has no alternative romantic partners available), the more P is threatened by R's presence. Data supporting this hypothesis were also found in the study I did with Severa (Mathes & Severa, 1981). To measure dependence, we used three different questions: (1) "Do you encourage your partner to engage in activities that interest him or her but do not interest you?" (2) "Do you and your partner do everything together?" (3) "Do you encourage your partner to maintain an identity separate from your own?" Responses were made on 7-point scales ranging from "Definitely false" to "Definitely true," and scoring was in the direction of independence (or separate identities). Negative and significant correlations between scores on the Interpersonal Jealousy Scale and responses to each of the items were predicted and found for both men ($-.27$, $-.32$, $-.39$) and women ($-.35$, $-.40$, $-.44$). Other researchers using other jealousy and dependence measures have found similar results (Bringle, Evenbeck, & Schmedel, 1977; Buunk, 1981; White, 1981b, 1981d).

## P's Values

A third aspect of the actual P-B-R triangle that enters into P's primary appraisal is that of P's values. If P values monogamy, exclusivity, and fidelity, R's presence is more threatening than if P values individual freedom or sharing. In fact, if P values individual freedom or sharing, P may evaluate R's presence as positive/benign because R's presence gives B a chance to be sexually free, P a chance to be sexually free (what is good for the goose is good for the gander, or vice versa), and P a chance to share B with R.

One factor that may determine the extent to which an individual believes in individual freedom is the individual's level of moral maturity. Let me explain. Imagine a newly married couple, P and B. P and B are trying to decide whether they want a marriage involving romantic fidelity (a P-B relationship) or a marriage involving romantic freedom (a P-B-R relationship). P would like romantic fidelity from B but would like variety for himself or herself. Similarly, B would like romantic fidelity from P but would like to fool around a bit on his or her own. What are P and B to do? They cannot both have their cake and eat it too. A compromise is necessary, and this is where morality enters the picture. Moralities specify what must be given up to make cooperation possible (Kohlberg, 1981).

What determines which morality, which compromise, a couple chooses? One factor is probably level of moral maturity. Kohlberg (1981) has suggested that there are three broad levels of moral maturity—"preconventional," "conventional," and "postconventional." The preconventional individual has no morality. He or she is selfish, concerned only with the satisfaction of his or her own needs. If P and B were both functioning at this level, each would demand fidelity from the partner, while cheating on the partner behind the partner's back. Neither P nor B would compromise, and thus such relationships are somewhat unstable, except if one of the individuals has a distinct power advantage. If this were the case, the more powerful individual would force fidelity onto the partner while retaining his or her own freedom. The medieval tower and chastity belt come to mind.

The conventional individual works in terms of cultural norms and laws. If P and B were working at this level, they would allow the conventions and laws of the United States (assuming that they are citizens of the United States) to guide them. Although the norms and laws of the United States concerning marital fidelity are not as clear as they once were, they generally link fidelity to formal commitment. Romantic freedom is prescribed for individuals engaging in casual dating, whereas romantic fidelity is prescribed for married individuals. If P and B were working at the conventional level of moral maturity, they would practice romantic fidelity.

The postconventional individual works in terms of individual rights and social contracts (Kohlberg calls this sublevel Stage 5) or universal ethical principles such as justice (Kohlberg calls this sublevel Stage 6). If P and B were working in terms of individual rights and social contracts, they would each retain their romantic freedom except if they mutually contracted to limit it. If P and B were working in terms of universal ethical principles, they would always retain their romantic freedom (though they might not exercise it), each being answerable only to universal ethical principles.

This suggests that postconventional individuals, because they value individual freedom, are more likely to evaluate R's presence as positive/benign (or at least as less stressful) than are conventional individuals. To test this thinking, Donna Deuger-Guldeck and I (Mathes & Deuger, 1985) had college students, who were dating someone at the time, fill out measures of moral maturity and the Interpersonal Jealousy Scale. To measure endorsement of conventional morality, we used the California F Scale (Adorno, Frenkel-Brunswik, Levinson, & Sanford, 1950) and the Attitudes Toward Women Scale (Spence & Helmreich, 1978). To measure endorsement of postconventional morality, we used the Defining Issues Test (Rest, Cooper, Coder, Masanz, & Anderson, 1974). We hypothesized that positive and significant correlations would be found between scores on the Interpersonal Jealousy Scale and scores on the California F and Attitudes Toward Women Scales, and that a negative and significant correlation would be found between scores on the Interpersonal Jealousy Scale and scores on the Defining Issues Test. The predicted correlations were found for women but not men. For women, scores on the Interpersonal Jealousy Scale correlated .35 with scores on the California F Scale, .28 with scores on the Attitudes Toward Women Scale, and −.26 with scores on the Defining Issues Test. For men, only one of the predicted correlations was found: Scores on the Interpersonal Jealousy Scale correlated .32 with scores on the California F Scale.

Other researchers have also found positive correlations between jealousy and various measure of conventional thinking. Bringle, Roach, Andler, and Evenbeck (1977) found positive correlations between jealousy and the Dogmatism and Attitudes Toward Women Scales, and White (1981d) found positive correlations between jealousy and the Attitudes Toward Women Scale for both men and women.

Buunk's (1981) study of Dutch open marriages offers support for the hypothesis that individuals who value individual freedom and sharing appraise the P-B-R triangle as benign/positive. He found that individuals with spouses who had had a sexual affair evaluated the affair as positive for the following four reasons: "I was pleased because it gave me freedom too," "I was pleased for my partner that he/she had an enjoyable experience," "I was pleased that my partner had sexual intercourse with someone I liked," and "I was glad that my partner did not direct his/her attention solely to me." The first two reasons seem to reflect the value of individual freedom, whereas the latter two seem to reflect the value of sharing.

Since an individual's values are to some extent culturally determined, culture enters the theory here. Hupka (1981) has shown that individuals who are members of cultures that (1) value private property, (2) make marriage a prerequisite to sexual gratification, and (3) make marriage a prerequisite to full adult status are more likely to evaluate the P-B-R situation as stressful (i.e., to experience jealousy) than individuals who are members of cultures that do not endorse these three practices.

Some individuals have gone so far as to argue that primary appraisal of the P-B-R triangle is exclusively a matter of cultural values, and that therefore it is possible to create a culture in which sexual intercourse between B and R is generally appraised as positive/benign (Francoeur & Francoeur, 1974; O'Neill & O'Neill, 1972). Thus in their book *Open Marriage*, the O'Neills (1972) state:

> To begin with we would like to lay to rest the idea that sexual jealousy is natural, instinctive, and inevitable. It is none of these things. Jealousy is primarily a *learned* response, determined by cultural attitudes. In many societies around the world, including the Eskimo, the Marquesans, and Lobi of West Africa, the Siriono of Bolivia and others, jealousy is a minimum; and in still others, such as the Toda of India, it is almost completely absent. If in other societies it is greatly reduced or hardly exists at all, then it cannot be regarded as "natural" to man's behavior. Why then is it so prevalent in our society? (p. 236)

Responding to their own question, they state: "The idea of sexually exclusive monogamy and possession of another breeds deep-rooted dependencies, infantile and childish emotions and insecurities. The more insecure you are, the more you will be jealous" (p. 237).

Others, however, disagree, stating that jealousy is inevitable and universal. Thus, Kingsley Davis (1936/1977) describes the characteristics of jealousy in various cultures as "variable but inevitable" because sexual affection is a universally desired but limited commodity. Davis (1936/1977) states:

> Yet sexual affection is, unlike divine grace, a distributive value. To let it go undistributed would introduce anarchy into the group and destroy the social system. Promiscuity can take place only in so far as society has broken down and reached a state of anomie. (pp. 132–133)

Similarly, Hupka (1981) states: "No society of past or present has been able to eliminate the appraisal of threat in a jealous situation. Each social design merely alters the situation in which it is induced" (p. 327).

To shed some light on this controversy, Deuger-Guldeck and I (Mathes & Deuger, 1982) studied cats and dogs, our rationale being that if jealousy is merely a learned emotion found in monogamous cultures, jealousy should not be found in cats or dogs, who have neither culture nor monogamy. Two hypotheses were tested. The first was that jealousy would be found in cats and dogs, and the second was that, as with people, a positive relationship would be found between the extent of the animals' affection and their jealousy. The owners of 58 cats and 70 dogs participated in this study by answering a five-item questionnaire:

1. How long have you had your pet?
2. Does your pet like you very much?
3. Does your pet show signs of distress when you leave it?
4. Has your pet ever shown signs of jealousy?
5. If your pet has shown signs of jealousy, does it have frequent episodes of jealousy?

Responses to questions 2, 3, and 5 were made on 7-point scales ranging from "No, definitely" (1) to "Yes, definitely" (7). Question 4 required a yes or no response.

Seventy-nine percent of the cat owners and 95% of the dog owners reported that their animals had shown signs of jealousy. Thus, support was found for the first hypothesis. (To rule out the possibility that these reports were simple projections, subjects filled out the Self-Report Jealousy Scale, and scores on it were correlated with answers to question 4. Significant correlations were not found, suggesting that the results cannot be explained in terms of projection.) Furthermore, for cats, frequency of jealousy was positively and significantly correlated with how much a cat liked its owner (.48) and the extent to which the cat showed signs of distress when it was left behind (.50). For dogs, frequency of jealousy was positively and significantly correlated with length of time with owner (.26), how much the dog liked the owner (.24), and the extent to which the dog showed signs of distress when it was left behind (.51). Thus, support was also found for the second hypothesis. The results of this study suggest that jealousy is not simply an emotion taught by monogamous cultures to preserve monogamy, but rather an inevitable and universal emotion found even in dogs and cats. Jealousy appears to be a universal distress response to the possibility of losing a loved one to a rival.

### P's Psychological Health

A fourth aspect of the actual P-B-R triangle that may enter into P's primary appraisal is P's mental health. If P is mentally healthy, P will appraise R's presence as less stressful than if P is neurotic. If P is healthy, P will be more optimistic about his or her chances of keeping B than if P is neurotic. Furthermore, if P is healthy, P will suffer less should P lose B to R than if P is neurotic—there are other fish in the sea.

Evidence supporting this thinking comes from a number of sources. In the 1981 study, Severa and I looked not only at jealousy and romantic love and dependence, but also at psychological health (Mathes & Severa, 1981). To measure psychological health, we gave subjects Maslow's Insecurity Scale (Maslow, Birsch, Stein, & Honigmann, 1945) and Rosenberg's (1965) Self-esteem Scale. Although we predicted a positive correlation between jealousy and insecurity, and a negative correlation between jealousy and self-esteem, only the former correlation was found for women (.26). However, other researchers have repeatedly found positive and significant correlations between jealousy and various kinds of psychopathology: neuroticism (Buunk, 1981; Rosmarin et al., 1979), anxiety (Bringle, Roach, et al., 1977; Bringle & Williams, 1979; Jaremko & Lindsey, 1979; White, 1984), low self-esteem (Buunk, 1982; Hupka & Bachelor, 1979; Jaremko & Lindsey, 1979; Rosmarin et al., 1979; Stewart & Beatty, 1985), and external locus of control (Bringle, Roach, et al., 1977; White, 1984).

Petra Roter, Steven Joerger, and I (Mathes, Roter, & Joerger, 1982) carried out a study in which we gave subjects six jealousy scales, two measures of neuroticism, two measures of romantic love, and the Maudsley Introversion–Extraversion Scale. The jealousy scales included the single-item measure of Pines and Aronson (1983), the Self-Report and Projective Jealousy Scales of Bringle, Roach, et al. (1977), White's

(1984) Chronic Jealousy and Relationship Jealousy Scales, and the Interpersonal Jealousy Scale. The measures of neuroticism included the Maudsley Neuroticism Scale and the Insecurity Scale of Fei and Berscheid (1977). The measures of romantic love included Rubin's (1970) Romantic Love Scale and the Dependency Scale of Fei and Berscheid (1977). These 11 scales were then factor-analyzed with sex as a dummy variable. The first factor, which accounted for 29.0% of the total variance, appeared to be a Jealousy–Neuroticism variable. The following scales loaded .30 or greater on this factor: the Pines–Aronson item, the Chronic Jealousy and Relationship Jealousy Scales, the Maudsley Neuroticism Scale, and the Insecurity Scale. In addition, the Dependency Scale loaded −.31 on this factor. Thus this study also supports the hypothesis that neurotics are more vulnerable to jealousy than normal individuals. The second factor, which accounted for 15.5% of the total variance, appeared to be a Normal Jealousy factor; the remaining three jealousy scales loaded .30 or greater on it. The third factor, which accounted for 10.1% of the total variance, appeared to represent Introversion–Extraversion, as the Maudsley Introversion–Extraversion Scale loaded −.70 on it. The fourth factor, which accounted for 9.7% of the total variance, appeared to represent Romantic Love; the Romantic Love and Dependency Scales loaded .30 or greater on it.

### P's Trait Jealousy

A fifth aspect of the actual P-B-R triangle that may enter into P's primary appraisal is P's level of trait jealousy. If P is high in trait jealousy, P will appraise R's presence as more stressful than if P is low in trait jealousy. There is some evidence that jealousy exists as a personality trait. In the factor-analytic study described above (Mathes, Roter, & Joerger, 1982), convergence was found among three measures of jealousy: the Self-Report and Projective Jealousy Scales of Bringle, Roach, et al. (1977), and the Interpersonal Jealousy Scale. These scales were also found to diverge from measures of neuroticism, romantic love, and introversion–extraversion, suggesting that jealousy is not merely another name for neuroticism or romantic love.

   In another study I carried out (Mathes, 1984), convergence over target persons and divergence from love, liking, and sexual attraction were demonstrated. Each subject filled out the Interpersonal Jealousy Scale, Rubin's Romantic Love and Liking Scales, and a Sexual Attraction Scale for his or her dating partner, a same-sex friend, and an opposite-sex friend. These measures were then factor-analyzed with sex as a dummy variable. Four factors were found. The first, which accounted for 24.8%

of the total variance, appeared to be a Liking–Love factor. All of the subscales of the Liking and Love Scales, regardless of target person, loaded .30 or greater on this factor. The second factor, which accounted for 18.0% of the total variance, appeared to be a Jealousy factor. All of the subscales of the Interpersonal Jealousy Scale, regardless of target person, loaded .30 or greater on this factor. The third factor, which accounted for 8.0% of the total variance, appeared to be a Sex Differences factor. In addition to sex of subject, which loaded .74 on this factor, three other measures loaded .30 or greater on it: Sexual Attraction for the opposite-sex friend (.75), Liking for the dating partner (−.34), and Love for the same-sex friend, (−.31). The fourth factor, which accounted for 10.0% of the total variance, appeared to be a Dating Partner factor; all of the dating partner measures loaded .30 or greater on it. The jealousy factor of this study provides evidence of convergence over target persons, and the fact that the Liking, Love, and Sexual Attraction Scales did not load on this factor provides evidence of divergence.

These two studies suggest that jealousy is a trait. Jealous people score high on jealousy, regardless of the instrument used to measure jealousy and regardless of the target of the jealousy (dating partner, same-sex friend, or opposite-sex friend). Nonjealous people score low on jealousy, regardless of the instrument used to measure it and regardless of the target of the jealousy.

## SECONDARY APPRAISAL

If, after taking these aspects of the actual P-B-R triangle (probability that R will take B, love for B, values, psychological health, and trait jealousy) into consideration, P's primary appraisal is that the P-B-R triangle is positive/benign, P will engage in secondary appraisal designed to maintain R's involvement with B or, possibly, to increase R's involvement with B. If P's primary appraisal is that the P-B-R triangle is irrelevant with regard to his or her well-being, P will not engage in further (i.e., secondary) appraisal. If P's primary appraisal of the P-B-R triangle is that it is stressful, P will engage in secondary appraisal designed to remedy the situation. It is probably only this last situation that qualifies as jealousy; a negative primary appraisal of the P-B-R triangle seems intrinsic to jealousy.

### Reward

If P's primary appraisal of the P-B-R triangle is that it is stressful, P's secondary appraisal will be oriented toward determining whether anything can be done to salvage his or her relationship with B. P finds himself or herself in competition with R, and must determine his or her own chances of winning. One line of inquiry that P may follow focuses on rewards. Who has the most to offer B—P or R? This calls for social comparison. White (1981c) has found that individuals tend to compare themselves with rivals along the following dimensions: physical/sexual attractiveness, intelligence, personality, career success, sensitivity to B, similarity to B, and willingness to make a commitment to B. B's wants enter into this appraisal. For example, if B cares only about money, comparison will focus primarily on the career success of P and R. White (1981a, 1981c) has found that P's attempts to determine what B wants, or more specifically why B is attracted to R, involve the following attributions: "because B is dissatisfied with me (P)," "because B is sexually attracted to R," "because B is generally attracted to R," "because B is testing our (P and B's) relationship and/or seeking attention," and "because B wants commitment from me (P)." If P feels that he or she has more to offer B than R has to offer B, especially if what P has to offer is what B really wants, P will probably conclude that his or her chances of keeping B are good. On the other hand, if R has more to offer and what R has to offer is what B wants, P will probably be forced to conclude that his or her chances of keeping B are poor.

## Punishment

Another line of secondary appraisal that P may follow focuses on punishment: P may ask whether punishment would be effective in causing B to stay. The punishments considered may involve withdrawal of affection, financial support, or sexual privileges; physical or emotional violence; divorce; or threats of any of these (Whitehurst, 1971). As with rewards, P will probably tailor punishments to B. For example, P will not threaten to divorce B if P and B are not married. P may also appraise the effectiveness of the use of punishment to drive R away from B. If P finds a punishment or set of punishments that he or she believes will persuade B to remain in the relationship, P will probably conclude that his or her chances of keeping B are good. On the other hand, if P can think of no effective punishment or set of punishments, he or she will probably conclude that B is lost.

## Moral and Legal Power

A third line of secondary appraisal that P may follow is that of moral and legal power over B. Is B legally married to P? If B is legally married to P, then P has legal and social rights to B. P may also ask whether B feels bound to P. Would B feel immoral and guilty if he or she left P for R? If P concludes that B is legally and morally bound to P, and that the legal and social systems and B's own conscience will support and enforce P's rights, P will probably conclude that the chances of keeping B are good. On the other hand, if P's claims are weak and unlikely to be supported, P will probably conclude that his or her chances of keeping B are not very good.

P will probably use secondary appraisal to examine other sources of power over B (discussion, marital therapy, etc.) to determine his or her chances of retaining B. The final product will be a rough estimate of his or her chances of keeping B. This probability, though, is not the only factor that enters into P's secondary appraisal. P probably also looks at cost. How much will it cost P (in terms of time, money, effort, etc.) to keep B or win B back from R? Are the benefits B provides worth the cost of keeping B from R or winning him or her back from R? How much does P really love B? Does P have alternative romantic possibilities? Cheaper alternative romantic possibilities? How much shame (loss of self-esteem) will P suffer if he or she loses B to R? The rational thing for P to do in deciding whether or not to fight for B would seem to be to multiply the probability of retaining B or winning B back by the benefits B has to offer. If this "figure" is greater than the costs and the best alternative deal available, P should implement the coping strategies that may keep B or win B back from R. On the other hand, if this figure is less than the costs or there is a cheaper alternative, P should let R have B and focus on salvaging his or her own self-esteem. Whether individuals actually make decisions in this manner is an empirical question.

If the conclusion of P's secondary appraisal is to fight for B, P will put into action those coping strategies that his or her secondary appraisal has indicated are most likely to work. If P feels that he or she has more to offer B than R has to offer B, P will attempt to make this clear to B. If P feels that giving B things previously withheld (attention, commitment, sex, a big diamond ring) will save B from R, P will give these things to B. If P feels that refusing to support B financially until B gives up seeing R may work, P will follow that course. If P feels that his or her greatest strength is moral, P will ask his or her pastor to talk to B about the sin of adultery.

## REAPPRAISAL

Once P has put one or more coping strategies into action, P will engage in reappraisal; that is, P will appraise the success of his or her coping actions. If the actions succeed—in other words, if they destroy the P-B-R triangle, leaving only P and B—P will probably move on to new problems. If the coping actions fail, P will have to reappraise the situation further and decide whether, in light of these new data, attempting to hold B is possible and/or worthwhile. Depending on the outcome of this appraisal, P will either decide to put new coping plans into action or give up on B and focus on saving face.

## COPING

I have carried out only a few studies on coping. The first study, which I conducted with John Phillips, Julie Skowron, and William Dick (Mathes, Phillips, Skowran, & Dick, 1982), was not specifically designed to investigate coping behavior. Its purpose was to investigate the validity of the Interpersonal Jealousy Scale by determining whether the scale could predict real-world behavior and not just responses on paper-and-pencil questionnaires. Inadvertently, however, we studied coping behavior. The coping behavior we studied would probably qualify as the exercise of moral power to prevent R from dating B. Specifically, we gave dating couples the Interpersonal Jealousy Scale. Several weeks later, a male stooge called the men and a female stooge called the women and asked for permission to date each subject's romantic partner. A typical conversation went something like the following (Mathes, Phillips, et al., 1982, p. 1229):

> Confederate: "Hello Subject, this is Confederate. I don't think that we have even met but the reason I am calling is that I was sitting in the Union earlier this week with a friend when Patsy (subject's girl friend) came along and sat down with us. She knew my friend. We talked for a while and I was impressed by what a nice girl Patsy is. After about ten minutes or so she left and I asked my friend whether Patsy was going out with anyone. My friend told me that she was going out with you. So, I decided to call you and ask you whether it is all right if I were to give Patsy a call and ask her out for a beer after class someday so that I can get to know her better. I'm calling you because I don't want to cause any trouble. Would you mind?"
> Subject: "Well we're engaged to be married so I don't think you had better ask her out."

The conversations were tape-recorded. We hypothesized that jealous subjects would be less likely to give the stooge permission than less jealous subjects would be. The tapes of the conversations were rated by three judges with respect to the extent to which each subject granted the stooge permission to date the subject's boyfriend or girlfriend. The judges used a 5-point scale ranging from "Definitely no, you may not go out with my partner" (1) to "Definitely yes, you may go out with my partner" (5), and their ratings were summed to create a composite rating. Support for the hypothesis was found. Scores on the Interpersonal Jealousy Scale were negatively and significantly correlated with permission for both men (−.40) and women (−.37). This study suggests that one coping strategy highly jealous individuals are likely to put into action is denying R permission to date B. Whether this coping behavior is effective or not is another question.

Another study I carried out (Mathes, 1988) investigated the effectiveness of coping with the loss of B to R by finding a new love. If the worst happens and P loses B to R, a reasonable strategy for coping with this situation would seem to be to find a new B who offers all or possibly more of the relationship rewards and self-esteem perks that the old B used to provide. To test this thinking, I had college students who had experienced the loss of a romantic relationship fill out a questionnaire concerning subsequent romantic relationships, entitled the Subsequent Relationships Questionnaire. I also had them fill out the Interpersonal Jealousy Scale with respect to current feelings for the lost romantic partner. Subjects filled out a copy of the Subsequent Relationships Questionnaire for each subsequent relationship. The first six items on the Subsequent Relationships Questionnaire focused on relationship rewards:

1. How many times have you dated this person?
2. While going with this person did you love him or her?
3. While going with this person did this person love you?
4. While going with this person was the relationship a sexual relationship?
5. While going with this person did your social life revolve entirely around him or her?
6. Are you dating this person now?

The last six items focused on self-esteem rewards:

7. While going with this person did he or she make you feel good about yourself?
8. While going with this person were you proud to be with him or her?

9. If this relationship has been terminated, did you terminate it?
10. If this relationship has been terminated, did your partner terminate it?
11. If this relationship has been terminated, was the termination due to your finding someone you liked better?
12. If this relationship has been terminated, was the termination due to your partner's finding someone he or she liked better?

Responses to all of the items, except the first one, were made on 7-point scales ranging from "No, definitely" (1) to "Yes, definitely" (7); the scoring of items 10 and 12 was reversed. If a subject had not had a subsequent relationship, item 1 was give a score of 0 and subsequent items were given scores of 1. If a subsequent relationship had not been terminated, items 9 through 12 were given scores of 7. If a subject had had more than one subsequent relationship, responses to each item were summed.

It was hypothesized that negative and significant correlations would be found between scores on the Interpersonal Jealousy Scale and the 12 items of the Subsequent Relationships Questionnaire. Support for this hypothesis was found for women but not for men. For women, negative and significant correlations were found between scores on the Interpersonal Jealousy Scale and responses to item 2, love for subsequent partner (−.29); item 3, subsequent partner's love for subject (−.25); item 4, sexual involvement (−.31); item 6, whether the subject was currently dating the subsequent partner (−.26); item 8, pride in subsequent partner (−.25); and item 11, subject's termination of subsequent partner in favor of someone better (−.23). For men, none of the correlations were significant. These data suggest that if P is a woman, a successful strategy for coping with the loss of B to R is to establish a successful relationship with a new B.

In a third study (Mathes, 1986), I investigated the long-range effects of jealousy on romantic relationships. If P is jealous, and presumably engages in coping activities designed to keep B from R, do P's jealous activities generally succeed or do they backfire and drive B away from P to R? To answer this question, I wrote in the fall of 1985 to 70 subjects who had filled out the Interpersonal Jealousy Scale as members of couples in 1978. (Sixty-five couples filled out the scale in 1978, but I was able to find addresses for only 70 of the individual subjects.) Of these subjects, 39 responded and 9 reported that they were still with their 1978 partners. Comparing the 1978 mean jealousy score of the 9 "successful" individuals (168.88, $SD = 36.55$) with the mean jealousy score of the 30 "unsuccessful" individuals (142.77, $SD = 36.55$), I found that the successful individuals had significantly higher 1978 jealousy scores than the unsuccessful individuals. This suggests that jealous people indeed do succeed in holding on to their partners.

## EMOTIONAL RESPONSES

P's primary appraisal of the P-B-R triangle will determine his or her initial emotional response. If P decides that R's presence is positive/benign, because P wants to get rid of B, P's emotional response will probably be positive—relief, joy, and so on. If P decides that R's presence is positive/benign because this situation allows for individual freedom and sharing, P's emotional response also will probably be positive—excitement (freedom), love (sharing), and so on. However, these positive emotions will probably not be unadulterated, because as long as P wants to keep B, P's appraisal of the P-B-R triangle must also be negative. There is always the possibility of losing B to R. And even though B may not physically leave P for R, B may do so emotionally: B may come to love R more than P. Thus the excitement and love will be tempered by negative emotions—anxiety, depression, and anger. Supporting this, Buunk's (1981) study of Dutch open marriages found that the P-B-R triangle generated not only positive but also negative primary appraisals.

If P's primary appraisal of the P-B-R triangle is that it is neutral with respect to P's well-being, there will probably be little emotional response. If P's primary appraisal of the P-B-R triangle is that it is stressful, P will probably experience negative emotions. Adams, Davies, and I (Mathes et al., 1985) investigated three negative emotions—depression, anxiety, and anger. We hypothesized that P would experience all three of these emotions if he or she lost B to R. Furthermore, we hypothesized that the depression would result from the loss of relationship rewards, whereas the anxiety and anger would result from the loss of self-esteem. To test these hypotheses, we presented the four loss conditions used in our earlier research ("fate," "lover's destiny," "rejection," and "rival") to subjects, and asked them how depressed, anxious, angry, and jealous they would feel:

1. If this happened to you would you feel depressed over the loss?
2. If this happened to you would you feel anxious concerning your own well-being?

3. If this happened to you would you feel angry toward your boyfriend (girlfriend)?
4. If this happened to you would you feel jealous?

Responses were made on 7-point scales ranging from "No, definitely" (1) to "Yes, definitely" (7).

It was hypothesized that depression would be high across all of the loss conditions, because they all involve the loss of relationship rewards. Paralleling the loss of self-esteem, anxiety and anger would be low in the fate condition, moderate in the lover's destiny condition, and high in the rejection and rival conditions. Following definition, jealousy would be low in all of the conditions except the rival condition.

The results are presented in Figure 3.3. As can be seen, the depression hypothesis was supported: Depression was high for all four loss conditions. The anger hypothesis was generally supported. Anger was low for the fate condition, moderate for the lover's destiny condition, and high for the rival condition. Contrary to prediction, anger was only moderate for the rejection condition. Apparently, losing B to R is more insulting than simply being rejected by B, possibly because both P and B are without a partner in the rejection situation, whereas only P is without a partner in the rival situation. The anxiety hypothesis was not supported: Anxiety was moderately high for all four conditions. This suggests that anxiety may be a function of the loss of relationship rewards (separation anxiety?) and not a function of the loss of self-esteem. Support was found for the jealousy hypothesis; the rival condition received the highest jealousy rating (22.34). The other means were all below the neither-true-nor-false midpoint of 16: fate, 7.07; lover's destiny, 13.46; and rejection, 15.50.

An examination of Figure 3.3 shows that the emotional response (other than jealousy) that most closely parallels jealousy is anger. This suggests that anger is especially characteristic of the P-B-R stress situation. Mullen and Maack (1985) also have suggested that anger is the primary emotional response to P-B-R stress. They suggest that infidelity causes pain and pain causes anger and the desire for revenge. Similarly, Davis (1936/1977) suggests that society encourages P to respond to B's infidelity with anger and punishment, so as to preserve the institution of marriage.

If B and R engage in a sexual encounter and P finds out, at whom is P angrier, B or R? Mullen and Maack (1985) suggest that it is B, because B has violated P's trust. To support their hypothesis, they examined the records of 138 patients admitted into Maudsley and Bethlem Hospitals between 1967 and 1980 who had been diagnosed as exhibiting patholog-

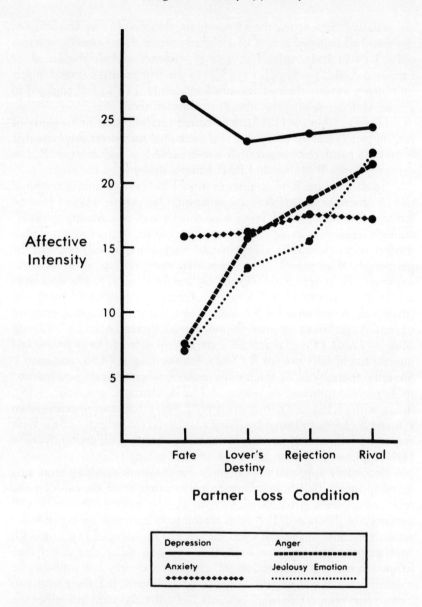

**FIGURE 3.3.** Depression, anxiety, anger, and jealousy as a function of type of partner loss. From "Jealousy: Loss of Relationship Rewards, Loss of Self-esteem, Depression, Anxiety, and Anger" by E. W. Mathes, H. E. Adams, & R. M. Davies, 1985, *Journal of Personality and Social Psychology, 42*, p. 1559. Copyright 1985 by the American Psychological Association. Adapted by permission.

ical jealousy. Supporting their hypothesis, they found that 48 (56%) of the men had engaged in acts of violence against their partners, whereas only 3 (4%) had engaged in acts of violence against the actual or supposed rivals. Twenty-three (43%) of the women had engaged in acts of violence against their partners, whereas only 4 (8%) had engaged in acts of violence against the actual or supposed rivals.

However, Mowat (1966), who found similar results in his study of pathologically jealous murderers and attempted murderers, suggests that B may be murdered instead of R not because P is less angry at R, but simply because P cannot find R, R being a delusion.

To shed further light on this question, I had college students respond to 135 variations of the following situation: "If a partner whom I (had no feelings for; liked; loved very, very much) and was (dating casually; dating exclusively; living with; engaged to; married to) had sex with a third party, I (would be angry; would punish; might kill) (myself; the partner; the third party)." Responses were made on 7-point scales ranging from "Definitely false" (1) to "Definitely true" (7). The data were analyzed by means of a 2 (sex of subject) $\times$ 3 (degree of love) $\times$ 5 (degree of commitment) $\times$ 3 (emotion or action) $\times$ 3 (target of emotion or action) analysis of variance. Supporting Mullen and Maack (1985) and Mowat (1966), I found that P felt most negative (would be angry; would punish; might kill) toward B (3.92), followed by R (3.55) and then P himself or herself (2.27). P felt most negative when he or she was married to B (3.72), followed by engaged (3.24), dating exclusively (3.19), living with (3.18), and dating casually (2.89). P felt most negative when P loved B (3.79), followed by liking (3.37) and no feelings (2.58). With respect to feelings and actions, P was most likely to respond with anger (4.49), followed by punishment (3.49) and killing (1.76).

Secondary appraisal may modify the emotions resulting from primary appraisal. If P finds reason to believe that he or she can save the relationship with B by getting rid of R, the negative emotions will probably be dampened. If P finds reason to believe that the relationship rewards are lost but that P's self-esteem can be salvaged (e.g., through sour grapes—"Losing that loser B is the best thing that could ever happen to me"), P's depression and separation anxiety will probably be amplified, but P's anger will probably be dampened. If P finds reason to believe that both relationship rewards and self-esteem are lost, all of the negative emotions will probably be amplified.

Ultimately, the success or failure of the coping strategies will determine whether the negative emotions are dampened or amplified. If the coping mechanisms succeed, the negative emotions will dampen and disappear; if the coping mechanisms fail, the negative emotions will be amplified.

## SUMMARY

The cognitive theory of jealousy I have presented in this chapter suggests that when confronted with a P-B-R triangle, P initially engages in primary appraisal to determine whether the situation is benign/positive, irrelevant, or stressful with respect to his or her well-being. P's primary appraisal takes into consideration the probability that R will succeed in taking B from P; P's love for B; P's values; P's mental health; and P's level of trait jealousy. If P's primary appraisal of the P-B-R situation is that it is stressful, we have a case of jealousy. Primary appraisal is followed by secondary appraisal. P attempts to determine whether there are strategies available that would eliminate R and restore the P-B relationship and that are not too costly. Such strategies may include reward, punishment, and moral and legal power. Secondary appraisal is followed by the implementation of coping strategies and reappraisal to determine the effectiveness of the coping strategies.

A negative primary appraisal of the P-B-R situation results in negative emotions (depression, anxiety, anger, etc.). P's anger is aimed at both B and R, though P's anger against B is greater than P's anger against R. Secondary appraisal often modifies these initial emotions. The discovery of a promising coping strategy dampens the negative emotions, whereas the failure to find a promising coping strategy amplifies the negative emotions. Reappraisal also often modifies the emotions. The success of a coping strategy dampens the negative emotions, whereas the failure of a coping strategy amplifies them.

## REFERENCES

Adorno, T. W., Frenkel-Brunswik, E., Levinson, P. J., & Sanford, R. M. (1950). *The authoritarian personality.* New York: Harper.

Bers, S. A., & Rodin, J. (1984). Social-comparison jealousy: A developmental and motivational study. *Journal of Personality and Social Psychology, 47,* 766–779.

Bringle, R. G., Evenbeck, S., & Schmedel, K. (1977). *The role of jealousy in marriage.* Paper presented at the 85th annual convention of the American Psychological Association, San Francisco.

Bringle, R. G., Roach, S., Andler, C., & Evenbeck, S. (1977). *Correlates of jealousy.* Paper presented at the 49th annual meeting of the Midwestern Psychological Association, Chicago.

Bringle, R. G., & Williams, L. J. (1979). Parent-offspring similarity on jealousy and related personality dimensions. *Motivation and Emotion, 3,* 265–286.

Buunk, B. (1981). Jealousy in sexually open marriages. *Alternative Lifestyles, 4,* 357–372.

Buunk, R. (1982). *Jealousy: Some recent findings and issues.* Paper presented at the First International Conference on Personal Relationships, Madison, WI.

Davis, K. (1977). Jealousy and sexual property. In G. Clanton & L. G. Smith (Eds.), *Jealousy* (pp. 129–135). Englewood Cliffs, NJ: Prentice-Hall. (Original work published 1936)

Fei, J., & Berscheid, E. (1977). *Perceived dependency, insecurity, and love in heterosexual relationships: The eternal triangle?* Unpublished manuscript, University of Minnesota.

Francoeur, A. K., & Francoeur, R. T. (1974).*Hot and cool sex: Cultures in conflict.* New York: Harcourt, Brace & Jovanovich.

Hupka, R. B. (1981). Cultural determinants of jealousy. *Alternative Lifestyles, 4,* 310–356.

Hupka, R. B., & Bachelor, B. (1979). *Validation of a scale to measure romantic jealousy.* Paper presented at the meeting of the Western Psychological Association, San Diego, CA.

Jaremko, M., & Lindsey, R. (1979). Stress-coping abilities of individuals high and low in jealousy. *Psychological Reports, 44,* 547–553.

Kohlberg, L. (1981). *The philosophy of moral development.* New York: Harper & Row.

Lazarus, R. S. (1966). *Psychological stress and the coping process.* New York: McGraw Hill.

Lazarus, R. S., & Averill, J. R. (1972). Emotion and cognition: With special reference to anxiety. In C. D. Spielberger (Ed.), *Anxiety: Current trends in theory and research* (Vol. 2, pp. 242–274). New York: Academic Press.

Lazarus, R. S., Kanner, A. D., & Folkman, S. (1980). Emotions: A cognitive–phenomenological analysis. In R. Plutchik & H. Kellerman (Eds.), *Emotion: Theory, research, and experience* (Vol. 1, pp. 189–217). New York: Academic Press.

Maslow, A. J., Birsch, E., Stein, M., & Honigmann, I. (1945). A clinically derived test for measuring psychological security-insecurity. *Journal of General Psychology, 33,* 21–44.

Mathes, E. W. (1984). Convergence among measures of interpersonal attraction. *Motivation and Emotion, 8,* 77–84.

Mathes, E. W. (1986). Jealousy and romantic love: A longitudinal study. *Psychological Reports, 58,* 885–886.

Mathes, E. W. (1988). *Dealing with romantic jealousy.* Paper presented at the 96th annual convention of the American Psychological Association, Atlanta.

Mathes, E. W., Adams, H. E., & Davies, R. M. (1985). Jealousy: Loss of relationship rewards, loss of self-esteem, depression, anxiety, and anger. *Journal of Personality and Social Psychology, 48,* 1552–1561.

Mathes, E. W., & Deuger, D. J. (1982). Jealousy: A creation of human culture? *Psychological Reports, 51,* 351–354.

Mathes, E. W., & Deuger, D. J. (1985). *Jealousy and moral development.* Paper presented at the 57th annual meeting of the Midwestern Psychological Association, Chicago.

Mathes, E. W., Phillips, J. T., Skowron, J., & Dick, W. E. (1982). Behavioral correlates of the Interpersonal Jealousy Scale. *Educational and Psychological Measurement, 42,* 1227–1231.

Mathes, E. W., Roter, P. M., & Joerger, S. M. (1982). A convergent validity study of six jealousy scales. *Psychological Reports, 50,* 1143–1147.

Mathes, E. W., & Severa, N. (1981). Jealousy, romantic love, and liking: Theoretical considerations and preliminary scale development. *Psychological Reports, 49,* 23–31.

Mowat, R. R. (1966). *Morbid jealousy and murder.* London: Tavistock.

Mullen, P. E., & Maack, L. H. (1985). Jealousy, pathological jealousy, and aggression. In D. P. Farrington & J. Gunn (Eds.), *Aggression and dangerousness* (pp. 103–126). New York: Wiley.

O'Neill, N., & O'Neill, G. (1972). *Open marriage.* New York: Avon.

Pines, A., & Aronson, E. (1983). Antecedents, correlates, and consequences of sexual jealousy. *Journal of Personality, 51,* 108–136.

Rest, J., Cooper, P., Coder, R., Masanz, J., & Anderson, D. (1974). Judging the important issues in moral dilemmas: An objective measure of development. *Developmental Psychology, 10,* 491–501.

Rosenberg, M. (1965). *Society and the adolescent self-image.* Princeton, NJ: Princeton University Press.

Rosmarin, D. M., Chambless, D. L., & LaPointe, K. (1979). *The survey of interpersonal reactions: An inventory for the measurement of jealousy.* Unpublished manuscript, University of Georgia.

Rubin, Z. (1970). Measurement of romantic love. *Journal of Personality and Social Psychology, 16,* 265–273.

Salovey, P., & Rodin, J. (1986). The differentiation of social-comparison jealousy and romantic jealousy. *Journal of Personality and Social Psychology, 50,* 1100–1112.

Shettel-Neuber, J., Bryson, J. B., & Young, L. E. (1978). Physical attractiveness of the "other person" and jealousy. *Personality and Social Psychology Bulletin, 4,* 612–615.

Smith, R. H., Kim, S. H., & Parrott, W. G. (1988). Envy and jealousy: Semantic problems and experiential distinctions. *Personality and Social Psychology Bulletin, 14,* 401–409.

Spence, S. T., & Helmreich, R. (1978). *Masculinity and femininity.* Austin: University of Texas Press.

Stewart, R. A., & Beatty, M. J. (1985). Jealousy and self-esteem. *Perceptual and Motor Skills, 60,* 153–154.

White, G. L. (1981a). Jealousy and partner's perceived motives for attraction to a rival. *Social Psychology Quarterly, 44*, 24–30.

White, G. L. (1981b). A model of romantic jealousy. *Motivation and Emotion, 5*, 295–310.

White, G. L. (1981c). *Social comparison, motive attribution, alternative assessment, and coping with jealousy.* Paper presented at the 89th annual convention of the American Psychological Association, Anaheim, CA.

White, G. L. (1981d). Some correlates of romantic jealousy. *Journal of Personality, 49*, 129–147.

White, G. L. (1984). Comparison of four jealousy scales. *Journal of Research in Personality, 18*, 115–130.

Whitehurst, R. N. (1971). Violence potential in extramarital sexual response. *Journal of Marriage and the Family, 33*, 683–691.

## Chapter Four

# Envy and the Sense
# of Injustice

RICHARD H. SMITH
*Boston University*

> Who dares to say that ever proud Salieri
> Could stoop to envy, like a loathsome snake
> Trampled upon by men, yet still alive
> And impotently gnawing sand and dust?
> No one! . . . But now—myself I say it—now
> I do know envy! Yes, Salieri envies,
> Deeply, in anguish envies.—O ye Heavens!
> Where, where is justice, when the sacred gift,
> When deathless genius come not to reward
> Perfervid love and utter denial,
> And toils and strivings and beseeching prayers,
> But puts a halo round a lack-wit's skull,
> A frivolous idler's brow? . . . O Mozart, Mozart!
> —*Pushkin (1832/1964, p. 430)*

The experience of envy typically involves both feelings of discontent brought about by another person's superiority and also a measure of hostility directed at the envied person. Discontent seems a natural result of noticing another's superiority. As many have argued (e.g., Festinger, 1954; Heider, 1958; Morse & Gergen, 1970; Nozick, 1974; Silver & Sabini, 1978; Smith & Insko, 1987; Tesser & Collins, 1988), self-esteem is often based on comparisons with others. To use Heider's words, "In evaluating one's own lot, *o*'s lot plays the role of background or surrounding, which, through the effects of contrast, can serve either to enhance $p$'s lot or impair it" (p. 285). In the case of envy, the background is another's advantage, and thus the result is often self-impairment and unhappiness (e.g., Salovey & Rodin, 1984; Silver & Sabini, 1978; Smith, Diener, & Garonzik, 1990; Tesser & Collins, 1988).

Although the discontent that is so much a part of envy appears easily explained, it is curious that envy should also include hostility. When, later in Pushkin's (1832/1964) short play about Antonio Salieri and Mozart, Salieri weeps as he listens to the first notes of Mozart's *Requiem*, it is because he knows that the music is so very fine in comparison to his own compositions. However, as Salieri weeps, Mozart is dying from the poison he has given him. Why should envy move a person to any degree of hostility, much less murder?

## ENVY AND HOSTILITY

One theoretical perspective that suggests a logic to envious hostility is provided by Campos, Barrett, Lamb, Goldsmith, and Stenberg's (1983) analysis of socioemotional development. Campos et al. argue that the "complex" emotion of envy, in addition to involving a response similar to sadness, should also produce anger. The anger should result from the envying person perceiving an obstacle to attaining a significant goal—the obstacle being represented by another person's advantage. The empirical work examining links between frustration and aggression is at least in part consistent with Campos et al.'s analysis (see Berkowitz, 1989, for a recent review of this work). The inability to obtain a desired attribute, highlighted by its presence in another, is a form of frustration (Berkowitz, 1972). In fact, frustration is usually defined as the blocking of a goal—a definition similar to Campos et al.'s (1983) description of the conditions leading to the anger component of envy. Some studies on frustration and aggression indicate that people need no more impetus than the blocking of a goal to act aggressively toward another person, even toward someone unassociated with the immediate frustrating event (Berkowitz, 1989). Still further research suggests that unpleasant, aversive experiences in general can produce a readiness to act aggressively; these findings have led some to propose that people are biologically disposed to feel hostility when confronted with such experiences (Berkowitz, 1989; Zillmann, 1979).

Does the theoretical analysis proposed by Campos et al. (1983), together with the research evidence linking frustration with aggression, provide a full explanation for hostile feelings in envy? What other typical features of the envy-producing situation might also be necessary to explain such hostile feelings, especially the intense and virulent kind portrayed by Pushkin in the person of Salieri?

## JUSTICE-RELATED FEELINGS IN ENVY

It is often noted, so much so that it can seem a trivial observation, that envy can masquerade as resentment (Rawls, 1971). That is, another's *legitimate* advantage will be construed by the envying person as *illegitimate*, so that envious feelings come across to oneself and to others as resentment or righteous indignation rather than envy. Thus, in his influential theory of justice, Rawls (1971) takes great care to avoid confusing envy with resentment; only the latter emotion, is a "moral" feeling in his view. According to Rawls, if we feel envy because of another person's advantage, we are *unable* to show that the other's advantage follows from unfair circumstances or improper actions. On the other hand, if unfair circumstances or improper actions can be shown, then the feeling evoked is *resentment*, not envy. In order to explain hostile feelings that do arise in envy (if these hostile feelings did not arise, then one would not have "envy proper" but rather "benign envy," a form of admiration), Rawls prefers to rely on the nonmoral yet aversive characteristics of the envy-producing situation (described as the blocking of an important goal by emotion theorists such as Campos et al., 1983): "[T]he better situation of others catches our attention . . . we are downcast by their good fortune and no longer value as highly what we have; and this sense of hurt and loss arouses our rancor and hostility" (p. 533).

Is Rawls correct in removing so thoroughly any trace of moral feelings from envy? Note in the quotation above from Pushkin's play that Salieri's envy is linked to the *injustice* of God's bestowing on the "frivolous idler" Mozart the sublime musical gifts that he, Salieri, deserves more. Earlier, he has said,

Men say: there is no justice upon earth.
But neither is there justice in the Heavens!
For I was born with a great love for art:
When—still a child—I heard the organ peal
Its lofty measures through our ancient church,
I listened all attention—and sweet tears,
Sweet and involuntary tears would flow. (p. 428)

Salieri continues, on and on, about the sacrifices he has made for music; these sacrifices and his keen, surpassing appreciation of music, he feels, make him the appropriate holder for musical genius. It is the injustice of Mozart's being granted this genius that fires Salieri's anger and motivates his committing murder, which, from Salieri's point of view, is vengeance.

It is my main purpose in this chapter to show that a full explanation for the hostile feelings in envy will indeed require the inclusion of a justice component in envious feelings. Most simply, I argue that the person feeling envy (in its typically hostile form) will believe that the envied person's advantage is to some degree unfair. Hostile feelings are an immediate, natural response to felt injustice, and thus such unfairness beliefs provide an explanation for these feelings.

## Theoretical Perspectives Linking Justice-Related Feelings to Envy

One problem with using the frustration–aggression perspective *alone* as an explanation for hostile feelings in envy is that research in this area has sometimes failed to find an increase in aggression as the result of frustration (Gentry, 1970; Taylor & Pisano, 1971). Furthermore, some studies, such as those by Rule and Nesdale (1976), Kulik and Brown (1979), and Worchel (1974), appear to indicate that a primary determinant of how a person reacts to frustration (or aversive experiences generally) will be the attribution made for its cause. For example, in the study by Kulik and Brown (1979), aggression was most likely to follow "illegitimate" frustration. In the Rule and Nesdale (1976) study, aggression was most likely if the frustration was caused by another deliberately. Thus, whether or not frustration is sufficient for producing aggression, a person's interpretation of the cause of this experience will enhance, in a *clearly* robust manner, the likelihood of hostility. The frustrated/aroused person's assumptions about the legitimacy or fairness of the aversive experience constitute one of the more important variables predicting an aggressive (and thus hostile) response. As is also clear from research on relative deprivation (e.g., Folger, 1987), equity theory (e.g., Walster, Walster, & Berscheid, 1978), and justice-related motives in general (e.g., Masters & Smith, 1987)—and, indeed, from almost anyone's personal experience—hostile feelings are an immediate, *natural* response to felt injustice. Again, including a justice component to envious feelings provides a good explanation for the hostility usually part of envy.

A number of scholars have argued that a sense of injustice is usually present in envy. Scheler (1915/1961), influenced greatly by Nietzsche (1886/1909), claims that envy results from desiring something possessed by another and being powerless to obtain it, joined with a hate-producing belief that the envied person is the *cause* of the deprived state. In Scheler's view, the causal belief is both delusional and usually unconscious, and yet it is a critical component of envy. Because one can interpret the offending comparison as being caused by another person's agency, hostility can now easily charge one's feelings. Implicit in Scheler's analysis is the sense that the envied person *deserves* such hostility, at least from the envying person's subjective and presumably deluded vantage point.

Another argument suggesting a justice-related aspect to envy is provided by Heider (1958). In his analysis of people's reactions to "the lot of the other," he describes what he calls an "ought force" often arising in the comparison of lots. Especially when an individual is similar to or in the same class as the advantaged, envied person it will seem natural and somehow fairer if their lots are equalized. Thus, even in cases where another's advantage may appear fair by objective, societal standard, deprivation may often "hurt certain of our natural sentiments of equality" (Ley & Wauthier, 1946, p. 137). Suppose that one's neighbor wins a lottery, and, as a result of this good fortune, disparities of wealth, possessions, and the like increase immensely. According to Heider, these disparities may create uneasiness and tension exactly because the ought force has been violated. Because local standards of "procedural" justice (Thibaut & Walker, 1975) have been met (the money having been obtained through fair means), the neighbor cannot be faulted openly for his or her good fortune. Nonetheless, the envious discontent evoked by the good fortune will often include a sense of injustice.

Consider how Cassius, another literary prototype of the envious person, complains to Brutus about Caesar's recent ascendancy in Shakespeare's *Julius Caesar*:

> I was born free as Caesar, so were you;
> We both have fed as well, and we can both
> Endure the winter's cold as well as he.
> For once, upon a raw and gusty day,
> The troubled Tiber chafing with her shores,
> Caesar said to me, "Dar'st thou, Cassius, now
> Leap in with me into this angry flood
> And swim to yonder point?" Upon the word,
> Accoutred as I was, I plunged in
> And bade him follow. So, indeed he did.
> The torrent roar'd, and we did buffet it
> With lusty sinews, throwing it aside
> And stemming it with hearts of controversy.

But ere we could arrive the point propos'd,
Caesar cried, "Help me, Cassius, or I sink!"
I, as Aeneas, our great ancestor,
Did from the flames of Troy upon his shoulder
The old Anchises bear, so from the waves of Tiber
Did I the tired Caesar. And this man
Is now become a god, and Cassius is
A wretched creature and must bend his body
If Caesar carelessly but nod on him. (Shakespeare, 1599/1934, p. 11)

Clearly, the prime reason why Cassius finds Caesar's elevated status so intolerable is that Cassius sees himself as Caesar's equal, if not his better. It is also clear that Cassius finds Caesar's advantage to be undeserved; it violates what "ought" to be. Interestingly, it is essentially Cassius's task to convince Brutus that Caesar is undeserving. Only then can he expect Brutus, who fancies that his own motivations are noble, to join in the conspiracy against Caesar. Again, it appears to be the sense of injustice evoked by the features of the situation that generates much of the hostility.

## DISTINGUISHING JUSTICE-RELATED FEELINGS IN ENVY FROM RESENTMENT PROPER

A troublesome problem with including a sense of injustice in envy is that one must now contend with the conceptual blur between envy and resentment that Rawls guards against. How can one claim that a sense of injustice is part what it means to feel envy (especially its typically hostile form), but also maintain the conceptual integrity of true resentment? And yet should the feelings of injustice ascribed to Salieri–feelings that appear to fuel Salieri's malice and rancor—be separated from his envy? Should Cassius's deep-seated bitterness over Caesar's undeserved and arrogantly accepted ascendence—a feeling that also appears to fuel his malice and rancor—be similarly separated from his envy?

One claim I wish to make in this chapter is that the sense of injustice potentially explaining the hostile feelings in envy is distinct from the sense of injustice leading to hostility in obvious cases of unfair treatment. In obvious cases of unfair treatment, there is a transparent consensus that the conditions leading to the hostile feelings are unfair. Furthermore, these hostile feelings, because of their consensual righteousness, will tend to be expressed with an undisturbed conscience and with candor. Such hostility is a function of what may be called in the present context "resentment proper." On the other hand, the hostile feelings that are part of envy may be qualitatively different *exactly because they have an unsanctioned, illegitimate character.* The sense of injustice leading to the envious hostility will have a more subjective, personal validity than the sense of injustice leading to full-blown, "legitimate" hostility. In the eyes of an objective observer, claims of unfairness leading to envious hostility will appear invalid, and the resulting hostility will appear inappropriate (Silver & Sabini, 1978). Indeed, one of the reasons why few people will admit to envy is that to do so betrays such inappropriate hostility. Ordinarily, unfair treatment is a good cause for anger and protest, but when the standard used to determine such unfairness is unsanctioned or dubious (as in the case of envy), open anger and protest are less likely. Furthermore, if others are likely to label the envious person's hostility as inappropriate (from some perspectives the feeling is considered a "sin"; e.g., see Silver & Sabini, 1978), then this form of hostility will remain concealed and harbored rather than openly expressed. Hostility of this concealed, unsanctioned kind (envy) may be distinct from open, sanctioned hostility (resentment proper). Heider's (1958) description of the paradox so characteristic of envious feelings is fitting:

[E]nvy, which is derived from what may be considered an ought tendency toward equalization of lots, is at the same time an emotion of which one is ashamed. . . . We have a right to be treated justly, but we are also reminded . . . that one should smile at the fortune of another. Envy is fraught with conflict, over the fact that these feelings should not be entertained though at the same time one may have just cause for them. (p. 289)

Thus, allowing a moral, justice-based component to consort with the other characteristics of envy may not necessarily impair the conceptual integrity of more straightforward feelings of injustice that follow from obviously unfair events. As suggested above, it may be that what makes envy different from righteous indignation, or resentment proper, is the subjective, unsanctioned nature of the sense of injustice in envy.

Although Salieri (as portrayed by Pushkin) believes that Mozart's genius has been unjustly bestowed on him, he well knows that few people will sympathize with this brand of moral sentiment. Therefore, Salieri's hostility is the result of a necessarily *private* grievance, and his killing of Mozart is a covert affair. Compare Salieri's moral sentiments and retributive actions with Hamlet's, when Hamlet learns that Claudius has poisoned his mother:

Here, thou incestuous, murderous, damned Dane,
Drink off this potion;—is thy union here?
Follow my mother. (Shakespeare, 1602/1963, p. 96)

Both Salieri and Hamlet feel vengeful, and both kill using poison, but Hamlet's feelings and actions are overt and unabashed. And even Laertes, with whom Hamlet has just been dueling, approves of the killing. Immediately after Hamlet forces the poison down his uncle's throat, Laertes says, "He is justly serv'd" (p. 96).

It is sometimes claimed that Hamlet himself is motivated in part out of envy (and Oedipal jealousy) (e.g., Weisberg, 1972). Whether reasonable or not, such an analysis is consistent with Hamlet's inability to carry through with a quick and open avenging of his father's murder during the *earlier* acts of the play, when he is still out to "catch the conscience of the king." However, in the final act, Hamlet returns to Denmark in a different frame of mind. He has shed his "antic disposition" and appears driven by calm, unfettered resolve. In the end, Claudius is a villain to one and all, and Hamlet finishes him off with unhesitating, sanctioned swiftness.

Again, Hamlet's sense of injustice and his moral outrage appear to have a different character from Salieri's. Hamlet, backed by friend and adversary alike, feels an open and justified "resentment proper" and finds acting on the feeling an easy task in the end. Salieri, lacking anyone's sympathy, feels a sense of injustice, but must hide the feeling, stew in it, and act in secret.

It is worth noting that other details of *Julius Caesar* provide another example of the distinction between the sense of injustice that I am arguing is inherent in envy and that is found in resentment proper. The planning of Caesar's murder is the result of conspiratorial (hence, private) efforts on the part of Cassius and the other senators and tribunes who share his sentiments. One of the questions often raised by the play is that of whether Caesar's murder is justified. In fact, it is often a high school student's first venture into Shakespeare criticism when the debate in a 10th-grade English class turns to whether the conspirators act with just cause. One fact is clear in the debate: The conspirators themselves must justify their actions to the Roman people. Brutus, relying on his rhetorical skills and on his reputation as a man of honor, addresses a crowd of citizens and lays out "the reason of" Caesar's death. Brutus successfully persuades the crowd of the righteousness of the murder, but, as we all know, his appeal is short-lived. Mark Antony, who has been loyal to Caesar, follows Brutus in addressing the crowd and, in what is perhaps the most famous persuasive speech in English literature, turns their sentiments against Brutus and the other conspirators. The righteousness felt by the conspirators is unable to withstand public scrutiny. Mark Antony, skillfully yet quite easily in point of fact, characterizes their motivations as ignoble rather than noble—born of "private griefs" rather than true injustice and legitimate complaint. He effectively portrays them as unkind and traitorous ingrates, and, in an ironic turn of events, argues convincingly that their actions are *un*justified. In the end, it is the crowd that is whipped into righteous indignation:

> Revenge! About! Seek! Burn! Fire! Kill!
> Slay! Let not a traitor live! (Shakespeare, 1599/1934, p. 66)

Cassius and Brutus, however, believe that they are acting appropriately and feel motivated by a sense of injustice. Caesar has grown more powerful than he deserves, and they feel that to allow Caesar's ambition to go unchecked will lead to tyrannical rule. Furthermore, it seems that Caesar has turned arrogant and smug toward his friends:

> Upon what meat doth this our Caesar feed,
> That he has grown so great? (p. 12)

But, as would be the case with envy, their complaints go unappreciated outside the ranks of the conspiracy. In contrast, Mark Antony and the crowd are the ones who are allowed the satisfaction of feeling a fully sanctioned righteous indignation and who feel unimpeded in seeking revenge.

## Experiment on the Private Nature of Envious Hostility

The private nature of envious hostility is indirectly supported by the results of a recent study of mine (Smith, 1990). Subjects read two-page scenarios describing individuals in situations that would bring about varying degrees of envy. They were asked to take the role of the disadvantaged individual in each story and then to indicate the extent to which they would feel envy. They were also asked to engage in a hypothetical task calling for them to allocate a valuable resource between themselves and the advantaged person in the scenario. They were given seven alternatives from which to choose, each alternative representing a distinct social orientation or motivation (Bornstein et al., 1983). One of these seven alternatives was unambiguously hostile in orientation (because by choosing it they would be indicating a willingness to give up resources for themselves, just so that the advantaged person could be maximally deprived). The subjects made their allocations in one of two ways: It was clear either that the advantaged person would know who was the source of the allocation (public allocation) or that the advantaged person would be unaware of the source (private allocation). A median split was performed on subjects' reports of envy, and then this measured variable was included in a 2 (allocation: public vs. private) × 2 (envy: high vs. low) analysis of variance, with the proportion of subjects choosing the hostile alternative as the dependent variable. There was a significant main effect only for publicity of allocation, $F$ (1, 315) = 7.91, $p < .05$. However, this main effect was qualified by a significant publicity of allocation × envy interaction, $F$ (1, 315) = 4.70, $p < .05$. The likelihood of subjects making hostile choices *was* associated reports of envy, but *only* in private-allocation conditions (see Table 4.1 for the proportions characterizing the interaction).

Although the results of this experiment are only suggestive, they are nonetheless consistent with the view that envy is associated with a hostile orientation toward the envied person, and, furthermore, that it operates in private realms of experience. The hostile yet private aspect of envy may be one of its more distinctive features. As argued above, despite a degree of ill will often directed at the person who is envied, social prohibitions prevent the expression of this ill will. In fact, the envying person may overcompensate by openly expressing attitudes suggesting the opposite of envy—excessive praise, for example. The lowest proportion of hostile choices occurred in the public-allocation/high-envy condition, as if subjects were forestalling the opportunity for envy to be attributed to them.

**TABLE 4.1. Percentage of Hostile Allocation Choices as a Function of Level of Reported Envy and Publicity of Allocation**

| Publicity of allocation | Reported envy | |
| --- | --- | --- |
| | High | Low |
| Public | 6.7% | 11.8% |
| Private | 30.6% | 14.5% |

*Note.* The hostile allocation alternative was one of seven options from which subjects could choose.

## THE POSSIBLE LEGITIMACY
## OF ENVIOUS HOSTILITY

It would seem impossible to eliminate entirely the experiential and conceptual similarity between the sense of injustice found in envy and resentment proper. Although envious hostility may be based on subjective, illegitimate beliefs of unfairness, whereas resentment proper is based on legitimate beliefs of unfairness, the quality of the hostile feelings in both cases is probably more similar than different. Furthermore, as the line between what is a legitimate grievance (producing resentment) and an illegitimate grievance (producing envious hostility) becomes obscure, the quality of these feelings may be much the same. Indeed, there may be many instances in which the envious person's sense of injustice borders on legitimacy.

Differences between people that evoke envy have what might be considered a mix of controllable and uncontrollable causes. Cinderella is envied by her sisters because she is beautiful and good. Presumably her sisters could choose to be as good, but could they control their lack of natural beauty? In fact, a host of differences between people are "natural" inequalities, in the sense that they occur from birth: differences in physique, health, intelligence, talents, and the like—even, arguably (e.g., Rawls, 1971), differences in temperament and personality. Although there is honest debate about the exact degree to which differences in such domains are entirely under a person's control (and certainly individual differences in perceptions of the malleability of such differences; see Dweck, 1986), one can safely claim that at least a fraction of each difference is congenital, unchangeable, or otherwise beyond a person's control. Furthermore, there are clearly envy-producing differences between people in many other domains, such as family resources and educational opportunities, that are certainly uncontrollable at birth and that vary in controllability across the life span.

The fact that many envy-producing comparisons between people are due to uncontrollable factors introduces a moral element into the way such differences are appreciated by the disadvantaged. The disadvantaged need not blame themselves for what is beyond their control and may have better and more persuasive cause to resent their compromised starting point. The envying person can reject the notion that the envied person *deserves* his or her advantage, even if societal norms dictate that one should not begrudge such an advantage. An advantage acquired arbitrarily seems an invalid basis for deservingness (Miller, 1982).

Even Rawls (1971) makes the point that the distribution of natural abilities, even those attributes that may enhance motivation and effort, is "arbitrary from a moral point of view" (pp. 311–312). This fact, together with the assumption that where people fall on the distribution of natural abilities affects their welfare, is a critical element in conceiving the appropriate way in which to form a just society. Decisions about a society's structure should be made under conditions whereby members of a society are unaware of their standing on this distribution—that is, "behind the veil of ignorance." Although it may sometimes appear that a person "deserves" favored treatment because of superior talent (and perhaps a person enjoying the superiority may be more disposed to believe this), Rawls notes:

> This view, however, is surely incorrect. It seems to be on the fixed points of our considered judgments that no one deserves his place in the distribution of native endowments, any more than one deserves one's initial starting place in society. The assertion that a man deserves the superior character that enables him to make the effort to cultivate his abilities is equally problematic; for his character depends in large part upon fortunate family and social circumstances for which he can claim no credit. The notion of desert seems not to apply to these cases. (p. 104)

## THE IMPORTANT CONSEQUENCES OF NATURAL INEQUALITIES

Perhaps it would be immaterial to claim that natural inequalities are unfair, if it were not also true that natural inequalities make a difference in people's lives. An unusual perspective on this view appears in Rousseau's *A Discourse on Inequality* (1754/1984). Rousseau takes as an unexplainable given that human beings differ in terms of physique, talents, and tempermant. The main purpose of his essay is to show how in the course of human history these inequalities have been enhanced many times over through the workings of society. In the relatively solitary "state of nature," human beings were unaffected by the unequal distribution of natural endowments. "What is intelligence to people who do not speak, or cunning to those who have no commerce with others?" (p. 105) However, as human society expanded and as human culture became more elaborate, these inequalities began to affect people's lives. People became "accustomed to judging different objects and to making comparisons," thus acquiring notions of merit which in turn produced "feelings of preference" (p. 114). Finally,

Each began to look at the others and to want to be looked at himself; and public esteem came to be prized. He who sang or danced the best; he who was the most handsome, the strongest, the most adroit or the most eloquent became the most highly regarded, and this was the first step towards inequality and at the same time towards vice. From those first preferences there arose, on the one side, vanity and scorn, on the other, shame and envy, and the fermentation produced by these new leavens finally produced compounds fatal to happiness and innocence. (p. 114)

Rousseau makes it clear that those who are favored in the distribution of natural inequalities are ultimately the preferred and the powerful, "for when a giant and dwarf walk the same road, every step each takes gives an extra advantage to the giant" (p. 105).

The uncontrollable origins of many inequalities among people and the powerful effects of these inequalities on people's lives would seem to give a keener edge to the envying person's sense of injustice and would provide a more robust validity to this sense of injustice. Although, again, societal norms and dictates may still work against the open expression of indignation (and thus the feeling would be characterized by others as envy rather than as resentment), the intensity and the righteousness of the subjectively held sense of injustice should be all the more present.

Recall Scheler's (1915/1961) claim that the envying person harbors the delusional belief that the advantaged person is the cause of his or her deprivation. According to Scheler, it is this belief that produces the ill will. Even here, one might question whether such a belief is entirely delusional. From the perspective of social comparison theory (Festinger, 1954; Suls & Miller, 1977), the presence of a superior person is indeed "the cause" of one's inferiority, self-evaluation being largely comparative. It is inappropriate to *blame* the superior person for one's inferiority, and yet it may still make sense to understand that this person's presence is at the root of one's perception of inferiority. Regardless of the actual validity of such beliefs, in comparison situations leading to envy, distinctions between cause and blame may become lost from the envious person's subjective and often self-serving perspective: What may actually be experienced is a sense of being wronged. Thus, delusional or not, these beliefs may give a certain character to the envying person's hostility; they suggest that the source of the hostility will be a sense of injustice and that retributive urges will result.

Given that many envy-producing differences are beyond a person's control, and given that it is at least possible to conceive of the envied person as "causing" the invidious difference, it would seem that many traditional cases of envy have particularly rich moral overtones. Again, although societal norms may prove unsympathetic to construing such differences in moral terms—for instance, doing so may call into question religious doctrine or moral codes (e.g., Sabini & Silver, 1982), appear to compromise the efficient and proper running of a society (e.g., Mora, 1987; Silber, 1989), or run counter to appropriate and mature ways of coping with these differences (e.g., Hartley, 1960; Kushner, 1981; Vonnegut, 1970)—such differences have the potential to produce a lasting and palpable sense of injustice nonetheless. People made envious by virtue of their poor relative standing, especially on important, nontransferable attributes, are hard-luck cases. They are behind the eight ball, or, to use Goffman's (1952) analogy, they are "marks." When children say to one another, "Where were you when the brains were handed out?" or "He got beaten with the ugly stick," these are expressions of the seemingly arbitrary plan operating behind natural inequalities and constitute testimony to the emotional pain that bad luck of this sort can bring. In an unconventional but arguable sense, people on the short end of the distribution have been unfairly treated by fate; short of malicious actions (e.g., Salieri's poisoning Mozart), they are powerless to change the essential features of the inequality, or, more precisely put, the inequity.

> The Moving Finger writes; and, having writ,
> Moves on: nor all your Piety nor Wit
> Shall lure it back to cancel half a Line,
> Nor all your Tears wash out a Word of it. (Khayyám, 1858/1952, p. 170)

Scheler (1915/1961) describes the feeling of *ressentiment* as having one source in repeated, repressed feelings of envy. As noted above, Scheler understands envy to result from a person's inability to acquire an attribute enjoyed by another person, together with a sense that the envied person is the cause of the deprivation. He claims that envy leads to *ressentiment* when it is experienced repeatedly "in the sphere in which we compare ourselves to others" and when forces work to block its full expression, as will often be the case with such an unsanctioned emotion. When the repression is complete, "the result is a general negativism—a sudden, violent, seemingly unsystematic and unfounded rejection of things, situations, or natural objects whose loose connection with the original cause of the hatred can only be discovered by complicated analysis" (p. 70). Interestingly, Scheler argues that the chief causes of *ressentiment* are "innate" attributes, such as beauty and hereditary character traits. Presumably, invidious comparisons on these characteristics are frequent, affecting, and mostly irreducible.

## *Summary*

The main goal of this chapter has been to argue that envious feelings are, at least in part, characterized by a sense of injustice. It appears that this form of moral feeling can be distinguished from resentment proper because, in general, it has a subjective, unsanctioned character. The likelihood of envy's containing a sense of injustice is also suggested by there appearing to be a legitimacy to the subjective appraisal of injustice in many instances of envy.

I have suggested that the sense of injustice present in envious feelings may explain the hostility that is typically part of these feelings. Indeed, one way of providing support for a justice-related component in envy would be to show that envy, without an accompanying sense of injustice, will not breed hostility. In other words, if another person's advantage only produces hostility when the advantage is construed as unfair on some level, then envy may in fact require a moral dimension. Envy is partly defined by its hostile features; otherwise, the feeling evoked by the unflattering comparison may be better labeled as one of its benign forms, such as admiration or simply discontent. In fact, there is considerable evidence suggesting that one response to unflattering social comparisons can be depression (see Alloy & Abramson, 1988, for a review), sometimes characterized as a form of hostility turned "inward." Even Rawls (1971) notes that, rather than hostility, an alternative response to severely unflattering comparisons is "to relapse into resignation and apathy" (p. 536), a form of depressed affect relatively *free* of ill will. However, he leaves unspecified what factors might predict each of these quite different alternatives—the depression-laden envy as opposed to the hostile kind. Possibly, depressive responses to unflattering comparison circumstances result when one is unable to construe the comparison as unfair, at least on some subjective level.

Thus, a full explanation of the hostile feelings typical of envy may require that the envying person must also feel a sense of injustice. In other words, a person feeling envy in its typically hostile form may have to believe that the envied person's advantage is, to some degree and on some subjective level, unfair.

## EVIDENCE FOR A JUSTICE COMPONENT IN ENVY

There is little empirical social-psychological research directly examining the possibility of a justice component in envy. Salovey and Rodin (1986) found in a multidimensional scaling analysis of a large number of envy and jealousy situations that a fairness dimension was one of the only two dimensions appearing to differentiate the situations. For both envy and jealousy situations, there were some that appeared to involve unfair circumstances and others that appeared to involve fair circumstances. Consistent with the present perspective, subjects' ratings of each situation indicated that unfairness was associated with anger and only marginally associated with sadness.

Research I have done with Jerry Parrott and Sung Hee Kim (1990) is also consistent with the present perspective. We asked 150 male and female undergraduates to write detailed accounts of an occasion when they had felt strong envy. After writing their accounts, they indicated for an extensive set of items how characteristic each was of their experience. These items described either (1) affective states (e.g., hostility and depression) or (2) situational conditions (i.e., brief descriptions of the general circumstances that may have produced the emotion).

### Situational Condition Items

First, we took the situational condition items and, through factor analysis, extracted a number of composite variables. Three variables were relevant for the present purposes.

1. *Subjective Unfairness items.* These items consisted of beliefs that the envied person's advantage was unfair. However, the validity of these beliefs had the subjective, unsanctioned character argued to be found in hostile envy. An example of this type of item was "It seemed unfair that the person I envied started out in life with certain superior talents, abilities, or physical attributes."

2. *Objective Unfairness items.* These items also consisted of beliefs that the envied person's advantage was unfair. However, the validity of these beliefs had an objective, sanctioned character of the type I have argued to be found in resentment proper. An example of this type of item was "An objective judge who knew the facts would agree that the person I envied did not deserve his or her good fortune."

3. *Inferiority items.* These items were straightforward statements indicating that the envied person's advantage evoked beliefs of personal inferiority. An example of this type of item was "The discrepancy between the person I envied and me was due to my own inferior qualities."

### Affective State Items

A similar factor analysis was performed on the affective state items. The main factors of interest to emerge in this analysis were a Hostility factor, containing items such as "feeling hostile" and "ill will," and a Depression factor, containing items such as "down" and "depressed."

## Results of Stepwise Regression

Consistent with the view that a sense of injustice may explain envious hostility, stepwise regression analysis revealed that hostility was predicted largely by the Subjective Unfairness factor, $t (146) = 63.04$, $p < .0001$, and to a lesser extent by the Objective Unfairness factor, $t (146) = 6.66$, $p < .05$. Consistent with the view that the absence of a sense of injustice will produce depressive envy, depressive feelings were largely predicted by the Inferiority factor, $t (146) = 146.33$, $p < .0001$. Interestingly, Inferiority was correlated with Subjective Unfairness but uncorrelated with Objective Unfairness. Without feelings of inferiority, there should be less cause for having subjective unfairness beliefs. However, objectively unfair treatment in general has no necessary relationship with inferiority. If a rival is unfairly given a promotion and thus enjoys an advantage, one might feel resentful but not necessarily inferior.

## CONCLUDING REMARKS

In discussing the envying person's sense of injustice, I have largely taken the subjective stance of the envying person, rather than the viewpoint of observers who may be in a position to give a different characterization to the emotion they see exhibited. In effect, I have argued that the envying person, if the feeling is hostile envy, will actually see his or her feelings as a form of resentment. Even Salieri (as depicted by Pushkin), who privately admits to feeling envy itself, claims that the basic problem is one of justice. How can this sense of injustice be called envy? Once again, I am arguing that because the envying person's complaint must usually remain private, the actual experience of the feeling will be distinct from more open, sanctioned forms of resentment proper. Furthermore, even if the quality of the experience of hostile envy is largely similar to the experience of resentment proper, if a subjectively held sense of injustice is necessary for hostile feelings to emerge, then it must necessarily be part of the envious response. Once again, envy in its prototypic form is partly defined by a measure of hostility.

I have focused for the most part on hostile envy. However, it may be useful to assume that there are varieties of envious experience, as Jerry Parrott outlines in Chapter 1 of the present volume. I have suggested, for example, that there may be a *depressive* form of envy that results from the envying person's preoccupation with his or her inferiority. As noted earlier, with this nonmalicious form of envy, hostile feelings may be turned inward.

There may also be more clearly *malicious* forms of envy, in which the envying person's hostility is more spiteful and less justified by any standard. The examples of envy that I have chosen in order to illustrate the sense of injustice often associated with the emotion have tended to fall on the borderline between ambiguously unfair circumstances (characteristic of envious hostility) and obviously unfair circumstances (characteristic of resentment proper). However, let us take yet another example from literature: Claggart's envy of Billy Budd (Melville, 1924/1961). Surely Billy Budd—an innocent, guileless, and cheerful figure, as he is portrayed by Melville—is undeserving of Claggart's hostility. Even if one could grant that Claggart has been unfairly treated by life and thus feels a kind of *ressentiment* like that described by Scheler (see Parrott's discussion of "global resentment" as well), how can Claggart, much less an observer, justify the ill will that he feels toward Billy Budd? Furthermore, it is one thing to feel a hostile envy and quite another thing to act on it (as Claggart does), as if the envied person truly were to blame for one's inferiority (Elster, 1989). And yet some of the accounts provided by our subjects in the second study described above involved cases where the envied person "had it all"—good looks, brains, and wealth. But the crowning advantage was that they were also *good* people. Their goodness did not always lessen the intensity of the hostile envy, and, for some subjects, appeared to fuel it. These subjects often admitted wishing that a misfortune would befall the envied person. Indeed, it is frequently argued that *Schadenfreude*, joy at the suffering of others, is a cousin to envy (e.g., Elster, 1989; Heider, 1958).

Clearly, much research is needed in order to sort out various manifestations of envious experience, its apparent overlap with a sense of injustice being only one issue. This chapter serves more to raise a number of important, empirically overlooked questions than to settle them. Understanding hostile envy seems a particularly important matter, because such feelings have the obvious potential to hamper social interaction (e.g., Sullivan, 1953), to create unhappiness (e.g., Russell, 1930), to compromise health (e.g., Sullivan, 1953), and, arguably, to handicap human excellence (e.g., Hartley, 1960; Mora, 1987; Schoeck, 1969; Silber, 1989). Understanding why some individuals can use unflattering social comparisons as a basis for more constructive, emulative impulses, whereas other seem overcome by destructive, hateful feelings, is an important social-psychological problem.

## REFERENCES

Alloy, L. B., & Abramson, L. Y. (1988). Depressive realism: Four theoretical perspectives. In L. B. Alloy (Ed.), *Cognitive processes in depression* (pp. 223–265). New York: Guilford.

Berkowitz, L. (1972). Frustrations, comparisons, and other sources of emotional arousal as contributors to social unrest. *Journal of Social Issues, 28,* 77–91.

Berkowitz, L. (1989). Frustration–aggression hypothesis: Examination and reformulation. *Psychological Bulletin, 106,* 59–73.

Bornstein, G., Crum, L., Wittenbraker, J., Harring, K., Insko, C. A., & Thibaut, J. (1983). On the measurement of social orientations in the minimal group paradigm. *European Journal of Social Psychology, 13,* 321–350.

Campos, J. J., Barrett, K. C., Lamb, M. E., Goldsmith, H. H., & Stenberg, C. (1983). Socioemotional development. In M. M. Haith & J. J. Campos (Vol. Eds.), *Handbook of child psychology* (4th ed.): *Vol. 2. Infancy and developmental psychobiology* (pp. 783–915). New York: Wiley.

Dweck, C. S. (1986). Motivational processes affecting learning. *American Psychologist, 41,* 1040–1048.

Elster, J. (1989). *The cement of society.* New York: Cambridge University Press.

Festinger, L. A. (1954). A theory of social comparison processes. *Human Relations, 7,* 117–140.

Folger, R. (1987). Reformulating the preconditions of resentment: A referent conditions model. In J. C. Masters & W. P. Smith (Eds.), *Social comparison, social justice and relative deprivation: Theoretical, empirical, and policy perspectives* (pp. 183–215). Hillsdale, NJ: Erlbaum.

Gentry, W. D. (1970). Effects of frustration, attack, and prior aggressive training on overt aggression and vascular processes. *Journal of Personality and Social Psychology, 16,* 718–725.

Goffman, I. (1952). On cooling the mark. *Psychiatry, 15,* 451–463.

Hartley, L. P. (1960). *Facial justice.* London: Hamish Hamilton.

Heider, F. (1958). *The psychology of interpersonal relations.* New York: Wiley.

Khayyám, O. (1952). *The rubaiyat of Omar Khayyam* (E. Fitzgerald, Trans.). Garden City, NY: Doubleday. (Original work published 1858)

Kulik, J. A., & Brown, R. (1979). Frustration, attribution of blame, and aggression. *Journal of Experimental Social Psychology, 15,* 183–194.

Kushner, H. S. (1981). *When bad things happen to good people.* New York: Avon Books.

Ley, A., & Wauthier, M. L. (1946). *Etudes de psychologie instinctive et affective.* Paris: Presses Univ. de France.

Masters, J. C., & Smith, W. P. (Eds.). (1987). Social comparison, social justice and relative deprivation: Theoretical, empirical, and policy perspectives. Hillsdale, NJ: Erlbaum.

Melville, H. (1961). Billy Budd, foretopman. In *Billy Budd and other tales* (pp. 7–88). New York: Signet. (Original work published 1924)

Miller, R. (1982). Rights or consequences. In P. A. French, T. E. Uehling, & H. K. Wettstein (Eds.), *Midwest studies in philosophy: Vol. 7. Social and political philosophy* (pp. 73–87). Minneapolis: University of Minnesota Press.

Morse, S., & Gergen, K. J. (1970). Social comparison, self-consistency, and the concept of the self. *Journal of Personality and Social Psychology, 16,* 148–156.

Mora, F. (1987). *Egalitarian envy.* New York: Paragon House.

Nietzsche, F. (1909). *Beyond good and evil: Prelude to a philosophy of the future* (H. Zimmer, Trans.). New York: T. N. Foulis. (Original work published 1886)

Nozick, R. (1974). *Anarchy, state, and utopia.* New York: Basic Books.

Pushkin, A. (1964). Mozart and Salieri. In A. Yarmolinsky (Ed.), *The poems, prose and play of Alexander Pushkin* (A. F. B. Clark, Trans.). New York: Modern Library. (Original work published 1832)

Rawls, J. (1971). *A theory of justice.* Cambridge, MA: Harvard University Press.

Rousseau, J. J. (1984). *A discourse on inequality* (M. Cranston, Trans.). Harmondsworth, England: Penguin. (Original work published 1754)

Rule, B., & Nesdale, A. (1976). Emotional arousal and aggressive behavior. *Psychological Bulletin, 83,* 851–863.

Russell, B. (1930). *The conquest of happiness.* New York: Liveright.

Sabini, J., & Silver, M. (1982). *The moralities of everyday life.* New York: Oxford University Press.

Salovey, P., & Rodin, J. (1984). Some antecedents and consequences of social-comparison jealousy. *Journal of Personality and Social Psychology, 47,* 780–792.

Salovey, P., & Rodin, J. (1986). The differentiation of social-comparison jealousy and romantic jealousy. *Journal of Personality and Social Psychology, 50,* 1100–1112.

Scheler, M. (1961). *Ressentiment* (L. A. Coser, Ed., W. W. Holdhein, Trans.). Glencoe, IL: Free Press. (Original work published 1915)

Schoeck, H. (1969). *Envy: A theory of social behavior.* New York: Harcourt, Brace & World.

Silber, J. (1989). *Shooting straight: What's wrong with America and how to fix it.* New York: Harper & Row.

Silver, M., & Sabini, J. (1978). The perception of envy. *Social Psychology Quarterly, 41,* 105–117.

Shakespeare, W. (1963). *The tragedy of Hamlet, prince of Denmark.* New York: Norton. (Original work published 1602)

Shakespeare, W. (1934). *The tragedy of Julius Caesar.* New York: Henry Holt. (Original work published 1599)

Smith, R. H. (1990). *The private nature of envious hostility.* Unpublished manuscript.

Smith, R. H., Diener, E., & Garonzik, R. (1990). The roles of comparison level and alternative comparison domains in the perception of envy. *British Journal of Social Psychology, 29,* 247–255.

Smith, R. H., & Insko, C. A. (1987). Social comparison choices during ability evaluation: The effects of comparison publicity, performance feedback, and self-esteem. *Personality and Social Psychology Bulletin, 13*, 111–122.

Smith, R. H., Parrott, W. G., & Kim, S. H. (1990). *Hostile and depressive responses to insidious comparisons.* Unpublished manuscript.

Sullivan, H. S. (1953). *The interpersonal theory of psychiatry.* New York: Norton.

Suls, J. M., & Miller, R. L. (1977). *Social comparison processes.* Washington, DC: Hemisphere.

Taylor, S. P., & Pisano, R. (1971). Physical aggression as a function of frustration and physical attack. *Journal of Social Psychology, 84*, 261–267.

Tesser, A., & Collins, J. E. (1988). Emotion in social reflection and comparison situations: Intuitive, systematic, and exploratory approaches. *Journal of Personality and Social Psychology, 55*, 695–709.

Thibaut, J. W., & Walker, L. (1975). *Procedural justice: A psychological analysis.* Hillsdale, NJ: Erlbaum.

Vonnegut, K. (1970). *Welcome to the monkey house.* New York: Dell.

Walster, E., Walster, G. W., & Berscheid, E. (1978). *Equity: Theory and research.* Boston: Allyn & Bacon.

Weisberg, R. (1972). Hamlet and *ressentiment. American Imago, 29*, 318–337.

Worchel, S. (1974). The effect of three types of arbitrary thwarting on the instigation of aggression. *Journal of Personality, 42*, 301–318.

Zillmann, D. (1979). *Hostility and aggression.* Hillsdale, NJ: Erlbaum.

# PART II

# THE EXPERIENCE OF JEALOUSY IN CLOSE RELATIONSHIPS

We are rarely moved to envy and jealousy in the context of relationships that are not meaningful to us. Sometimes, for example, we use jealousy as a gauge to assess the importance of close relationships. When we care little about someone, are we likely to feel jealous when that person might be taken from us? Although there is a considerable body of research on the experience of jealousy in the context of relationships—much of it contributed by the authors of the next four chapters—there is very little work on envy at this level. Hence, the next four chapters deal only with jealousy; they focus on the characteristics of personal relationships, especially romantic ones, that give rise to jealousy.

The idea that jealousy is the result of transactions between individuals and their social environments is the theme of the first chapter in this part of the book, by Robert Bringle. Bringle argues that there are no *a priori* circumstances that evoke jealousy; rather, jealousy is a social construct embedded within a cultural context. An individual's beliefs, values, expectations, past history, and personality characteristics within this context determine what is jealousy-provoking.

Gordon Clanton and David Kosins then argue that adult jealousy is not a defect rooted in childhood conflicts with siblings and parents. Based on the results of a large-scale survey they conducted, which unearthed little support for these psychodynamic formulations, they contend instead that a sociological view emphasizing jealousy's role as a protector of valued relationships is a theoretical framework with greater utility.

In Chapter 7, Bram Buunk first defines jealousy as the aversive emotional reactions evoked by the real, imagined, or expected attraction between one's current or formal partner and a third person. Buunk discusses the importance of norms and rules in generating romantic jealousy. He argues especially that understanding when jealousy is likely to be provoked will be facilitated by a theoretical perspective emphasizing the exchange of rewards and potential rewards in romantic relationships. Buunk suggests that Kelley's interdependence theory provides a particularly useful vantage point.

The final chapter of this section is contributed by Jeff Bryson, who identifies nine different ways in which individuals react to jealousy-provoking experiences. These nine jealousy reactions are compared with Caryl Rusbult's four classic responses to declines in relationship satisfaction: exit, voice, loyalty, and neglect. Bryson provides some data suggesting that jealous reactions may vary across cultures. As he says, "It appears that, when jealous, the French get mad, the Dutch get sad, the Germans would rather not fight about it, the Italians don't want to talk about it, and the Americans are concerned about what their friends think!" Bryson's chapter thus provides an obvious link to the third section of this volume.

*Chapter Five*

# Psychosocial Aspects of Jealousy: A Transactional Model

## ROBERT G. BRINGLE
*Purdue University at Indianapolis*

## *A TRANSACTIONAL MODEL OF JEALOUSY*
### *General Perspective*

*Transactional theory of perception*: a functionalistic theory of perception which holds that our fundamental perceptions are learned reactions on the basis of our transactions or interactions with the environment. The transactional functionalists hold that we build up probabilities of what to expect perceptually on the basis of our experiences and that we bring these probabilities to each new situation. (Chaplain, 1975, p. 549)

The transactional perspective has been reflected in theories and research on object perception (e.g., Ames, 1953; Brunswik, 1947), social perception (e.g., Heider, 1958), and social cognition (e.g., Markus & Zajonc, 1985). Applied to jealousy, the model implies that there are no *a priori* circumstances that are jealousy-evoking. Jealousy is a social construct embedded within a cultural context. Individuals go through their social worlds making judgments about events precipitated by and related to their relationships. An individual's beliefs, value system, expectancies, past history, and personality characteristics relevant to social relationships and jealousy define where interpersonal events are perceived to be located on a continuum from "benign" to "catastrophic." Perception of these events is a *constructive process* in which an individual's perceptual expectancies combine with sensory information from the social environment to construct or form the final perception. Thus, perception of events in the social environment is a "transaction" between the person and the social environment; both the person and the stimulus contribute to the final outcome, but *to varying degrees*.

Jealousy can be defined as any "aversive emotional reaction that occurs as the result of a partner's extradyadic relationship that is real, imagined, or considered likely to occur" (Bringle & Buunk, 1985, p. 242). Individuals have numerous extradyadic relationships (e.g., with family members, friends, coworkers) that do not typically evoke jealousy. What contributes to the perception of jealousy and elicits the negative emotional reactions? The common core is any extradyadic event or behavior by the partner or other persons that is appraised as potentially reducing relationship outcomes will produce jealousy. Perception of threat of loss of the partner to a rival is one eventuality that will precipitate jealousy, but it is not the only possibility. Many other losses can occur in the absence of relationship termination. Buunk and I (Buunk & Bringle, 1987) have suggested organizing these into short-term losses and long-term losses. Short-term consequences include arguments, strained communications, loss of status, loss of time together, self-deprecation, violation of specialness, social embarrassment, the imposition of negative emotions, and possibly envy of the partner. Long-term consequences include interpreting the partner's motives and the implications this has for continued relationship distress or dissolution.

According to this definition, jealousy is not limited to sexual or romantic relationships. Nonromantic as well as romantic relationships hold the potential for eliciting jealousy; however, the actual events that trigger jealousy will be very different in romantic, work, family, and social relationships. Romantic jealousy, in contrast to nonromantic jealousy, is more prevalent, more powerful, more significant, more stressful, more complex, and more salient to both researchers and the general population.

### The Role of Commitment, Insecurity, and Arousability

The transactional model of jealousy identifies three constructs as being critical in determining jealous responses: commitment, insecurity, and arousability. No one of these constructs is sufficient; all are necessary for a jealous response to occur. Furthermore, higher levels of each variable are posited to increase the intensity and frequency of jealous responses.

In addition, the model postulates that each one of these constructs (commitment, insecurity, and arousability) is a function of variables from three different loci:

1. *Person.* There are attributes of the individual that mediate appraisals by defining what constitutes commitment in a relationship and violations of exclusivity. These include stable qualities (such as the cultural context and norms distilled into a belief system, personality characteristics, temperament, and values), as well as less stable aspects of the person (such as moods and sexual excitement).

2. *Relationship.* The nature of the existing relationship with the partner includes stable relationship properties (e.g., history, interaction styles) and transitory states (e.g., a recent fight).

3. *Situation.* The nature of the social circumstances impinging on the individual (including both contextual factors and specific events) which imply that past relationship outcomes may be depreciated, current outcomes may diminish, and future outcomes may be thwarted because of the partner's extradyadic behavior.

## Commitment

"Commitment," within this model, refers to interdependence. Commitment need not be explicit, as in a marriage; however, it is a precondition for jealousy. Before jealousy can occur, one must first be involved in a relationship that represents an investment, that has the potential and expectation for future outcomes, and that has the potential for loss of outcomes if the relationship is abridged or terminated. Thus, some level of commitment may occur as a result of a brief encounter or a first date. To the degree that outcomes attained from the relationship are particularistic (Foa & Foa, 1980), and norms of exclusivity for certain outcomes (e.g., sexual gratification) are established, commitment to the relationship will be heightened. Other things being equal, the greater the commitment, the greater the emotional reaction to jealousy-evoking events.

According to exchange theory (Rusbult, 1980, 1983; Thibaut & Kelley, 1959), commitment is a positive function of relationship satisfaction, investment, and the degree to which the individual's outcomes exceed outcomes from any other possible relationship, including no relationship at all (comparison level for alternatives, or CLalt). Commitment can be heightened either by increasing outcomes and investments or by depressing CLalt. Stable and transient aspects of the person, relationship, and situation that heighten commitment will be positively related to emotional reactions in jealousy-evoking circumstances. These include chronic or relatively stable attributes of the person (e.g., need for affiliation, need for approval) and the relationship (e.g., love, sexual satisfaction). In addition, situational variables (e.g., availability of alternative relationships, children) and transient or acute person variables (e.g., recent failure) and relationship variables (e.g., resolved conflict) affect commitment.

### Insecurity

As previously detailed, "commitment" is defined as being a function of the jealous person's appraisal of the relationship. In contrast, "insecurity" is a function of the jealous person's appraisal of the *partner's* commitment to the relationship. Jealousy will occur when commitment is accompanied by uncertainty concerning the continuation of outcomes that have established the commitment. Commitment without insecurity will not result in jealousy; however, insecurity is never zero. As Duck and Sants (1983, p. 37) note, "One of the great human dilemmas appears to be the problem of deciding how much real affection a partner has for oneself." Because insecurity is heightened to the extent that the partner's commitment to the current relationship is perceived as being diminished, circumstances that are perceived by the jealous person as depressing the partner's commitment (i.e., decreasing outcomes and investments in the current relationship or raising the partner's CLalt) will increase insecurity. Insecurity refers to uncertainty of the following types:

1. Predisposing and background factors that generate uncertainty in the person about the partner's intentions. Both chronic person variables (e.g., low self-esteem, low attractiveness), chronic relationship variables (e.g., low involvement by partner, partner's attractiveness), and chronic situational variables (e.g., partner works around attractive others) can contribute to an enduring sense of vulnerability and uncertainty for the person and can be the precursors of jealousy.

2. A shift in the partner's commitment. This might be a function of a transformation from appraisals of outcomes that are based on the couple's joint outcomes (Kelley, 1979; Pruitt, 1981) to appraisals of individualistic outcomes that are independent of concerns for the other person's outcomes.

3. Precipitating factors that have traditionally been referred to as "jealousy-evoking events." These are acute events that cause the per-

ceiver to sense a decrease in the stability of the relationship because they call into question the partner's commitment. Jealousy-evoking events are threatening to the extent that they represent a sign that changes may have already taken place for the partner. That is, it is not that the partner spent the evening with someone else that is so threatening; what is threatening is that such an event represents (a) changes in the partner's commitment to the prior-existing relationship and (b) the partner's decision to put his or her outcomes in front of the prior-existing relationship's outcomes.

## Arousability

Finally, jealousy generates emotional responses. As such, both acute and chronic variables that affect arousal are also related to the intensity and frequency of jealous responses, particularly fear and anger (Plutchik, 1980, p. 346). Pre-event arousal will increase the emotional reaction when one is jealous; however, one can be emotional as a result of jealousy in the absence of pre-event arousal. The term "arousability" (rather than "arousal") is specified in the model to indicate that a predisposition to arousal (e.g., emotionality, temperament; Derryberry & Rothbart, 1988) will heighten the intensity of emotional reactions that persons experience as a result of initial appraisals of a jealousy-evoking event. Arousal may result from a jealousy-evoking event, and this arousal will influence subsequent states and cognitions. Thus, even if pre-event arousal is low, individuals with more emotional temperaments will experience and express more intense jealous reactions than those with less emotional temperaments.

## Types of Jealousy

The transactional model specifies that a jealous reaction is the result of a transaction between endogenous variables (i.e., person variables) and exogenous variables (i.e., relationship and situational variables) that affect commitment, insecurity, and arousability. However, the endogenous and exogenous variables are not always equally important in determining the jealous reactions. When the relative importance of each varies systematically for individuals, then it is possible to differentiate types of jealousy. There is some evidence (Buunk, 1989; Hupka, 1989; Pfeiffer & Wong, 1989; White & Mullen, 1989) converging on the position that it may be useful to identify two types of jealousy: (1) "suspicious jealousy," in which the endogenous variables are primarily important in determining jealous responses; and (2) "reactive jealousy," in which exogenous variables are primarily important (see Figure 5.1). (See also

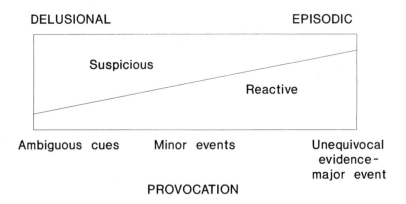

FIGURE 5.1. Suspicious and reactive jealousy as a function of provoking circumstances.

Parrott, Chapter 1, this volume, for a similar distinction between "suspicious jealousy" and "*fait accompli* jealousy.")

*Suspicious Jealousy*

Suspicious jealousy encompasses the following attributes:

1. Anxiety, fear, doubt, suspiciousness, and upset that accompany excessive worrying about what the partner might have done or is intending to do that would elicit jealousy. The anxiety and worrying is considered excessive if it is disproportionate to any known incidents that would consensually be considered violating exclusivity (e.g., a major jealousy-evoking event).
2. Obsessive mistrust of the partner.
3. Behaviors that include regular snooping, checking for clues that might confirm suspicions, and attempts to control the partner's behavior.
4. High, stable levels of insecurity that are primarily controlled by person variables (and possibly some chronic relationship variables such as high relative involvement).
5. High levels of emotional responding to consensually minor jealousy-evoking cues in the absence of any major jealousy-evoking events. In keeping with past distinctions (Bringle & Buunk, 1985), the emotional reactions constitute suspicious jealousy, and the cognitive and behavioral responses constitute the "coping strategies" of suspicious jealousy.

For the person experiencing suspicious jealousy, even if the partner may not have engaged in extradyadic sexual behavior, minor cues become the basis for elaborating scenarios that are assumed by the jealous person to confirm suspicions. Thus, suspicious jealousy is not independent of external cues. For example, the person experiencing suspicious jealousy may have a partner who cheats on tax returns. This evidence, though not directly related to the relationship, may generate concerns about the integrity of the partner's social values and interpersonal behavior. Or the person may know that the partner "cheated" in a previous relationship. Declarations by the partner of commitment to the present relationship and no evidence of extradyadic sexual behavior in the current relationship may do little to abate mistrust and decrease vigilance. The heightened vigilance, agitation, worrying, and emotional responses of suspicious jealousy can be understood in terms of characteristic tendencies (1) to perceive ambiguous cues as self-referential (personalization); (2) to focus on the emotion-provoking aspects of the event (selective abstraction); and (3) to assume that an isolated event implies a more extensive set of unobserved events (overgeneralization) (Beck, 1976; Larsen, Diener, & Cropanzano, 1987).

Delusional systems that have jealousy as a theme constitute the clearest example of extreme suspicious jealousy. However, it should be noted that an occurrence of infidelity by the partner does not mean that the person is not delusional.

*Reactive Jealousy*

Reactive jealousy occurs as events take place that clearly jeopardize or reduce outcomes from the relationship. For most persons in our society, proscriptive extradyadic sexual intimacy by the partner represents a serious violation of exclusivity and commitment, serves as an unequivocal inducement for a jealous response, and leads to an extensive reappraisal of the relationship's future. Across a consensually heterogeneous set of jealousy-evoking events ranging from benign through moderate, persons demonstrating reactive jealousy will show a pattern of emotional responses that is more moderate in intensity and more varied than those experiencing suspicious jealousy, for whom a higher level of emotional intensity is expected. This quantitative distinction serves as the basis for defining and measuring "dispositional jealousy," which is discussed later.

The following qualities would be expected to influence levels of emotional reactions for reactive jealousy:

1. *Intentionality.* Intentional extradyadic behavior by the partner (e.g., flirting with someone else) will produce greater upset than unintentional behavior or the behavior of others (e.g., someone flirting with the partner).

2. *Sexuality.* Extradyadic sexual behavior by the partner (e.g., petting, intercourse) will produce greater upset than nonsexual intimacy (e.g., self-disclosure) (e.g., Thompson, 1984).

3. *Specificity.* The partner's behavior directed at a specific other (e.g., regular and prolonged intimate talk with the same person) will produce greater upset than general, diffuse behaviors (e.g., the partner talks intimately with numerous persons).

4. *Contemporaneous behaviors.* Current extradyadic behaviors by the partner will produce greater upset than behaviors in previous, terminated relationships.

5. *Overt behaviors.* Extradyadic behaviors by the partner that are public and are observed by others will produce greater upset than behaviors that are discreet.

6. *Control.* Situations in which the jealous person perceives a lack of self-control over circumstances surrounding the jealousy-evoking event will produce greater upset than those in which perceptions of control are greater.

7. *Responsibility.* When the jealous person assumes some responsibility for the jealousy-evoking event, less upset will result than when less responsibility is attributed to self.

8. *Aggressiveness.* Behaviors that are perceived to have the intention of hurting the jealous person (i.e., lowering the jealous person's outcomes) will produce greater upset than extradyadic behaviors that are not perceived as having this intent (i.e., the intent is to increase the partner's outcomes, not primarily to decrease the person's outcomes) (Buunk, 1984).

Numerous analyses of people's emotional responses when jealous have been conducted, although the stimulus has not always been limited to reactive jealousy (Bush, Bush, & Jennings, 1988; Bryson, 1976; Buunk, 1989; Hupka, 1984; Mathes, Adams, & Davies, 1985; Salovey & Rodin, 1986). Anger, fear (and anxiety), and sadness appear regularly in these studies, and they may constitute the core of reactive jealousy. Anger can be understood as occurring in reactive jealousy to the extent that, from the jealous person's point of view, the evoking behavior represents a voluntary act by the partner that is unjustifiable, serious in implication, and morally reprehensible (Averill, 1982, 1983). Fear and anxiety result from questioning the adequacy of one's resources to cope with the threat and uncertainties concerning the future of the relationship. Sadness results from the combination of high levels of commitment and relationship losses that are irretrievable or the possibility of relationship termination.

During reactive jealousy, cognitive and behavioral responses will include protests over the transgressions, punishments to deter future transgressions, and reappraisals of the relationship. These constitute the coping strategies of reactive jealousy (see also Buunk, 1982b; Salovey & Rodin, 1988).

## The Relationship between Suspicious Jealousy and Reactive Jealousy

Differentiation between suspicious jealousy and reactive jealousy is clearest in extreme cases, but becomes blurred if the circumstances are more moderate (i.e., minor jealousy-evoking events). A partner who develops close friendships at work with opposite-sex coworkers, spends more time away, and engages in animated conversations at parties with others of the opposite sex are types of cues that may be benign. Or the pattern may suggest that the partner's outcomes in the current relationship have diminished and/or that appraisals of outcomes from alternative relationships have increased. Given the base rates of extradyadic sexual relationships and divorces (e.g., Blumstein & Schwartz, 1983; Thompson, 1983), vigilance may be prudent. Determining when concerns are justified and when suspicions are inordinate can be difficult in ambiguous situations. For most individuals, unequivocal evidence of extradyadic sexual intimacy by the partner is a clear benchmark; however, the occurrence of sexual behavior is not always easy to document. Furthermore, ambiguity can exist because the sexual behavior can vary along a gradient from touching to light kissing to heavy kissing to fondling to intercourse.

The overlap between suspicious and reactive jealousy is blurred further when reactive jealousy spawns suspicious jealousy. Even when a person is certain that a minor violation of exclusivity has occurred, there are still many uncertainties. Why did it occur? What actually happened? What is the rival like? How do they behave when together? What do they talk about? These questions generate many of the thoughts, feelings, and behaviors that have been delineated for suspicious jealousy. Shrestha, Rees, Rix, Hore, and Faragher (1985) found that the mean response on an index of jealousy, which included many items indicative of suspicious jealousy, was higher for a group identified as "justifiably jealous" (i.e., reactive jealousy) than for a group identified as "morbidly jealous" (displaying sexual jealousy during a clinical interview, but not reporting any substantial evidence of infidelity by the partner). Although not demonstrated in this research, it seems reasonable to presume that the high suspicious jealousy score for the justifiably jealous group was, indeed, reactive; it was episodic. They were searching, snooping, worrying, mistrustful, and accusatory *because* of the affair and the questions it raised. What is crucial to differentiating this (reactive jealousy causing suspicious jealousy) from suspicious jealousy alone is that persons displaying suspicious jealousy show the characteristic thoughts, feelings, and behaviors *regularly*, whether or not there is clear evidence to justify jealousy.

Finally, in addition to the possibility that reactive jealousy results in suspicious jealousy, it is also possible that suspicious jealousy can generate reactive jealousy. Suspiciousness that transcends warranted vigilance and includes constant checking, accusations, attempts to control the partner's behavior, nagging, and confrontations and emotional displays over "little things," rather than establishing firmness and ground rules, may be counterproductive when it attempts to deter what a partner had no intention of doing anyway. Accusations and threats can lead to reactance, resentment, counteraccusation, counterthreat, and provocation; all may reduce outcomes for the partner and make alternative relationships more attractive.

## Summary

The transactional model specifies that greater commitment, insecurity, and arousability will lead to higher levels of emotional upset and constitute jealousy:

$$\text{Jealousy} = (\text{Commitment}) \times (\text{Insecurity}) \times (\text{Arousability})$$

Levels of commitment, insecurity, and arousability are all influenced by qualities of the person, relationship, and situation. Within these domains, variables may be organized in terms of stable and transient qualities.

Suspicious jealousy is characterized by a person's searching for the partner's alleged jealousy-evoking behaviors, whereas reactive jealousy is a reaction to actual jealousy-evoking events. Suspicious and reactive jealousy may be differentiated on the basis of precursors (chronic person variables for suspicious jealousy and acute situational variables for reactive jealousy) and their respective response profiles (quantitative and qualitative).

Thus, according to the transactional model, Jealousy is not determined by a single cause. It results from the joint effects of commitment, insecurity, and arousability. Furthermore, a jealousy-evoking event can influence subsequent appraisals of commitment and insecurity, and subsequent levels of arousal. This conceptual framework is amenable to analyses of jealousy from different points of view, including cultural differences, personality, social cognition, emotions, social exchange, social comparison, and communications.

## SUPPORTING EVIDENCE FOR
## THE TRANSACTIONAL MODEL
### The Measurement of Dispositional Jealousy

It was within this broad transactional context that my colleagues and I initiated research on jealousy. The first efforts were guided by the casual observation that interpretations of jealousy-evoking events differed both within persons and across persons. The presumption was that these differences were not random. How then could we best document these differences? Open-ended questions were used to generate a heterogeneous set of jealousy-evoking events. On the first scale, the Self-Report Jealousy Scale (SRJS-I), most items were low and moderate in jealousy-evoking potential in order to accentuate the measurement of individual differences (Bringle, Roach, Andler, & Evenbeck, 1979). The scale included romantic, social, family, and work items. Only one item specifically referred to a partner's sexual involvement (having an affair), because it was thought that similar items would add little variability in responses. Respondents indicated how "jealous" they had been if the event had occurred, or would be if the event had not occurred, on a 9-point scale ranging from "Not at all jealous" to "Very jealous."

This measurement approach produced a data matrix that could be collapsed across respondents to examine differences among jealousy-evoking events, and that could be collapsed across events (items) to examine differences among individuals. The expectation was that two types of systematic variance would be documented: (1) a reliable rank order of persons across jealousy-evoking circumstances, relationships, and partners, *and* (2) a reliable rank order of jealousy-evoking circumstances across persons, relationships, and partners. This conceptualization of regularity in persons and situations was called "dispositional jealousy" (see Argyle & Little, 1976). The person component of dispositional jealousy was assumed to capture the quantitative distinction (but not the qualitative or behavioral differences) between suspicious jealousy (higher-intensity emotional reactions across a heterogeneous set of jealousy-evoking events) and reactive jealousy (lower-intensity emotional reactions). That is, it was assumed that high dispositional jealousy scores would reflect suspiciously jealous persons' reporting higher-intensity emotional reactions across a variety of minor jealousy-evoking events, in contrast to reactively jealous persons, who would generally score lower.

## Correlates of Dispositional Jealousy

The early research demonstrated that there were clear differences among items in reported jealousy; as would be expected, one's partner having an affair was rated more intensely than someone flirting with one's partner. Furthermore, the factor structure of the SRJS-I reflected the types of social relationships referred to in the items, with major factors for Social, Romantic, Family, and Work (Bringle et al., 1979).

The differences in items, however, were of less interest to us than the differences in respondents (Bringle & Evenbeck, 1979). What do these individual differences mean? Are they related to other aspects of the person? What is the jealous person like, in contrast to those who report less jealous reactions? Because the scale items were heterogeneous in content and general in nature (i.e., not specific to a particular partner or relationship), the responses were assumed to reflect reliable and stable tendencies to be jealous. We thought that measuring this global aspect of jealousy (as opposed to reactions to a specific incident of jealousy) would be the aspect of jealousy most likely to be related to personality attributes. Numerous studies were subsequently conducted in which dispositional jealousy scores were correlated with various personality dimensions. Persons scoring high on the measure of dispositional jealousy, in contrast to dispositionally less jealous persons, were more likely to have less positive self-esteem, to have a less benevolent attitude toward the world, to report lower life satisfaction, to have a more external locus of control, to be more dogmatic, to be more easily aroused, and to be more sensitive to threatening stimuli in their social environments (Bringle, 1981; Bringle & Williams, 1979; Jaremko & Lindsey, 1979; Manges & Evenbeck, 1980; White, 1984).

## Discussion of the Personality Findings

A number of interpretations and responses to these findings deserve comment.

1. *The findings have not been consistently replicated by others.* Some studies have not confirmed correlations reported in our research. For example, concerning the relationship with self-esteem and jealousy, several studies have found only partial support (e.g., for one gender of respondents; Buunk, 1986; Hansen, 1985; White, 1981b), whereas others have failed to find any significant correlations (Buunk, 1982a; Mathes & Severa, 1981; White, 1981a). However, in contrast to measuring the global aspect of jealousy that dispositional jealousy represents, some of these studies obtained relationship-specific and/or event-specific measures of jealousy, which would have lower correspondence (Fishbein & Ajzen, 1975) to global personality attributes. Multiple operationalization is not advantageous if the presumed underlying construct that is being measured varies. In addition, there have been other differences (ages of respondents, types of relationship) that confound interpretation of differing results. What is clear is that significant correlations between jealousy and self-esteem have been more consistently obtained if the SRJS-I is used (Bringle, 1981, Jaremko & Lindsey, 1979, and Manges & Evenbeck, 1980, all found significant correlations; no studies are known to have failed to find a significant correlation with the SRJS-I) than if it is not used.

2. *The amount of variance explained is small.* The correlations obtained are quite modest, ranging from .25 to .45. However, we never expected a single personality correlate to explain a great deal of variability in jealousy responses. We did expect personality qualities to be *related to the perception of jealousy-evoking events*, and that was confirmed. It is important that the results obtained yield a rather *consistent* pattern (see Bringle, 1981). Furthermore, variables from other domains (e.g., relationship variables such as dependency or relative dependency) seldom show higher bivariate correlations to jealousy. Finally, there is this question: To what extent are common method variance and response sets inflating these moderate correlations and leading to an overestimation of actual effect size? In comparing various jealousy scales, including the SRJS-I, White (1984) concluded that the convergence among the scales significantly exceeded common method variance and that social desirability response set was only a minor problem.

3. *There is more to jealousy than dispositional jealousy.* We never assumed that dispositional jealousy was the only perspective from which to view jealousy. We did assume that it was a perspective particularly relevant to certain questions about jealousy (e.g., a general measure of jealous tendencies for answering questions such as "What is the jealous person like?"). There is ample room within the transactional model for additional conceptualizations of jealousy (e.g., relationship-specific mea-

sures, event-specific measures, analyses of types of emotions, cognitions, and behaviors).

In order to evaluate the presumption that dispositional jealousy is a meaningful perspective, we designed a test of the dispositional perspective versus the interactionist perspective (Bringle, Renner, Terry, & Davis, 1983). The dispositional model predicts that there will be a main effect for persons and a main effect for situations (e.g., a reliable rank order of each) when a heterogeneous sample of persons responds to a heterogeneous sample of jealousy-evoking events (see Figure 5.2). The interactionist model predicts that an interaction of person and situational determinants will account for the pattern of reactions, *and* it predicts that neither person nor situation main effects will be important (Argyle & Little, 1976).

The results of Study 1 indicated that the person × situation interaction accounted for the single largest proportion of variance (estimates ranged from 16% to 19%, depending on assumptions employed). In addition, persons (15%–16%) and situations (11%–12%) explained substantial variability in responses. In Study 2, when situational differences were intentionally attenuated, persons accounted for approximately 35% of the variance. Thus, the results were inconsistent with the prediction of the interactionist model that the main effects would be negligible. Individual differences were found to be reliable across situations, and situations showed reliable differences across persons. However, the interaction term was not negligible. An additional finding from Study 2 demonstrated that within the reliable rank order of persons, respondents reported that the intensity of their reaction was different for different partners. For example, Joe reported himself as being a rather jealous person, but he was more jealous in his relationship with Mary than he was with Sue.

This research provides empirical support for two important points. First, the dispositional perspective is a viable one from which to analyze jealousy. Second, it is not the only one. Future empirical and conceptual work will need to maintain a balance among the person, relationship, and situational domains in order to provide a comprehensive and ecologically valid analysis of the phenomenon of jealousy.

4. *Dispositional jealousy is counterproductive because it stereotypes and stigmatizes jealous persons, and leads to the conclusion that they are "profoundly and irretrievably jealous"* (Clanton, 1981, p. 264). Perhaps it will now be clearer that in describing dispositional jealousy, we hypothesized that there are two testable patterns of responses—in other words, that both persons and situations can be reliably rank-ordered. The person component does have some trait-like qualities. For example, there is evidence of

cross-sectional stability across ages (Bringle, 1989a), cross-situational stability (Bringle et al., 1983; Mathes et al., 1985, Study 1), and longitudinal stability (2-week test–retest reliability = .73; Bringle et al., 1979). There is other evidence of cross-situational consistency, though it is confined to a paper-and-pencil assessment procedure. When the factor analysis on the SRJS-I was conducted with an oblique rotation, the four factors were substantially correlated with one another (Bringle et al., 1979). Finally, dispositional jealousy has demonstrated a consistent pattern of associations with other stable characteristics of personality. The degree to which dispositional jealousy encompasses other trait-like qualities (e.g., Buss & Craik, 1985) should be a matter of empirical assessment rather than conjecture or dogma. Equally important, it should be noted that dispositional jealousy is a *conceptual perspective* that may be useful in analyzing the nature of jealousy and should be considered part of a larger picture; it is not a clinical label of behavioral pathology.

5. *The word "jealousy" is used in the response format; some have argued that reporting or labeling feelings as jealous may not be strongly related to the actual experiences of jealousy.* For example, Clanton and Smith (1977) state, "The person who will admit to feeling jealous may in fact be *less* jealous than one who denies feeling jealous" (p. xi). This point never concerned me much. My impression from personally conducting some of the research studies was that most respondents were being open and honest in their responses. The concern may have applied to a small proportion of the sample, but I assumed that it was probably negligible and that we were getting useful responses from the vast majority of respondents. Furthermore, I thought that it was trivial whether the response format used "jealous," "upset," or "bothered." Finally, no one has presented any evidence to support Clanton and Smith's concern.

It was as a result of revising the SRJS-I to correct some inherent problems that data bearing on this issue were collected. The revision was initiated, first, because the SRJS-I contained some items that were more "envy items" than "jealousy items." Although it is difficult to write items that are "pure" jealousy items (particularly in the nonromantic domains), the items in the Revised Self-Report Jealousy Scale (SRJS-II) pertain more clearly to jealousy than to envy (Bringle, 1982). The second problem was that some items on the SRJS-I implied particular types of partners and relationships; for example, an item might refer to "date" or "spouse." The items on the SRJS-II were written so that they can refer to a wider range of relationships (e.g., heterosexual, homosexual, cohabiting, dating, marriage). Finally—and this is the change that is relevant to the current discussion—the response anchor "jealous" was replaced by "upset." We had observed anecdotally that some subjects

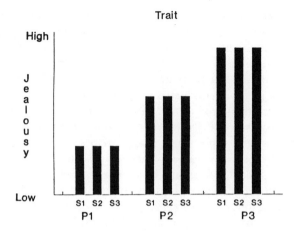

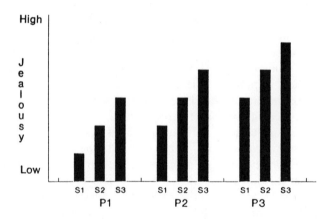

**FIGURE 5.2.** Four models of behavior (persons P1, P2, P3 reacting to the same three jealousy situations S1, S2, S3). From "An Analysis of Situation and Person Components of Jealousy," by R. G. Bringle, P. Renner, R. Terry, and S. Davis, 1983, *Journal of Research in Personality, 17,* pp. 354–368. Copyright 1983 by Academic Press, Inc. Adapted by permission.

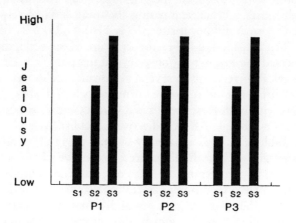

**Behavioral**

**Interactional**

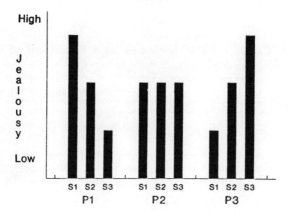

**FIGURE 5.2.** (continued)

reported difficulty in referring to "jealousy" when responding to some of the items. They often commented, "I wouldn't be jealous, but I would be angry or mad!" What really caught my attention was that two unpublished studies failed to replicate the correlation between self-esteem and dispositional jealousy when the SRJS-II was used.

Using the SRJS-II, which also presents romantic, work, social, and family jealousy-evoking circumstances, two groups of subjects responded to the items with one of the following two response formats: "Not at all jealous" to "Extremely jealous," or "Not at all upset" to "Extremely upset." When comparing the mean level of responses, the difference in format did not matter, $F$ (1, 116) = .33, $p > .05$ (Bringle, 1989c). When considering the factor structure of the scale, the response format affected the loadings of only several items.

The scales' correlations to several personality scales were also examined. The difference in response format labels did affect the scales' correlations with both Rosenberg's and Coopersmith's measures of self-esteem and the Multiple Affect Adjective Checklist (MAACL) Anxiety score (see Table 5.1). This apparently was not the result of differences in social desirability. These findings are provocative. They suggest that inconsistencies in past research findings on personality correlates may, in part, be attributable to different operationalizations of jealousy. More fundamentally, they suggest new research issues concerning the difference between using "upset," which is an operationalization consistent with our definition of jealousy, and "jealous," which is a self-labeling operationalization.

**TABLE 5.1. Correlates of Jealousy as a Function of Response Anchors**

| | Response anchors on SRJS-II | |
|---|---|---|
| | "Not at all upset" to "extremely upset" | "Not at all jealous" to "extremely jealous" |
| Rosenberg's Self-Esteem | .04 | −.44** |
| Coopersmith's Self-Esteem | −.04 | −.36** |
| Crowne–Marlowe Social Desirability | −.11 | −.09 |
| Exclusivity | .04 | .11 |
| Rubin's Love Scale | .28* | .28* |
| Relative Involvement | −.06 | −.12 |
| MAACL—Anxiety | −.03 | .34** |
| MAACL—Hostility | −.12 | .11 |
| MAACL—Depression | −.09 | .17 |

*Note.* SRJS-II, Revised Self-Report Jealousy Scale; MAACL, Multiple Affect Adjective Checklist. From "Some Thoughts on Critical Issues in Jealousy" by R. G. Bringle, 1989.
*$p < .05$.
**$p < .01$.

6. *The measure of dispositional jealousy is a measure of what some individuals expect to happen in a hypothetical situation, and respondents are likely to feel or act very differently from those expectations* (Clanton, 1981, p. 265). More generally, this point raises questions about the validity of self-report measures. My position is not that self-report measures are valid; nor is it that they are invalid. Self-report measures should be considered as having some situation-specific validity for certain aspects of the conceptual domain of jealousy experiences, and they are appropriate for some research questions. Specifically, these include (a) phenomenological representations of the respondent's current state; (b) expectations of future responses (but they are not a substitute for other measures of actual feelings, cognitions, and behaviors); and (c) cognitive representations of past events and responses (but they are not a substitute for those actual events, feelings, cognitions, and behaviors).

In order to evaluate the point that expectations of reactions to an event are very different from reports of actual reactions to the event, after responding to each item on the SRJS-II, respondents indicated whether or not something like it had happened in their life. There were no significant mean differences between responses that were anticipated and responses that were based on actual experience for 19 of the 25 items (Bringle, 1989c). Having actually experienced the event led to less extreme responses for two romantic items and led to more extreme responses for four nonromantic items (see Table 5.2). Thus, at least at the nomothetic level, the differences were few, and the direction of the difference depended on the domain of jealousy being measured.

## Conceptual Utility of the Transactional Model

At the conceptual level, variables that have been found in past research to be related to jealousy are easily organized within the transactional model's framework. Commitment has been demonstrated to be a joint function of satisfaction, investment, and the degree to which these are perceived as different from expected outcomes in alternative relationships (Rusbult, 1983). These and related variables (e.g., love, relationship length) have all been found to be related to jealousy (see reviews by Bringle & Buunk, 1985; Buunk & Bringle, 1987; White & Mullen, 1989). Person variables (e.g., need for affiliation, self-actualization, attachment styles) and situational variables (moods, children, anniversaries) affecting commitment have not received as much attention in research.

Variables related to insecurity have also received attention. Most research has been directed at jealousy-evoking events as causes of

**TABLE 5.2. Mean Jealousy Responses as a Function of Events'
Having Occurred**

| Event | $F$ | Has something like this happened to you? | |
| --- | --- | --- | --- |
| | | Yes | No |
| At a party, your partner kisses someone you do not know. | 7.83* | 6.23 | 7.18 |
| At a party, your partner dances with someone you do not know. | 8.09* | 5.24 | 6.08 |
| Your brother or sister is given more freedom. | 7.22* | 6.50 | 5.75 |
| Your brother or sister seems to be receiving more affection or attention from your parents. | 8.17* | 6.11 | 5.37 |
| The group to which you belong appears to be leaving you out of plans, activities, etc. | 9.36* | 7.07 | 6.31 |
| Your best friend suddenly shows interest in doing things with someone else. | 13.87* | 6.30 | 5.36 |

*Note.* From "Some Thoughts on Critical Issues in Jealousy" by R. G. Bringle, 1989.
*$p < .01$.

jealousy. However, other research has examined how relative dependency (who is more involved), inequity, and changes in the partner's circumstances (e.g., working around attractive persons of the opposite sex; Bringle & Buunk, 1989) can breed jealousy (see Bringle & Buunk, 1985; Buunk & Bringle, 1987; White & Mullen, 1989).

The importance of a variable conceptually related to arousability, "screening–nonscreening," was investigated in one study (Bringle & Williams, 1979). Nonscreeners, who do little stimulus screening, maintain diffuse and complex stimulus environments. They are not likely to rank the stimulus inputs, and therefore fail to filter out unimportant or irrelevant stimuli. Screeners show the opposite tendencies by being more selective and thereby reducing stimulus load. Most importantly, Mehrabian (1976) has shown that when subjects were faced with similar situations, the amplitude and duration of responses to novel stimuli were both greater for nonscreeners than for screeners. We (Bringle & Williams,

1979) found that screening–nonscreening was significantly correlated with dispositional jealousy, frequency of jealousy, diversity of feelings when jealous, and diversity of behaviors when jealous. In all cases, the correlations were consistent with the prediction that the more easily aroused nonscreeners reported greater emotional responsivity than did screeners.

Jealous reactions have also been related to anxiety (Bringle, 1981; Jaremko & Lindsey, 1979) and neuroticism (Buunk, 1981; Mathes, Roter, & Joerger, 1982). Although these variables are conceptually representative of emotionality and arousability, it is also probably the case that they are related to issues of insecurity as well.

## The Origins of Dispositional Jealousy

A popular theme in discussing jealousy is that adult jealousy has its roots in childhood sibling conflict (e.g., Clanton & Smith, 1977; Freud, 1922/1948; Levy, 1940). Given the popularity of this belief, it is interesting that there is no evidence to support it. Research has documented that sibling conflict is more common in children from small families and in children in earlier ordinal positions (e.g., Bossard & Boll, 1966; Koch, 1960; Sears, Maccoby, & Levine, 1957). Is adult jealousy related to these covariates of childhood conflict?

In order to answer this and other questions concerning the developmental origins of jealousy, we (Bringle & Williams, 1979) asked college students and their parents to complete questionnaires containing measures of dispositional jealousy, jealous feelings and behaviors, and two personality dimensions: (1) "repression–sensitization," a measure on which repressors are individuals who avoid threatening material by avoiding or denying, are highly defensive, and experience little manifest anxiety (Byrne, 1961; Byrne, Barry, & Nelson, 1963); and (2) screening–nonscreening, which is described above.

The results found essentially no support for the assumption that structural characteristics of the family (birth order and family size) were related to dispositional jealousy, jealous feelings, jealous behaviors, or frequency of jealousy (Bringle & Williams, 1979). Measures of screening and repression were both consistent predictors of dispositional jealousy and jealous feelings, with more jealous persons demonstrating both less screening and greater sensitization. The results also demonstrated parent–child continuity for dispositional jealousy; they showed that personalities of the offspring and parents, and the nature of the parent–child relationship, were more useful in understanding the origins of jealousy (especially for females) than were family structural characteristics.

## Groups Reporting Low Jealousy

Although there is wide consensus that a partner's extradyadic sexual behavior is upsetting, there are groups of individuals that permit their partners to have sexual relationships with others. Research has studied how they react to and manage these circumstances. These groups have included "swingers" (Gilmartin, 1977), members of communes (Pines & Aronson, 1981), and partners in open marriages (Buunk, 1981, 1982b). Studies of all these groups highlight how individuals select situations and tailor circumstances in ways that are compatible with existing dispositions and attitudes, *or* how individuals enter situations in order to change themselves so that they will be more like that to which they aspire (Synder & Ickes, 1985).

We conducted studies on two other groups that also constitute exceptions to the traditional pattern. The first group, male homosexuals, reported more relationships in the immediate past, more relationships of shorter duration, greater frequency of going to bars, and greater likelihood of having partners who saw others on a romantic basis than did a sample of heterosexual males (Bringle, 1989b). Given the higher rate of jealousy-evoking events for homosexual males, it is interesting that they reported *lower* levels of upset on the SRJS-II than did heterosexual males. The two groups did not differ in self-esteem, nor did they differ on relationship qualities such as involvement, relative involvement, satisfaction, and control and power in the relationship. Although this possibility was not directly measured in the research, homosexual males appear to have developed norms and ground rules that prevent feelings of insecurity and that attenuate emotional upset when they are faced with events that those in traditional heterosexual relationships find upsetting.

A second study (Bringle & Boebinger, 1990) compared persons who had been in one of three different types of relationships: a traditional dating relationship, a relationship with someone who was simultaneously dating someone else, or a relationship with someone who was married. Individuals who are knowingly involved with partners who have *collateral* relationships are exposing themselves to higher levels of jealousy-evoking events than those in traditional relationships. Interestingly, in comparison to traditional dating relationships, respondents from both types of collateral relationships reported less upset if their partners were to engage in jealousy-evoking sexual behavior with the other person (e.g., kissing, fondling). In contrast to the study on male homosexuals, which found no relationship differences, this study found that these "third persons" in triangles characterized their relationships as less involved (e.g., less love, commitment, need fulfillment) than did those in traditional relationships. This was the case even though the lengths of the relationships were not different. Thus, such individuals may be limiting the level of involvement (i.e., commitment) as a means of managing jealousy in the face of jealousy-evoking behaviors by the partner. For all members of special groups, self-selection into types of relationships is probably as important as managing circumstances in a particular type of relationship.

## Dispositional Jealousy and Marital Quality

Jealousy has the potential to contribute positively to a relationship. For example, high jealousy has been found to be associated with strong love (Buunk, 1981; Mathes et al., 1982; Mathes & Severa, 1981; White, 1984), with establishing "ground rules" (Buunk, 1981), and with attempts to test the relationship and increase commitment (White, 1980). However, there is also a negative side to jealousy. Unlike the negative emotional reactions, relationship growth and improvement are not *necessary* consequences of jealousy. Sommers (1984) found among an American sample that jealousy was viewed by no one as being "useful and constructive," but was endorsed by 62% as being "dangerous and destructive." Jealousy has also been strongly implicated in domestic violence (e.g., Daly, Wilson, & Weghorst, 1982; Roy, 1977; White & Mullen, 1989, Ch. 8; Whitehurst, 1971).

Thus, past research suggests both positive and negative effects of jealousy on relationships, but fails to answer this broad question: what kinds of relationships do chronically and intensely jealous persons have? A study on married couples (Bringle, 1989a) found that a couple's total dispositional jealousy had a small negative relationship to marital quality. In addition, when both dispositional jealousy and subscale scores (Romantic, Social, Work, and Family jealousy) were examined, intensity of jealousy and perceived and actual heterogamy (differences in husband's and wife's jealousy) were related inversely to marital quality. Social and Romantic jealousy scores were found to be more strongly related to marital quality than were Work and Family jealousy scores.

These findings bear on a persistent issue—whether jealousy is good, bad, or both good and bad, depending on the circumstances. Although the conclusions are preliminary, results from the research on personality correlates and adjustment of jealous couples suggest three points: (1) At the broadest level, less jealous persons and relationships "look better" than more jealous ones; (2) these correlations are small to moderate, suggesting that there are many exceptions to that general characterization; and (3) we need a better understanding of moderating effects in those cases that do and do not fit that conclusion.

## POSTSCRIPT

Why are people jealous? The transactional model of jealousy emphasizes the necessary interdependency between the person and the social environment in determining the meaning extracted from the stream of events in a relationship. This view stresses the importance of commitment, insecurity, and arousability in determining jealous responses. These are seen not only as causing jealousy, but also as being influenced and changed by jealousy. The nature of this reciprocal influence highlights that both relationships and jealousy are *processes* (Duck & Sants, 1983; Hupka, 1989), not steady states.

Although jealousy can assume a constructive role in a relationship, why do people respond in ways that are so punishing to themselves and to their relationships? Embedded in the fabric of jealousy are two fundamental values. First, there is the desire to be liked. Humans are gregarious, benefit from social relations, and desire the acceptance and approval of others. Human relationships define the very soul of the self. Second, there is the desire for self-integrity. People want to know that their view of the world is reasonable and meaningful. They want to believe that they are the way they want to be. Ideally, individuals create for themselves social environments in which self-enhancement and self-verification are supported by their most significant relationships (Swann, 1987). When jealousy occurs, these two fundamental values collide. A partner who is highly important to the definition of the individual behaves in a way that jeopardizes the integrity of the person and the relationship. The emotional energy released by jealousy can be understood as a struggle between these two central values; the need to preserve one domain threatens the existence of the other. The dilemma is simple, yet wrenching: "In what way do I compromise 'me' for the maintenance of 'we,' or sacrifice 'we' for the preservation of 'me'?" It is not surprising that jealousy is so painful, yet so unavoidable, compelling, and powerful.

## ACKNOWLEDGMENTS

I gratefully acknowledge the comments of Bram Buunk, Peter Salovey, and John Kremer on a draft of this chapter.

## REFERENCES

Ames, A., Jr. (1953). Reconstruction of the origin and nature of perception. In S. Ratner (Ed.), *Vision and action* (pp. 251–274). New Brunswick, NJ: Rutgers University Press.

Argyle, M., & Little, B. R. (1976). Do personality traits apply to social behavior? In N. S. Endler & D. Magnussen (Eds.), *Interactional psychology and personality* (pp. 30–57). Washington, DC: Hemisphere.

Averill, J. (1982). *Anger and aggression: An essay on emotion.* New York: Springer-Verlag.

Averill, J. (1983). Studies on anger and aggression: Implications for theories of emotion. *American Psychologist, 38,* 1145–1160.

Blumstein, P., & Schwartz, P. (1983). *American couples.* New York: William Morrow.

Beck, A. T. (1976). *Cognitive therapy and the emotional disorders.* New York: International Universities Press.

Bossard, J., & Boll, E. (1966). *The sociology of child development.* New York: Harper & Row.

Bringle, R. G. (1981). Conceptualizing jealousy as a disposition. *Alternative Lifestyles, 4,* 274–290.

Bringle, R. G. (1982). *Preliminary report on the Revised Self-Report Jealousy Scale.* Unpublished manuscript.

Bringle, R. G. (1989a). *Dispositional jealousy, homogamy, and marital quality.* Manuscript submitted for publication.

Bringle, R. G. (1989b). *The nature of jealousy in the relationships of homosexual and heterosexual males.* Unpublished manuscript.

Bringle, R. G. (1989c, May). Some thoughts on critical issues in jealousy. In G. L. White (Chair), *Themes for progress in jealousy research.* Symposium conducted at the Second Iowa Conference on Personal Relationships, Iowa City.

Bringle, R. G., & Boebinger, K. L. G. (1990). Jealousy and the 'third' person in the love triangle. *Journal of Social and Personal Relationships, 7,* 119–133.

Bringle, R. G., & Buunk, B. (1985). Jealousy and social behavior: A review of person, relationship and situational determinants. In P. Shaver (Ed.), *Review of personality and social psychology: Vol. 6. Self, situations, and social behavior* (pp. 241–264). Beverly Hills, CA: Sage.

Bringle, R. G., & Buunk, B. (1989). *Perceptions of threat in jealousy-evoking situations.* Unpublished manuscript.

Bringle, R. G., & Evenbeck, S. (1979). The study of jealousy as a dispositional characteristic. In M. Cook & G. Wilson (Eds.), *Love and attraction* (pp. 201–204). Oxford: Pergamon Press.

Bringle, R. G., Renner, P., Terry, R., & Davis, S. (1983). An analysis of situational and person components of jealousy. *Journal of Research in Personality, 17,* 354–368.

Bringle, R. G., Roach, S., Andler, C., & Evenbeck, S. (1979). Measuring the intensity of jealous reactions. *JSAS: Catalog of Selected Documents in Psychology, 9*(1832), 23–24.

Bringle, R. G., & Williams, L. J. (1979). Parental–offspring similarity on jealousy and related personality dimensions. *Motivation and Emotion, 3,* 265–286.

Brunswik, E. (1947). *Systematic and representative design of psychological experiments.* Berkeley: University of California Press.

Bryson, J. B. (1976, August). *The nature of sexual jealousy: An exploratory study.* Paper presented at the meeting of the American Psychological Association, Washington, DC.

Bush, C. R., Bush, J. P., & Jennings, J. (1988). Effects of jealousy threat on relationship perception and emotions. *Journal of Social and Personal Relationships, 5,* 285–303.

Buss, D. M., & Craik, K. H. (1985). Why not measure that trait? Alternative criteria for identifying important dispositions. *Journal of Personality and Social Psychology, 48,* 934–946.

Buunk, B. (1981). Jealousy in sexually open marriages. *Alternative Lifestyles, 4,* 357–372.

Buunk, B. (1982a). Anticipated sexual jealousy: Its relationship to self-esteem, dependency and reciprocity. *Personality and Social Psychology Bulletin, 8,* 310–316.

Buunk, B. (1982b). Strategies of jealousy: Styles of coping with extramarital involvement of the spouse. *Family Relations, 31,* 13–18.

Buunk, B. (1984). Attributions and jealousy. *Social Psychology Quarterly, 47,* 107–112.

Buunk, B. (1986). Husband's jealousy. In R. A. Lewis & R. E. Salt (Eds.), *Men in families* (pp. 97–114). Beverly Hills, CA: Sage.

Buunk, B. (1989, May). Types and manifestations of jealousy: An exchange-theoretical perspective. In G. L. White (Chair), *Themes for progress in jealousy research.* Symposium conducted at the Second Iowa Conference on Personal Relationships, Iowa City.

Buunk, B., & Bringle, R. G. (1987). Jealousy in love relationships. In D. Perlman & S. Duck (Eds.), *Intimate relationships: Development, dynamics, and deterioration* (pp. 123–147). Beverly Hills, CA: Sage.

Byrne, D. (1961). The Repression–Sensitization Scale: Rationale, reliability, and validity. *Journal of Personality, 29,* 334–339.

Byrne, D., Barry, J., & Nelson, D. (1963). The relation of revised Repression–Sensitization Scale to measures of self-description. *Psychological Reports, 13,* 323–334.

Chaplain, J. P. (1975). *Dictionary of psychology* (rev. ed.). New York: Dell.

Clanton, G. (1981). Frontiers of jealousy research. *Alternative Lifestyles, 4,* 259–273.

Clanton, G., & Smith, L. G. (Eds.). (1977). *Jealousy.* Englewood Cliffs, NJ: Prentice-Hall.

Daly, M., Wilson, M., & Weghorst, S. J. (1982). Male sexual jealousy. *Ethology and Sociobiology, 3,* 11–27.

Derryberry, D., & Rothbart, M. K. (1988). Arousal, affect and attention as components of temperament. *Journal of Social and Personality Psychology, 55,* 958–966.

Duck, S., & Sants, H. (1983). On the origin of the specious: Are personal relationships really interpersonal states? *Journal of Social and Clinical Psychology, 1,* 27–41.

Fishbein, M., & Ajzen, I. (1975). *Belief, attitude, intention, and behavior: An introduction to theory and research.* Reading, MA: Addison-Wesley.

Foa, E. B., & Foa, U. G. (1980). Resource theory: Interpersonal behavior as exchange. In K. J. Gergen, M. S. Greenber, & R. H. Willis (Eds.), *Social exchange: Advances in theory and research* (pp. 77–94). New York: Plenum.

Freud, S. (1948). Certain neurotic mechanisms in jealousy, paranoia, and homosexuality. In S. Freud, *Collected papers* (Vol. 2, pp. 232–243). London: Hogarth Press. Originally published in 1922.

Gilmartin, B. (1977). Jealousy among the swingers. In G. Clanton & L. G. Smith (Eds.), *Jealousy* (pp. 152–158). Englewood Cliffs, NJ: Prentice-Hall.

Hansen, G. L. (1985). Perceived threats and marital jealousy. *Social Psychology Quarterly, 48,* 262–268.

Heider, F. (1958). *The psychology of interpersonal relations.* New York: Wiley.

Hupka, R. (1984). Jealousy: Compound emotion or label for a particular situation? *Motivation and Emotion, 8,* 141–155.

Hupka, R. (1989, May). Components of the typical response to romantic jealousy situations. In G. L. White (Chair), *Themes for progress in jealousy research.* Symposium conducted at the Second Iowa Conference on Personal Relationships, Iowa City.

Jaremko, M. E., & Lindsey, R. (1979). Stress coping abilities of individuals high and low in jealousy. *Psychological Reports, 44,* 547–553.

Kelley, H. H. (1979). *Personal relationships: Their structure and processes.* Hillsdale, NJ: Erlbaum.

Koch, H. (1960). The relation of certain formal attributes of siblings to attitudes held toward each other and toward their parents. *Monographs of the Society for Research in Child Development, 25*(4, Serial No. 78).

Larsen, R. J., Diener, E., & Cropanzano, R. S. (1987). Cognitive operations associated with individual differences in affect intensity. *Journal of Personality and Social Psychology, 5,* 767–774.

Levy, D. M. (1940). Jealousy. *Journal of Pediatrics, 16,* 515–518.

Manges, K., & Evenbeck, S. (1980, May). *Social power, jealousy, and dependency in the intimate dyad.* Paper presented at the meeting of the Midwestern Psychological Association, St. Louis.

Markus, H., & Zajonc, R. B. (1985). The cognitive perspective in social psychology. In G. Lindzey & E. Aronson (Eds.), *The handbook of social psychology* (3rd ed., Vol. 1, pp. 137–230). New York: Random House.

Mathes, E. W., Adams, H. E., & Davies, R. M. (1985). Jealousy: Loss of relationship rewards, loss of self-esteem, depression, anxiety, and anger. *Journal of Personality and Social Psychology, 48,* 1552–1561.

Mathes, E. W., Roter, P. M., & Joerger, S. M. (1982). A convergent validity study of six jealousy scales. *Psychological Reports, 50,* 1143–1147.

Mathes, E. W., & Severa, N. (1981). Jealousy, romantic love and liking: Theoretical considerations and preliminary scale development. *Psychological Reports, 49,* 23–31.

Mehrabian, A. (1976). *Manual for the questionnaire measure of stimulus screening and arousability.* Los Angeles: University of California at Los Angeles.

Pfeiffer, S. M., & Wong, P. T. P. (1989). Multidimensional jealousy. *Journal of Social and Personal Relationships, 6,* 181–196.

Pines, A., & Aronson, E. (1981). Polyfidelity: An alternative lifestyle without jealousy? *Alternative Lifestyles, 4,* 373–392.

Plutchik, R. (1980). *Emotion: A psychoevolutionary synthesis.* New York: Harper & Row.

Pruitt, D. G. (1981). *Negotiation behavior.* New York: Academic Press.

Roy, M. (1977). A current survey of 150 cases. In M. Roy (Ed.), *Battered women: A psychosociological study of domestic violence* (pp. 25–44). New York: Van Nostrand Reinhold.

Rusbult, C. E. (1980). Commitment and satisfaction in romantic associations: A test of the investment model. *Journal of Experimental Social Psychology, 16,* 172–186.

Rusbult, C. E. (1983). A longitudinal test of the investment model: The development (and deterioration) of satisfaction and commitment in heterosexual involvements. *Journal of Personality and Social Psychology, 45,* 101–117.

Salovey, P., & Rodin, J. (1986). The differentiation of social-comparison jealousy and romantic jealousy. *Journal of Personality and Social Psychology, 50,* 1100–1112.

Salovey, P., & Rodin, J. (1988). Coping with envy and jealousy. *Journal of Social and Clinical Psychology, 7,* 15–33.

Sears, R., Maccoby, E., & Levine, H. (1957). *Patterns of child rearing.* Evanston, IL: Row & Peterson.

Shrestha, K., Rees, D. W., Rix, J. B., Hore, B. D., & Faragher, E. B. (1985). Sexual jealousy in alcoholics. *Acta Psychiatrica Scandinavica, 72,* 283–290.

Snyder, M., & Ickes, W. (1985). Personality and social behavior. In G. Lindzey & E. Aronson (Eds.), *The handbook of social psychology* (3rd ed., Vol. 2, pp. 883–947). New York: Random House.

Sommers, S. (1984). Adults evaluating their emotions: A cross-cultural perspective. In C. Z. Malatesta & C. E. Izard (Eds.), *Emotion in adult development* (pp. 319–338). Beverly Hills, CA: Sage.

Swann, W. B. (1987). Identity negotiations: Where two roads meet. *Journal of Personality and Social Psychology, 53,* 1038–1051.

Thibaut, J. W., & Kelley, H. H. (1959). *The social psychology of groups.* New York: Wiley.

Thompson, A. P. (1983). Extramarital sex: A review of the research literature. *Journal of Sex Research, 19,* 1–22.

Thompson, A. P. (1984). Emotional and sexual components of extramarital relations. *Journal of Marriage and the Family, 46*, 35–42.

White, G. L. (1980). Inducing jealousy: A power perspective. *Personality and Social Psychology Bulletin, 6*, 222–227.

White, G. L. (1981a). Jealousy and partner's perceived motives for attraction to a rival. *Social Psychology Quarterly, 44*, 24–30.

White, G. L. (1981b). Relative involvement, inadequacy and jealousy: A test of a causal model. *Alternative Lifestyles, 4*, 291–309.

White, G. L. (1984). Comparison of four jealousy scales. *Journal of Research in Personality, 18*, 115–130.

White, G. L., & Mullen, P. E. (1989). *Jealousy: Theory, research, and clinical strategies.* New York: Guilford Press.

Whitehurst, R. N. (1971). Violence potential in extramarital sexual spouses. *Journal of Marriage and the Family, 33*, 683–691.

*Chapter Six*

# Developmental
# Correlates of Jealousy

GORDON CLANTON
*San Diego State University*

DAVID J. KOSINS
*Seattle, Washington*

Conventional wisdom assumes, as do many approaches to clinical psychology, that early conflicts with parents and siblings make one more likely to experience intense jealousy in adult relationships. Our research fails to support this assumption. We found no statistically significant relationships between the self-report of jealousy and several developmental variables—namely, childhood conflicts with siblings, separations and losses during childhood, harshness of parental discipline, quality of early parent–child relations, and emotional support from peers in childhood. Furthermore, there was no significant difference in the intensity of jealousy reported by college students (representing the "normal" or nonclinical population), psychotherapy outpatients, and a small group of psychiatric inpatients. These findings suggest that jealousy is *not* best viewed primarily as an emotional disorder and that therapists treating clients with jealousy problems ought *not* to assume that jealousy is always rooted in disrupted attachment history and early sibling conflicts. Additional discussion relates adult jealousy to social desirability, demographic variables, and family constellation.

The purpose of the study reported in this chapter was to examine the relationship between adult jealousy and a number of developmental variables. Despite much speculation, no empirical literature on adult jealousy prior to this research had assessed the impact of developmental correlates. Furthermore, previous research had studied *either* pathologically jealous cases *or* jealousy in a normal sample (usually college students). The present study set out to *compare* results across three samples: (1) college students, representing a "normal" or nonclinical population; (2) psychotherapy outpatients; and (3) psychiatric inpatients.

For present purposes, jealousy may be defined as a protective reaction to a perceived threat to a valued relationship or to its quality (Clanton, 1981, p. 260; Clanton & Smith, 1977/1986, pp. vi, 239). The protective reaction can involve thoughts, feelings, and/or actions. Although jealous behaviors sometimes damage relationships, the *intention* of jealousy is the protection of the relationship and/or the protection of the ego of the threatened partner. Adult jealousy typically results when one believes that a romantic relationship is threatened by a real or imaginary rival.

We tested the psychoanalytic speculation that early sibling conflicts may increase the intensity of jealousy in adult romantic relationships (Freud, 1922/1955; Reik, 1945; Schmideberg, 1953). We also measured the relationship between adult jealousy and several developmental variables central to the attachment theory of John Bowlby (1969, 1973, 1980). Psychoanalytic formulations are notoriously difficult to test empirically, but Bowlby's work has resulted in instruments to *measure* disrupted attachment history. Such instruments were employed in this research. We acknowledge that we have not devised an empirical test of psychoanalytic theory. Our goal was much more modest.

Bowlby postulated that ill-formed or disrupted attachments with early caretakers often result in the condition of "anxious attachment." The anxiously attached person remains "excessively sensitive to the possibility of separation or loss of love" (Bowlby, 1973, p. 238) throughout the lifespan. Attachment theory suggests that individuals whose affectional bonds with primary caretakers have been disrupted would be especially susceptible to adult jealousy. As Bowlby (1977) put it:

A man who during childhood was frequently threatened with abandonment can easily attribute such intentions to his wife. He will then misinterpret things she says or does in terms of such intent, and then take whatever action he thinks would best meet the situation he believes to exist. Misunderstanding and conflict must follow. (p. 142)

On the basis of Bowlby's concept of anxious attachment, one would expect that a disrupted attachment history would increase vulnerability to adult jealousy by heightening perception of threat. In particular, intensity of adult jealousy was hypothesized to covary positively with number of separations and losses during childhood and harshness of parental discipline, and to covary negatively with quality of parent–child relations and degree of emotional support from peers during childhood.

This study was an unusual collaboration between a psychologist and a sociologist—two investigators guided by different theoretical frameworks,[1] but agreeing on how to test hypotheses of interest to both. As the research was undertaken, the psychologist (Kosins) anticipated that adult jealousy would correlate with disrupted attachment history and formed his hypotheses accordingly. The sociologist (Clanton) anticipated that the correlations would be weak or nonexistent, thus supporting the null hypothesis. As we shall see, the psychological hypotheses were *not* supported by the results. A sociological perspective will inform the discussion of why the hypotheses were not supported.

## METHOD

The original subjects in the data-collection phase of this study were 86 men and 165 women between the ages of 18 and 50, representing three separate voluntary populations: 85 undergraduate students enrolled in introductory psychology classes; 129 nonpsychotic, nonsociopathic psychotherapy outpatients; and 37 nonpsychotic, nonsociopathic psychiatric inpatients living on open wards of two private psychiatric hospitals. Table 6.1 presents more detailed demographic information on this sample.

The inpatient sample was later dropped from the hypothesis testing because of an insufficient number of males in this group; this left 77 men and 137 women in the sample. After the data of several participants who reported their ages as over 50 were excluded, only nine male subjects remained in the inpatient group. Deleting subjects with missing data further reduced the inpatient group to a size judged inadequate for inclusion in the analysis. Answers to many questions raised by this research must await its replication with a study that includes a larger sample of male inpatients.

Six self-report instruments were employed:

1. The dependent variable, intensity of jealousy, was assessed by the Romantic Relationship Scale (RRS), developed in a pilot study for this investigation (Kosins, 1983). It is described below.

2. The Sibling Relationship Scale (SRS), adapted from Cattell (1953), measured degree of early sibling conflict, including early rivalry, envy, and jealousy among siblings, as well as parental comparisons and favoritism that might foster such feelings.

3. The Attachment History Questionnaire (AHQ), based on the work of Kessler and Pottharst (1982), assessed number of separations and losses during childhood (AHQ1); harshness of parental discipline, including threats of abandonment (AHQ2); quality of parent–child relations (AHQ3); and quality of peer relations in childhood (AHQ4). The AHQ asks about hospitalizations and boarding school, family conflict and dissolution, parental support and criticism, types of punishment, and relationships with friends while still living with one's parents.

4. A demographic questionnaire was used to collect background data.

5. The Edwards Social Desirability Scale (Edwards, 1957) was administered to identify the extent to which the social desirability response set biased self-report on the variables under study.

6. Finally, subjects were given the Interpersonal Relationship Scale (IRS; Hupka & Rusch, 1977), a measure of jealousy and envy previously used in several research studies (Hupka & Bachelor, 1979; Rosmarin, Chambless, & LaPointe, 1979). This was included to generate an index of convergent validity of the RRS.[2]

Our jealousy measure, the Romantic Relationship Scale (RRS), presented subjects with 15 hypothetical situations that might produce jealousy (e.g., "At a party, your partner hugs another man/woman," and "Your partner tells you he/she is sexually attracted to a mutual friend of yours"). Respondents were asked to indicate on a 5-point Likert scale how they would feel: "very pleased," "pleased," "neutral," "displeased," or "very displeased." In addition, subjects were asked to indicate on a 5-point Likert scale the extent to which they agreed or disagreed with 13 statements such as "I frequently check up to see if my partner has been where he/she says he/she has been," and "I often worry that I'll lose my partner to another man/woman." Whereas some jealousy measures assess reaction to betrayal or relationship loss, we sought to include a range of situations in which the threat was more ambiguous and the outcome more dependent on the interpretation of the individual. See Appendix 6.1 for the full text of the RRS.

Because jealousy is viewed pejoratively by many people, the development of the RRS, our jealousy measure, included numerous steps to

**TABLE 6.1. Demographic Characteristics of the Research Sample**

| Characteristic | College students | | Outpatients | | Inpatients | | Total |
|---|---|---|---|---|---|---|---|
| | Males ($n = 30$) | Females ($n = 55$) | Males ($n = 47$) | Females ($n = 82$) | Males ($n = 9$) | Females ($n = 28$) | ($n = 251$) |
| Age | | | | | | | |
| M | 25.2 | 25.3 | 32.6 | 31.5 | 36.6 | 34.7 | 30.12 |
| SD | 7.9 | 7.6 | 7.5 | 6.9 | 9.8 | 7.4 | 8.27 |
| Education (years) | | | | | | | |
| M | 13.2 | 12.9 | 14.5 | 14.4 | 12.4 | 12.8 | 13.7 |
| SD | 1.4 | 1.1 | 2.5 | 2.2 | 2.4 | 2.4 | 2.1 |
| Marital status (%) | | | | | | | |
| Never married | 66.7 | 56.4 | 30.4 | 30.5 | 11.1 | 8.0 | 37.7 |
| Married | 20.0 | 27.3 | 37.0 | 40.2 | 77.8 | 68.0 | 38.5 |
| Divorced | 10.0 | 7.3 | 26.1 | 22.0 | — | 16.0 | 16.6 |
| Separated | 3.3 | 9.0 | 6.5 | 6.1 | 11.1 | 4.0 | 6.5 |
| Widowed | — | — | — | 1.2 | — | 4.0 | .8 |
| Annual income (%) | | | | | | | |
| Less than $10,000 | 25.0 | 23.1 | 8.7 | 13.6 | 11.1 | — | 14.5 |
| $10,000–$19,999 | 10.7 | 26.9 | 34.8 | 30.9 | — | 20.8 | 26.3 |
| $20,000–$29,999 | 32.1 | 23.1 | 21.7 | 13.6 | 66.7 | 41.7 | 24.2 |
| $30,000–$39,999 | 7.1 | 11.5 | 13.0 | 22.2 | 11.1 | 16.7 | 15.4 |
| $40,000–$49,999 | 10.7 | 7.7 | 4.3 | 6.2 | — | 4.2 | 6.3 |
| $50,000 or more | 14.3 | 7.7 | 17.4 | 13.6 | 11.1 | 16.7 | 13.3 |

| | | | | | | | |
|---|---|---|---|---|---|---|---|
| Race (%) | | | | | | | |
| Caucasian | 78.6 | 74.1 | 86.7 | 97.6 | 88.9 | 69.6 | 85.1 |
| Hispanic | 3.6 | 14.8 | 11.1 | 2.4 | 11.1 | 17.4 | 8.7 |
| Black | 3.6 | 1.9 | — | — | — | 13.0 | 2.1 |
| Oriental | 10.7 | 7.4 | — | — | — | — | 2.9 |
| Other | 3.6 | 1.9 | 2.2 | — | — | — | 1.2 |
| Religion (%) | | | | | | | |
| Protestant | 35.7 | 40.7 | 39.1 | 38.3 | 37.5 | 29.2 | 37.8 |
| Catholic | 25.0 | 29.6 | 21.7 | 23.5 | 25.0 | 62.5 | 28.6 |
| Jewish | — | 1.9 | 2.2 | 3.7 | — | — | 2.1 |
| Atheist/agnostic | 10.7 | 3.7 | 28.3 | 16.0 | 25.0 | — | 13.7 |
| Other | 28.6 | 24.1 | 8.7 | 18.5 | 12.5 | 8.3 | 17.8 |

*Note.* Missing cases for these variables are as follows: education, 4; marital status, 4; income, 11; race, 10; religion, 10.

reduce distortion from participants' trying to answer in socially desirable ways. One such step was to avoid the use of the word "jealousy" in the instrument.[3] The RRS in this study had adequate internal consistency (coefficient alpha = .90) and test–retest reliability ($r = .82$, $p < .001$) established over a 2-week interval. The convergent validity coefficient with the IRS (Hupka & Rusch, 1977) was .69 ($p < .001$). See Kosins (1983, pp. 112–122) for a more thorough discussion of construct and content validity of the RRS and the other scales.

Procedures for data collection differed for each subject group. The college students completed the batteries in class. The outpatients received the packets from one of 57 participating psychotherapists and mailed them to the principal investigator (Kosins). The inpatients completed their packets during their regular community meetings. For each group, all data gathered remained anonymous.

Treatment of the data involved multiple-regression analyses, with five predictor variables (corresponding to the five hypotheses described above) and one outcome variable (the intensity of adult jealousy). Four control variables were also included in the regression model: group membership, gender, the interaction of group and gender, and social desirability as measured by the Edwards Scale. We then tried to identify the degree to which the predictor variables were associated with adult jealousy, after taking into account the control variables.

## RESULTS

Neither sibling conflict during childhood nor any of the four hypothesized attributes of attachment history was associated with adult jealousy, after controlling for group membership, gender, the interaction of group and gender, and social desirability. No statistically significant relationships were found between the predictor variables and the outcome variable, adult jealousy (see Table 6.2.)

Confirming our sense that the self-report of jealousy is distorted by the desire to deny personal experience of what is perceived as a negative emotion, the Edwards Social Desirability Scale was the variable most strongly associated with jealousy in this study (see Table 6.3). Those people with low scores on the Edwards Scale obtained higher scores on the RRS, $F (1, 136) = 6.51$, $p = .012$. In other words, the less a person tended to give socially desirable responses in self-description, the more jealousy he or she admitted. Put differently, the willingness to admit one's weaknesses correlated more strongly with the self-report of jealousy than did any other variable considered in this study. This

**TABLE 6.2. Partial *F* Tests for Prediction of RRS from SRS and AHQ, Controlling for Group, Gender, Group × Gender, and Edwards Scores**

| Source | SS | df | MS | F | p |
|---|---|---|---|---|---|
| SRS | 10.82 | 1 | 10.82 | 0.07 | .799 |
| AHQ1 | 85.28 | 1 | 85.28 | 0.51 | .475 |
| AHQ2 | 16.24 | 1 | 16.24 | 0.10 | .755 |
| AHQ3 | 162.25 | 1 | 162.25 | 0.98 | .325 |
| AHQ4 | 245.56 | 1 | 245.56 | 1.48 | .226 |
| SRS and AHQ1–AHQ4 | 538.91 | 5 | 107.78 | 0.65 | .663 |
| Residual | 22,608.82 | 136 | 166.24 | | |

*Note.* The inpatient group was excluded from this analysis. RRS, Romantic Relationship Scale, a measure of jealousy; SRS, Sibling Relationship Scale; AHQ, Attachment History Questionnaire (AHQ1, separations and losses during childhood; AHQ2, harshness of parental discipline, threats of abandonment; AHQ3, quality of parent–child relations; AHQ4, quality of peer relations in childhood).

finding suggests that jealousy is very hard to assess by self-report, no matter how subtle the instrument.

It is important to remember that most of the scales social scientists use to measure jealousy are in fact measures of the ability to acknowledge and the willingness to disclose jealousy. In a time when jealousy is widely viewed in pejorative terms, we should not be surprised by the finding of Bringle (1981) that college students who were self-deprecating and dissatisfied with their lives were more likely to report that they would be jealous in a series of hypothetical jealousy-provoking situations. This finding does not demonstrate that jealous people are necessarily self-deprecating and dissatisfied with themselves. It does suggest, however, that people who are more willing to admit to dissatisfaction with themselves are also more likely to admit to jealousy.

With regard to gender differences, no significant differences between men and women were noted when they were compared directly. However, in all three subject groups, there was a *tendency* for women to respond with more jealousy than men to the hypothetical situations presented by both the RRS and the IRS. In addition, women in each group scored slightly lower than their male counterparts on the Edwards Scale. When social desirability and other control and independent variables were included in the full model regression analysis, the contribution of gender was still significant, with higher jealousy scores for women.

**TABLE 6.3. The Full Model for the Prediction of RRS Scores from Group Membership, Gender, the Edwards Covariate, and the Five Predictors**

| Variable | Raw score coefficient | Standard error of coefficient | Beta |
|---|---|---|---|
| Constant | 108.09 | | |
| Group | 2.19 | 2.90 | .08 |
| Gender | −4.47 | 2.89 | −.16 |
| Group × gender | −0.93 | 4.66 | −.02 |
| Edwards | −0.49 | 0.19 | −.24 |
| SRS | 0.03 | 0.11 | .02 |
| AHQ1 | −0.23 | 0.32 | −.06 |
| AHQ2 | −0.02 | 0.07 | −.04 |
| AHQ3 | 0.08 | 0.08 | .10 |
| AHQ4 | 0.17 | 0.14 | .12 |

Standard error of estimate = 12.89

Multiple $R$ =   .37

Multiple $R^2$ S =   .14

*Note.* RRS, Romantic Relationship Scale, a measure of jealousy; SRS, Sibling Relationship Scale; AHQ, Attachment History Questionnaire (AHQ1, separations and losses during childhood; AHQ2, harshness of parental discipline, threats of abandonment; AHQ3, quality of parent–child relations; AHQ4, quality of peer relations in childhood).

Given the strong relationship between self-reported jealousy and the social desirability response set noted above, the tendency in this study for women to report more jealousy than men may reflect women's greater willingness to disclose negative experiences and feelings (cf. Jourard, 1964).

A supplemental analysis found no relationship between adult jealousy and subjects' reports of whether or not their partners had ever been unfaithful. However, subjects who reported never having a sexual affair during their current relationship scored significantly higher on the jealousy measure than subjects who had experienced sex with others. In other words, fidelity was associated with increased jealousy over one's partner. (For further discussion of these results, see Kosins, 1983, pp. 195–197.)

Apart from gender, discussed above, none of the demographic variables (age, marital status, length of relationship, race, religion, income, and educational level) was found to correlate significantly with scores on the RRS. Birth order, age spacing, and family size were found to have no significant relationship to the intensity of adult jealousy, even though early research demonstrated associations between family constellation and *childhood* jealousy (e.g., Foster, 1927; Ross, 1931; Sewall, 1930). Thus, individuals may compensate in adulthood for early experiences that might otherwise influence the development of adult jealousy.

Although the small number of valid questionnaires required that we drop the inpatient group from the hypothesis testing, our findings in this connection are at once provocative and congruent with other outcomes of this study. Contrary to what many would expect, the small inpatient group scored no higher on the jealousy measure than did the "normal" college students. This finding constitutes provisional, circumstantial evidence that jealousy may be no more prevalent in clinical populations (inpatient as well as outpatient) than in nonclinical populations (represented by the student group). (An exception may be the presence of pathological or delusional jealousy in patients with paranoid disorders. Such patients were not included in this study.) If psychiatric inpatients are no more jealous than "normal" people, doubt is cast on the widespread assumption that jealousy usually grows out of some psychological defect. Certainly this matter is worthy of further research.

## DISCUSSION

Although the developmental hypotheses tested here were not supported by the data,[4] this study is useful precisely because it provides *an empirical basis for questioning the widespread view that jealousy is a psychological defect rooted in early experience.* The hypothesized relationship between jealousy and disrupted attachment history might well be found in a sample of pathologically jealous subjects, such as individuals with paranoid disorders or prisoners convicted of "crimes of passion." In our less pathological samples, however, jealousy did *not* correlate with disrupted relationships with parents, siblings, and peers during childhood.

The finding of the null hypothesis supports the sociological view that a great deal of jealousy is nonpathological, or even functional, behavior. The universal social function of jealousy is the protection of marriage and other valued relationships (Davis, 1936). In every culture, people marry and form other valued relationships in accordance with prevailing norms. Jealousy protects whatever kinds of relationships cultures teach people to value. Specific jealous behaviors vary enormously across cultures (Hupka, 1981) because of the great diversity of human beliefs concerning (1) what constitutes a valued relationship, (2) what constitutes a threat to such a relationship, and (3) what one ought to do to protect a threatened relationship. Across cultures, jealousy is a protective reaction to a perceived threat to a valued relationship or to its quality (Clanton, 1981, p. 260; Clanton & Smith, 1977/1986, pp. vi, 239).

The general social usefulness of jealousy is easily overlooked in contemporary American culture, because the word "jealousy" is used primarily to describe inappropriate and unconstructive expressions of the emotion. Beginning in the late 1960s, the growing emphasis on personal freedom and self-actualization in love relationships led to a devaluation of jealousy and to a greater readiness to see jealousy as a personal defect rooted in low self-esteem (Clanton, 1989; Clanton & Smith, 1977/ 1986). The sexual conservatism and the emphasis on "togetherness" in the period before 1965 produced a relatively positive view of jealousy. The liberalization of the late 1960s and 1970s produced a generally negative appraisal of jealousy. Insofar as norms encourage personal freedom in relationships, many jealous behaviors will be seen as inappropriate and undesirable. The view that jealousy is evidence of personal defects has persisted through the 1980s and into the 1990s, obscuring the fact that many jealous behaviors are appropriate and constructive ways of protecting valued relationships from real threats.

Awareness of the social usefulness of jealousy helps explain why this study found no relationship between adult jealousy and disrupted attachment history as theories based on the work of Freud or Bowlby would lead one to expect. If jealousy were a pathological condition, then most jealous adults probably would report disrupted attachment histories (conflict with parents and siblings, fear of abandonment, etc.). However, if much jealousy were actually functional and most jealous individuals were "normal," jealous adults would be no more likely than other "normal" people to report disrupted attachment histories. The failure of this study to find a relationship between adult jealousy and disrupted attachment history supports the view that jealousy is useful to individuals, couples, and groups. Because most jealousy is not pathological, jealous adults ought not to be expected to report disrupted attachment histories.

The findings of this study suggest that therapists working with clients who express concerns regarding jealousy would do well to focus on etiological factors other than attachment history and early sibling relations. Other antecedent conditions that affect the experience of jealousy and that may provide the therapist with useful clues include social, cultural, and subcultural influences; situational and environmental factors; individual personality characteristics; and the nature of current and previous romantic relationships (cf. Bringle & Williams, 1979). In general, therapists should give more attention to *context* and to socially constructed *meanings*, rather than focusing on jealous *behaviors* per se. Jealousy is more often an interactional problem of a couple rather than a personality defect of an individual.

Very often, jealousy is a sign that something is wrong with the *relationship* rather than with one of the partners (Margolin, 1981).

Because of the wide range of clients' attitudes and values regarding relationship boundaries, threats to relationships, and protective strategies, it is difficult for therapists to determine objectively whether a particular expression of jealousy is appropriate or inappropriate, constructive or destructive. Therapists' judgments in such matters often reflect their own values and lifestyle choices, as well as the widespread but erroneous belief that *all* jealousy is inappropriate and destructive.

In summary, this study challenges the widespread assumption that adult jealousy is correlated with disrupted attachment history. It thereby calls into question the common practice of viewing jealousy primarily as an emotional disorder. Given the counterintuitive findings, however, further research will be needed to substantiate the results.

## NOTES

1. This chapter is based on the Ph.D. dissertation of David J. Kosins, submitted to the California School of Professional Psychology, San Diego. Gordon Clanton, a sociologist at San Diego State University, was on the committee that supervised the dissertation.
2. The IRS uses the word "jealousy" in all but a few of its items. Factors assessed include (a) threat to exclusive companionship, (b) self-deprecation/envy, (c) dependency, (d) sexual possessiveness, (e) competition and vindictiveness, and (f) trust.
3. Self-report instruments that ask how "jealous" one is or how "jealous" one would be in a hypothetical situation are of limited usefulness. To pose the questions this way is to assume (a) that everyone knows what jealousy is (when, in fact, different people have different definitions of it); (b) that people always know when they are jealous (when, in fact, they may be jealous and not be aware of it); and (c) that people always tell the truth about their feelings (when, in fact, they often relabel or even lie about them). Although these assumptions make possible a methodological shortcut, they also place limits on the usefulness and generalizability of the findings. A measure of the self-report of "jealousy" is not necessarily a good measure of jealousy (cf. Bringle, 1982, p. 1). In our one use of the word "jealousy," our questionnaire eliciting background information asked: "In comparison to other people, how jealous of a person do you think you are?" Respondents indicated their responses along a 5-point Likert scale from "much less" to "much more." Our jealousy measure, the RRS, showed a significant positive correlation ($r = .62$, $p < .01$) with these self-ratings of jealousy.
4. For a discussion of methodological problems and limitations of the research design, see Kosins (1983, pp. 171–184). Attention is given to social desirability response set, problems associated with self-report and retrospective

reporting, instrument reactivity, missing data, biased administration, nonrandom sampling, and the limitations of correlational research.

## REFERENCES

Bowlby, J. (1969). *Attachment and loss: Vol. 1. Attachment.* New York: Basic Books.

Bowlby, J. (1973). *Attachment and loss: Vol. 2. Separation.* New York: Basic Books.

Bowlby, J. (1980). *Attachment and loss: Vol. 3. Loss.* New York: Basic Books.

Bringle, R. G. (1981). Conceptualizing jealousy as a disposition. *Alternative Lifestyles, 4,* 274–290.

Bringle, R. G. (1982). *Preliminary report on the revised Self-Report Jealousy Scale.* Unpublished manuscript, Indiana University–Purdue University at Indianapolis.

Bringle, R. G., & Williams, L. J. (1979). Parental–offspring similarity on jealousy and related personality dimensions. *Motivation and Emotion, 3,* 265–286.

Cattell, R. B. (1953). *A guide to mental testing* (3rd ed.). London: University of London Press.

Clanton, G. (1981). Frontiers of jealousy research: Introduction to the special issue on jealousy. *Alternative Lifestyles, 4,* 259–273.

Clanton, G. (1989). Jealousy in American culture, 1945–1985: Reflections from popular literature. In D. D. Franks & E. D. McCarthy (Eds.), *The sociology of emotions* (pp. 179–193). Greenwich, CT: JAI Press.

Clanton, G., & Smith, L. G. (Eds.). (1986). *Jealousy.* Lanham, MD: University Press of America. (Original work published 1977)

Davis, K. (1936). Jealousy and sexual property. *Social Forces, 14,* 395–405. (Reprinted in Clanton & Smith, 1977/1986.)

Edwards, A. L. (1957). *The social desirability variable in personality assessment research.* New York: Dryden Press.

Foster, S. (1927). A study of the personality makeup and social setting of fifty jealous children. *Mental Hygiene, 10,* 61–69.

Freud, S. (1955). Some neurotic mechanisms in jealousy, paranoia and homsexuality. In J. Strachey (Ed. and Trans.), *The standard edition of the complete psychological works of Sigmund Freud* (Vol. 18, pp. 221–232). London: Hogarth Press. (Original work published 1922)

Hupka, R. B. (1981). Cultural determinants of jealousy. *Alternative Lifestyles, 4,* 310–356.

Hupka, R. B., & Bachelor, B. (1979, April). *Validation of a scale to measure romantic jealousy.* Paper presented at the meeting of the Western Psychological Association, San Diego.

Hupka, R. B., & Rusch, P. A. (1977, April). *Development and validation of a scale to measure romantic jealousy.* Paper presented at the meeting of the Western Psychological Association, Seattle.

Jourard, S. M. (1964). *The transparent self.* Princeton, NJ: Van Nostrand.

Kessler, R. P., & Pottharst, K. (1982). *An instrument for measuring affectional bonding: The Attachment History Questionnaire.* Unpublished manuscript, California School for Professional Psychology, Los Angeles.

Kosins, D. J. (1983). *Developmental correlates of sexual jealousy.* Unpublished doctoral dissertation, California School for Professional Psychology, San Diego.

Margolin, G. (1981). A behavioral–systems approach to the treatment of jealousy. *Clinical Psychology Review, 1,* 469–487.

Reik, T. (1945). *Psychology of sex relations.* Westport, CT: Greenwood Press.

Rosmarin, D. M., Chambless, D. L., & LaPointe, K. (1979). *The survey of interpersonal reactions: An inventory for the measurement of jealousy.* Unpublished manuscript, University of Georgia.

Ross, B. M. (1931). Some traits associated with sibling jealousy in problem children. *Smith College Studies in Social Work, 1,* 364–376.

Schmideberg, M. (1953). Some aspects of jealousy and feeling hurt. *Psychoanalytic Review, 40,* 1–16.

Sewall, M. (1930). Some causes of jealousy in young children. *Smith College Studies in Social Work, 1,* 6–22.

# APPENDIX 6.1
## ROMANTIC RELATIONSHIP SCALE (RRS)

This is the female form of the jealousy measure used in this study. The male form substitutes the words "man" for "woman," "male" for "female," "he" for "she," "him" for "her," and "boyfriend" for "girlfriend."

## Part I: Instructions

Below are some situations in which you may have been involved. Please rate how you would feel if you were confronted with the situation by placing a check mark in a space on the scale. Do not answer in terms of how you think you *should* feel, but rather how you would *actually* feel. Answer as if you were in a serious relationship. If you have not been involved in a particular situation, then *imagine* how you would feel in that situation and reply to the item accordingly. Be sure to answer each item—even if you have to guess. Your first reaction to the item is what matters. There is no time limit, but work quickly. There are no right or wrong answers.

Scale of how you would *actually* feel:

    1—Very pleased
    2—Pleased
    3—Neutral
    4—Displeased
    5—Very displeased

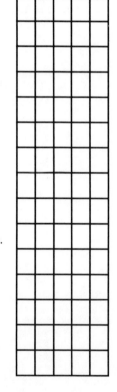

1. At a party, your partner dances with another woman.

2. Your partner comments to you on how attractive another woman is.

3. Another woman kisses your partner on the cheek at a New Year's party.

4. You see a picture in your partner's wallet of a woman he used to date.

5. At a party, your partner hugs another woman.

6. Someone flirts with your partner.

7. Your partner sees an old girlfriend and responds with a great deal of happiness.

8. Your partner pays more attention to another woman besides you at a party.

9. You hear your partner enjoying a conversation with another woman on the telephone. When he sees you he hangs up.

10. At a party, your partner disappears for a long period of time.

11. Your partner flirts with another woman.

12. Your partner goes to a bar several evenings without you.

13. Your partner tells you he is sexually attracted to a mutual friend of yours.

14. Your partner receives a letter from a former lover and refuses to tell you what it says.

15. At a party, your partner passionately kisses a woman you do not know.

## Part II: Instructions

Below you will find a list of statements. After reading each statement, place a check mark in a space on the scale to indicate how true the statement is for you. As before, answer as though you were in a serious romantic relationship. Say how you would *actually* feel, not how you think you *should* feel. Be sure to answer each one.

Scale of how you would *actually* feel:

    1—Strongly disagree
    2—Disagree
    3—Neutral
    4—Agree
    5—Strongly agree

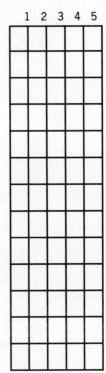

1.  If my partner admired another woman, I would feel irritated.
2.  I wouldn't worry or become suspicious if a female stranger called my partner.
3.  I frequently check up to see if my partner has been where he says he has been. '
4.  I wouldn't mind if my partner were accidentally to call me by the wrong name.
5.  I seldom worry about where my partner is or what he is doing with his time.
6.  I like to find fault with my partner's former girlfriends.
7.  If I thought that my partner was interested in another woman, I would get very upset.
8.  I feel inferior when my partner talks to an attractive stranger.
9.  I often worry that I'll lose my partner to another woman.
10. It wouldn't bother me if my partner flirted with another woman.
11. If my partner becomes close to another woman, I feel happy for him.
12. If I thought my partner was seeing another lover, I would feel angry or hurt.
13. If my partner went out with another woman, I would get intensely upset.

## Chapter Seven

# Jealousy in Close Relationships: An Exchange-Theoretical Perspective

BRAM P. BUUNK
*University of Groningen, The Netherlands*

The overwhelming and controversial nature of jealousy has long attracted the attention not only of clinicians such as Freud (1922/1940), but also of sociologists and social psychologists. For instance, more than 50 years ago, the well-known family sociologist Ernest Groves (1934) related jealousy to infantile habits and to feelings of inferiority, and noted that "The great enemy of love is jealousy. When jealousy creeps into the home, love packs up and gets ready to depart, for it cannot thrive under the perpetual tyranny of a jealous spouse" (p. 295).

Jealousy has not escaped the attention of social psychologists either. In his textbook *Elements of Social Psychology*, Gurnee (1936) described jealousy as arising whenever another person receives attention or recognition that one feels rightfully belongs to oneself, and offered some surprisingly timely observations about the attitude toward jealousy:

> It is customary nowadays to look upon it as something weak and undesirable, and no doubt some of its forms ought to be suppressed. On the other

hand, it is well to remember that it is normal in certain situations, and that it acts in the direction of ensuring fairness and impartiality in those important social relations upon which the strength of the family depends. (p. 110).

Although Gurnee may have referred here in part to envy, this quote would suggest that jealousy may already have been viewed with some ambivalence early in this century, even though it is common to observe that only with the advent of the "sexual revolution" did a negative view of jealousy become manifest (Clanton & Smith, 1977; see Clanton & Kosins, Chapter 6, this volume).

Notwithstanding such early observations of jealousy, theoretical and empirical work within social psychology on this phenomenon was virtually nonexistent until recently. The work of Kurt Lewin (1948) constituted an exception, as he was probably the first social psychologist to make a theoretical analysis of jealousy. Lewin applied his field theory to jealousy and noted that jealousy is easily aroused in marital relationships because of the overlapping "regions" in the "life spaces" of the partners, and because of the tendency for love to be all-inclusive. After Lewin's early theorizing, however, social psychologists seemed to forget about jealousy for decades. The strongly experimental focus of social psychology in the 1950s and 1960s was not very conducive to the study of such a volatile and strong emotion. It was not until the rise of more "relevant" research in the 1970s and the "emerging science of personal relationships" in the 1980s (Kelley, 1986) that jealousy became a legitimate and flourishing area of research. This is apparent from the publication of review articles (Bringle & Buunk, 1985), program overviews (Bringle & Buunk, 1986; Salovey & Rodin, 1989), and books (White & Mullen, 1989), and, of course, from the appearance of the present volume.

In this chapter, I present a selection of published and unpublished findings from my own research program on jealousy. This program has several distinctive features. First, divergent types of jealousy are studied. All these types concern aversive emotional reactions evoked by the real, imagined, or expected attraction between one's current or former partner and a third person (Buunk & Bringle, 1987). Originally, the program focused primarily upon "reactive" jealousy—that is, jealousy that occurs in response to actual extramarital relationships. Recently, however, the program has been expanded to other forms and manifestations of jealousy: (1) jealousy that arises out of rather innocent behaviors, such as simply looking at pictures of someone of the opposite sex in a magazine; and (2) jealousy that occurs without an apparent trigger.

A second feature of the program is the strong emphasis on relationship variables. Although the importance of personality factors is not

denied, jealousy is supposed to arise from certain features of relationships, to lead to certain types of conflicts in relationships, and to affect
the quality of relationships. As can be seen in Table 7.1, a third characteristic of the program is that the most important studies were conducted in
heterogeneous samples, including mostly married individuals varying in
age and educational background. Moreover, in several studies subjects
reported on their own experience with rather dramatic examples of actual
jealousy, instead of their reactions to hypothetical situations. Finally,
social exchange theory—in particular, interdependence theory as formulated by Kelley (1979)—has influenced this program to a substantial
degree and constitutes the organizing framework for this chapter.

## AN EXCHANGE-THEORETICAL PERSPECTIVE

Exchange theories offer a broad perspective on human behavior and
share a basic premise that individuals form and continue close relationships in light of the rewards these relationships offer (Burgess & Huston,
1979; La Gaipa, 1977). To obtain rewards, individuals have to provide
rewards themselves and to make sure that the costs of providing rewards
by the other are not too high. Relationships are more satisfying and
stable when the outcomes for each partner (rewards, punishments, and
costs) are more or less equal. In the first stages of a relationship, each
partner may produce rewards for the other without expecting immediate
returns, so as to show altruistic interest in the other (Mills & Clark,
1982). At the same time, however, both partners usually monitor the
degree of overall fair exchange rather closely, and attend to the possibilities for better outcomes elsewhere. In the course of the relationship, the
outcomes of both partners become intertwined, and positive experiences
of the one may vicariously become rewards for the other ("I am happy
because he or she is happy"). Furthermore, through the process of
commitment, each partner becomes more willing to suppress his or her
responsiveness to certain outcomes to be obtained outside the relationship. Moreover, feelings of obligation develop, which make individuals
tolerant of temporary inequities, and which make it more and more
difficult and often destructive to be concerned too deeply with reciprocity and equality (Milardo & Murstein, 1979; Scanzoni, 1979; Walster,
Walster, & Berscheid, 1978).

Among the various social exchange theories, the theory of Thibaut
and Kelley (1959, 1986) has occupied a central place within social
psychology, and is especially relevant for the present chapter. Thibaut
and Kelley (1959) went beyond the simple notion that people are at-

**TABLE 7.1. Overview of the Research Program**

| Number and label of sample | Description of sample |
|---|---|
| Study 1: General sample | 125 men and 125 women more or less representative of general population; average age, 35 years. |
| Study 2: Extramarital sample | 125 men and 125 women with extramarital experience; relatively high educational level; majority (78%) between 27 and 46 years of age. Included 44 divorced individuals. |
| Study 3: Open marriage sample | 50 couples with a positive attitude toward extramarital relationships (a subsample of Study 2), questioned 3 months later. |
| Study 4: Student sample | 242 male and 138 female undergraduate students; most (88%) between 18 and 24 years of age. |
| Study 5: Self-concept/jealousy sample | 109 American and 35 Dutch students who had experienced a jealousy-evoking event; 60% male, 40% female. |
| Study 6: Follow-up | Follow-up of Study 3, consisting of 70 respondents. |
| Study 7: Jealousy types sample | 855 women who had experience with jealousy; average age, 29 years. |

tracted to those who reward them; they were especially concerned with the interdependency between two individuals, which rests upon the ability each has to *control* the outcomes (rewards and punishments) of the other. Partners have "fate control" over each other to the extent that each cares about what the other does for him or her (e.g., one partner needs support from the other). They have "behavioral control" to the extent that their rewards depend upon a certain *combination* of the actions of both (e.g., both partners prefer the situation that they either clean the house together, or do not clean the house at all, above the situation that one of them does the cleaning). Kelley (1979, 1988) developed this theory further, applied it specifically to personal relationships, and elaborated upon the original notions of Thibaut and Kelley (1959) by including Heider's (1958) ideas on the attribution of dispositions. Although Thibaut and Kelley (1986) are not very comfortable with the label "exchange theory" for their theory, their interdependence theory can be viewed as part of the exchange tradition.

## General Assumptions from Social Exchange Theory

This chapter organizes various findings from the present research program under the following general assumptions derived from social exchange theory.

1. *Exchange and coordination.* Partners in an intimate relationship need each other in order to obtain valued outcomes, including instrumental support, affection, sexual fulfillment and emotional support. To realize such outcomes, the partners face two tasks, according to Kelley (1979): (a) They have to work out a mutually rewarding *exchange* of rewards, based upon the earlier-mentioned fate control they have over each other; and (b) they have to *coordinate* certain activities and behaviors, since many outcomes can only be achieved when the partners take each other's behaviors and actions into account. For instance, for one partner the preferred situation may be that *both* refrain from any type of personal friendships with others, whereas the other wants freedom to maintain some nonsexual friendships and would feel better if the partner would do the same. This is an example of behavioral control, since one partner's rewards depend upon a certain combination of the actions of both partners.

2. *Norms and rules.* To ensure a satisfying exchange of benefits, as well as coordination of behaviors in a relationship, norms and rules develop in the relationship that both partners accept and feel obligated to adhere to. Norms and rules can be developed by the couple ("Let's both not flirt with others"), or they can be self-evidently adapted from the larger social environment ("Of course we think that extramarital relationships are wrong no matter what"). Norms guarantee predictability, eliminate unsatisfactory behaviors from the relationship, enhance the cohesion of the relationship, reduce uncertainty, and often increase the outcomes attained by both partners. Moreover, they prevent the unrestrained use of power strategies (Thibaut & Kelley, 1959, pp. 130–147).

3. *Attributional analyses.* In the development of a relationship, an individual will scan the behavior of the partner to assess the extent to which he or she is sensitive to the individual's own outcomes. Can the partner be counted upon? Is the partner genuinely considerate and thoughtful? In making such attributional analyses, there is a strong inclination to attribute events in the relationship to stable dispositions. If the partner behaves in a way that clearly reflects his or her own interest

(such as flirting with someone else), and he or she knows that this is not appreciated, then this behavior is interpreted as reflecting a negative attitude. The foregoing implies that the degree of satisfaction or dissatisfaction with the relationship reflects two processes: (a) the *direct rewards* or *punishments* generated by the specific actions of the other ("It is painful when he or she pays so much attention to others and spends so little time with me"), and (b) the affective reactions that result from the *attributions* made for the partner's behaviors, and thus from the perceived dispositional causes of his or her actions ("He or she does not really care for me") (Thibaut & Kelley, 1986).

4. *Self's outcomes versus partner's outcomes.* When individuals are involved in interaction and conflict, the behaviors of each individual can be described along two dimensions: (a) the degree to which each take his or her own outcomes into account, and (b) the extent to which each pays attention to the outcomes of the other. For instance, the main concern of an individual can be that his or her outcomes are put ahead of the partner's, that both outcomes are as high as possible, or that both outcomes are as equal as possible. Loosely based on these two dimensions (care for one's own outcomes and care for partner's outcomes), a typology of conflict styles (such as aggression/pushing, problem solving, and soothing) has been developed and is described later in the chapter. An important assumption of interdependency theory is that during the course of a relationship, one progresses from being only responsive to one's own outcomes to also being responsive to the outcomes of the other. However, in the case of the partner's being seriously interested in a third person, such transformation is usually reversed. Furthermore, according to Kelley (1979), attributional conflict is likely to arise, especially with respect to negative or unpleasant behavior. This would apply in particular to the situation in which one partner commits adultery. The offended partner will tend to generalize from the event to a disposition of the actor, and will attribute the behavior to bad intentions and a negative attitude ("You did it to hurt me," "You have a weak personality"), while the adulterous actor may make either (a) excuses ("I couldn't help becoming involved with him or her") or (b) justifications ("I have the right to flirt with others: there is nothing wrong with it").

5. *Aspects of interdependence.* There are three important dimensions of interdependence (Kelley, 1979) that are all relevant for understanding jealousy.

a. *Correspondence of outcomes.* "Correspondence of outcomes" is the degree to which the relationship is characterized by cooperativeness and commonality of interest, as apparent from the frequency with which the partners engage in the exchange of rewards (including love and support), the extent to which they make positive attributions for each other's behavior, and the degree to which the coordination of behavior results in mutually rewarding outcomes (including satisfying joint leisure activities and smooth task and role division). To measure this construct, a short though reliable scale for relational satisfaction was developed in the present research program to assess the frequency with which the *interaction* with the partner is rewarding (Buunk, 1990a). This operationalization is in line with Kelley's (1979, p. 42) suggestion that the number of pleasurable activities shared by a married couple is a reasonable index of frequency of experienced correspondence of outcomes.

Satisfaction conceptualized in this manner must be distinguished from the cognitive process through which individuals evaluate their relationship as a whole. They make such evaluation by comparing their outcomes to their "comparison level" (CL), the level of outcomes they believe they deserve from the relationship. The outcomes obtained by one's peers, as well as the partner's outcomes (e.g., his or her extradyadic activities), may figure prominently in the individual's CL. CL also depends upon the outcomes that are salient to a person—the ones that are vivid and perhaps implicitly rehearsed as someone makes an evaluation of his or her circumstances. "The CL is subject to situation-to-situation and moment-to-moment variations" (Thibaut & Kelley, 1959, p. 82). It is not unlikely that even superficial sexual or romantic involvement (such as flirting) by a married individual with a third person may already raise his or her CL, since such behaviors entail a type of reward that usually has disappeared from long-term relationships.

b. *Degree of dependency.* "Degree of dependency" is the degree to which the partners have the ability to control and influence each other's outcomes. Stated differently, this variable refers to the extent to which an individual needs his or her partner to obtain rewards and to engage in certain activities. Dependency is affected by the cognitive process in which the current outcomes are compared to the "comparison level for alternatives" (CLalt), the lowest level of outcomes someone will accept in light of available alternative opportunities. These opportunities include the best alternative relationship to the present relationship, the appeal of living alone, and factors that are simultaneously available in addition to the present relationship (e.g., an interesting job, good friends, or an extramarital relationship). Degree of dependency is assumed here to be directly related to the degree of jealousy. In the present research program, this variable has been measured by a reliable scale for emotional dependency (Buunk, 1981a, 1982a), which includes items referring to the degree to which the behavior of the partner affects one's feelings, as well as to the CLalt.

c. *Relative dependency.* "Relative dependency" is the degree to which one is more or less dependent upon the relationship than the partner is. An individual is less dependent than the other when he or she has more rewarding activities outside the present relationship, has more actual relationships with others, or perceives the loss of the relationship as less serious because attractive alternatives to the current relationship can be expected. The less dependent partner needs the rewards of the other to a lesser extent, can more frequently control the outcomes of the other, and is the one who has more power. The more dependent person may have to tolerate poorer outcomes at higher costs, and will be the one who is more jealous (Kelley, 1988; White, 1981a).

## Some Implications for the Nature of Reactive Jealousy

Before I discuss in greater detail findings from my research program related to these five issues, I should note some general implications of this perspective for the feelings and perceptions involved in reactive jealousy. When the partner becomes involved with someone else, it is likely that the amount of rewards provided by the partner decreases. However, as noted above, satisfaction or dissatisfaction reflects not only the outcomes generated by the specific behaviors of the other, but also the meaning attached to these behaviors (Thibaut & Kelley, 1986). In intimate relationships, the value of various rewards and activities is raised by the fact that one partner provides these rewards only to the other, and that the partners engage in these activities only with each other. The implication of this is that jealousy may still be present even when the partner spends as much time in the relationship as before he or she met the rival, and is as warm and caring as before. If an extradyadic relationship is known to exist, not only will such positive behavior of the partner probably be interpreted in a negative way ("My partner does it only to relieve his or her guilt"), but by virtue of the fact that the partner shows romantic interest in someone else, certain rewards *are* lost. When the partner provides similar rewards to a third person, these rewards may lose much of their meaning. In addition, the partner's behavior may make it more difficult to engage in jointly rewarding activities, as the partner now spends time with another person. Finally, the attraction to the rival may be interpreted in the sense that in some ways the current relationship lies below the partner's CL, or even below his or her CLalt. This may induce the perception that the partner will not be very motivated to put energy into the primary relationship, and may even end this relationship.

Data obtained in Study 2 (the extramarital sample) and Study 3 (the open marriage sample) illustrate these analyses: In addition to uncertainty about the future, major perceptions reported by the respondents as a response to their partners' extramarital behavior included (1) affective deprivation—receiving less love and attention than before (direct loss of rewards); (2) the feeling of being excluded from the activities of the partner (fewer interdependent rewarding activities); (3) the perception that the partner enjoyed certain things more with the other (current relationship below partner's CLalt); and (4) the idea of no longer being the only one for the partner (loss of exclusive rewards) (Buunk, 1981a; Bringle & Buunk, 1986; Buunk & Bringle, 1987).

## EXCHANGE, RECIPROCITY, AND REACTIVE JEALOUSY

From a social exchange perspective, the most satisfying situation probably exists when partners can coordinate their degree of extradyadic involvement. This would be the case when a certain degree of involvement (whether occasionally dancing with someone at a party or having friends of the opposite sex) is preferred by both partners, and when each partner feels comfortable with accepting that level of extradyadic involvement in the other. It seems likely that such a situation will in general be perceived as most fair. Not only will one's own CL be affected by the outcomes obtained by the partner; in addition, what one feels the partner "deserves" will be determined by what one obtains oneself. Thus, the more individuals themselves feel a need to be involved in certain extradyadic behaviors with others, or have actually done so, the less jealously they will react. It can therefore be hypothesized that jealousy with respect to a given extradyadic behavior and one's own tendency to engage in the same behavior will be negatively related. When someone, for instance, regularly flirts with others, he or she will feel that it is quite unjustified to react jealously when the partner does the same. Conversely, when someone refrains from certain extradyadic behaviors, he or she will be upset if the partner engages in that behavior. Not only considerations of fairness may play a role in this regard. By adhering to a norm of reciprocity, a couple can also prevent unequal dependence, which will arise when one partner is more involved in extradyadic relationships than the other.

On the basis of the foregoing, it can be expected that when the partner becomes involved with another, an individual will be more jealous to the extent that the individual has not been involved in extramarital relationships of his or her own. This hypothesis was tested in Study 2 (Buunk, 1980, 1983). In this study, each subject was asked to focus upon the spouse's most significant (or only) extramarital past or current affair. The 20-item Actual Sexual Jealousy Scale (Buunk, 1990c) was administered, measuring the degree of jealousy in response to this affair. The reliability of this short version was .93. In addition to this scale, the respondents were asked to indicate whether they themselves were at that moment involved in an affair, and how many affairs they had been involved in before that relationship of their partners. As expected, men ($r = -.33$, $p < .01$) as well as women ($r = -.36$, $p < .01$) reacted with more jealousy if they themselves had been involved in fewer affairs. Moreover, jealousy was more intense when a subject did not have an extramarital relationship of his or her own at the same moment (correlations between jealousy and having a relationship: among men, $r = -.26$, $p < .01$; among women, $r = -.40$; $p < .01$).

The same hypothesis was also tested in a different way in this study, as well as in Study 1 (the general population sample) and Study 4 (the student sample). In all of these studies, the Anticipated Sexual Jealousy Scale (Buunk, 1988a, 1990b) was used to measure the extent to which the idea of sexual attraction between the partner and a rival evoked a negative emotional response. Five types of sexual attraction to someone of the opposite sex are covered by the scale: flirting, light petting, falling in love, sexual intercourse, and a long-term sexual relationship. This scale correlated very highly, and negatively, with the Extramarital Behavioral Intentions Scale, a scale measuring one's own desire to be involved in the same extradyadic behaviors described in the Anticipated Sexual Jealousy Scale (Buunk, 1988b). The correlations ranged from $-.55$ to $-.79$, and various alternative explanations for these data could be ruled out, such as becoming used to the partner's extradyadic behaviors and self-presentational bias (Buunk, 1982a).

It must be noted that these findings were established in samples varying considerably in their normative approval of extramarital behaviors. This would suggest that considerations of reciprocity with respect to extradyadic behaviors lead individuals with divergent values to adjust their own extradyadic intentions to their ability to tolerate similar behaviors from their partners. In addition, it is possible that during the process of mate selection, those relationships in which the needs for extradyadic involvement are too far apart are terminated relatively more often.

## NORMS, RULES, AND REACTIVE JEALOUSY

Given the fact that many jealousy studies have examined reactive jealousy, it is remarkable how little attention has been paid to the norms and rules surrounding extradyadic relationships. The focus in most studies has been upon the emotional responses characteristic of jealousy, and upon the personality and relationship characteristics associated with jealousy. The extent to which jealousy arises out of the perceptions that norms or rules are being violated, and the functions of norms and rules in preventing jealousy, have seldom been taken into account. As mentioned earlier, norms and rules increase predictability within a relationship, prevent negative outcomes, minimize uncertainty, prevent abuse of power by one's partner, and foster the cohesiveness of a relationship (Thibaut & Kelley, 1959, p. 147). Peplau (1983) has noted that norms can arise in two major ways. They can develop during a relationship as a result of the interaction between the partners, but they can also be imported from the larger social environment.

### Norms Imported from the Larger Social Environment

Societal norms with respect to extramarital relationships that individuals bring into their marriages often reflect strongly held moral values. A large majority of the American population unequivocally disapproves of extramarital sex (Glenn & Weaver, 1979). Nevertheless, there still exists considerable variety in the degree of disapproval. Even the casual observer will notice that within certain ethnic and religious groups, attitudes toward extramarital relationships are more strict than in other groups (Buunk & Van Driel, 1989). Whereas only very small minorities have a positive attitude toward extramarital sexual relationships, there are more individuals who find such behavior understandable under certain circumstances, and even more individuals who will have a tolerant attitude toward less serious transgressions such as flirting.

From a social exchange perspective, an individual's problem is often to influence the partner without making his or her own dependency upon the relationship too apparent. This can be done by an appeal to a supraindividual value. "The enforcement of norms often involves appeals to impersonal values or suprapersonal agents" (Thibaut & Kelley, 1959, p. 135). Thus, a spouse in a social context where norms against adultery prevail has a strong power strategy at his or her disposal to obtain compliance from the partner who is flirting or who seems inclined to "play around." The spouse can induce feelings of guilt by bringing up various moral arguments—emphasizing the breaking of trust, the betrayal, and the lack of loyalty that extramarital inclinations imply. This may reduce the extent to which giving up the extradyadic behavior is viewed as a matter of compliance to the other, and may thereby soften resistance. If the partner actually commits adultery, the individual with norms condemning such behavior will feel very justified in reacting jealousy and blaming the partner for his or her moral transgression, especially when the spouse has always agreed on these norms and when the reference group is preceived as disapproving of extramarital relationships.

In Study 1 (the general population sample), the influence of moral norms upon reactive jealousy was examined. A scale for the normative disapproval of extramarital sex was developed (alpha = .93) that contained eight items such as "Extramarital sex is always wrong," "Extramarital relationships cannot be excused," and "Extramarital relationships can be good for a marriage" (reverse scoring on this last item). As expected, this scale correlated very highly with the Anticipated Sexual Jealousy Scale ($r = .77$, $p < .001$; Buunk, 1988a). Moreover, unpublished data from the same study showed that this jealousy scale was highly correlated with an item measuring the perceived disapproval of extramarital sex among friends ($r = .70$, $p < .001$). Thus, an important factor accounting for reactive jealousy seems to be the degree to which this reaction is considered to be normatively *justified*. It is therefore not surprising that additional data from this study showed that the main emotional reaction in such a situation is a feeling of being treated unjustly. Each subject was asked to imagine a situation in which the spouse would disclose that he or she had had an affair. A list of 18 emotional reactions to this situation was presented to the subjects, with the request to indicate the applicability of each of the items. A factor analysis over these items showed a very strong first factor, explaining no less than 56% of the variance. It included emotions such as angry and mad, as well as anger-evoking cognitions and perceptions such as feeling betrayed, humiliated, cheated, and unjustly treated (Buunk, 1986b). Unpublished data from Study 1 showed that a scale based upon this factor (alpha = .94) correlated highly with the scale for normative disapproval ($r = .79$, $p < .001$). These findings illustrate quite clearly that reactive jealousy is related to a sense that central norms and values are being violated.

## Norms Developed in the Relationship

It is also possible that the couple will develop specific norms and rules in the relationship with respect to extradyadic involvements, which will be designated as "ground rules." Such rules specify under what concrete circumstances extramarital relationships are permissible. Transgression of such rules will evoke a response such as "I am upset that you did this, because we agreed not to act like this." Ground rules are behavioral rules that specify under what circumstances extradyadic relationships are allowed. Such ground rules are usually arrived at in a relationship after protracted negotiation and discussion, and may be changed whenever both partners agree to do so. Sometimes norms are implicitly taken on; sometimes they are only adopted only after extensive discussion and negotiation. Indeed, ground rules with respect to extradyadic relationships are assumed by the participants to protect the marriage from the possible negative consequences of extramarital relationships, including jealousy and threats to the relationship. Various ground rules were identified in Study 3 (the open marriage sample). These included marriage primacy (e.g., "You always put your own marriage first," "You are completely honest with your spouse"), restricted intensity (e.g., "There are only brief contacts"), visibility (e.g., "Your spouse knows the outside partner") and invisibility (e.g., "Your spouse is not too aware of it"), and mate exchange (Buunk, 1980).

Despite the claims of proponents of "open" marriages (Knapp & Whitehurst, 1977), it appeared that these ground rules were in themselves no guarantee against jealousy. The majority of the open marriage sample (about 80%) had been jealous at one time or another, and none of these ground rule patterns was correlated negatively with the frequency of jealousy (Buunk, 1981a). Nevertheless, a follow-up study of the same sample 5 years later (Study 6) showed three important things. First, these ground rules appeared to be quite stable over time: The correlations between Time 1 and Time 2 ranged from .26 to .50 (Buunk, 1987b), which is rather high, given the 5-year gap. Second, there was no temporal stability of jealousy: The correlation between Time 1 and Time 2 for scores on the Anticipated Sexual Jealousy Scale was .04. This was all the more striking, since not only were the various ground rules quite stable, but so were relational satisfaction, sexual satisfaction, and emotional dependency. Apparently, jealousy was a quite unstable characteristic in this sample. Third, a decrease in jealousy over time was significantly more likely when the couple was adhering at Time 1 to the ground rules of marriage primacy, visibility, and mate exchange. Thus, although the establishment of ground rules is not an antidote against jealousy, in the long run such rules seem to help in reducing the occurrence of jealousy among partners who are open to rather far-reaching levels of extradyadic involvement.

## ATTRIBUTIONAL ANALYSES AND JEALOUSY

According to interdependence theory, an individual scans the behavior of the partner for its responsiveness to the partner's versus his or her own interests (Kelley, 1979). Behavior of the partner that has or may have negative consequences for the individual or the relationship is especially likely to invoke attributional activity. Thus, when the partner becomes involved in an extramarital relationship, the individual will be particularly concerned with the question of *why* the partner engaged in this relationship, in order to assess the implications of that behavior for the relationship. On the basis of interdependency theory, it can be predicted that the more dependent the individual is on the relationship, the more likely he or she is to wonder why the partner does what he or she does (Kelley, 1988). Furthermore, since attributional activity will be stronger as the partner's behavior deviates more sharply from expectations (cf. Jones & Davis, 1965), an individual who disapproves strongly of extramarital relationships will be more likely to engage in a search for attributions for the partner's behavior.

Study 1 (the general population sample) offers support for these predictions. As described earlier, in this study subjects were asked to indicate how they would react if their spouses would have an extramarital affair. Among 18 reactions (such as becoming angry, taking revenge, and blaming oneself), the wish to identify the causes for the partner's behavior appeared to be the most common (Buunk, 1986a). Additional data showed that this attributional need was positively correlated with the earlier-mentioned scales for normative disapproval ($r = .50$, $p < .001$) and for emotional dependency ($r = .39$, $p < .01$) (Buunk, 1989). Thus as expected, individuals who feel dependent upon their partners and those who disapprove of extramarital relationships are more inclined to egage in looking for reasons for the partners' behavior.

When an individual is making attributions for the partner's behavior, the extent to which this behavior manifests a positive or negative attitude toward the individual will be a central dimension along which the partner's behavior is evaluated (Kelley, 1979). It is clear that people will seldom see extradyadic relationships of their partners as reflecting a positive attitude. To the contrary, it is painful for one to realize that a partner is seeking other rewarding relationships at the expense of, or with disregard for, the interdependencies within the current relationship. Nevertheless, people differ in the extent to which they attribute their partners' behavior to dissatisfaction with their primary relationships, and it can be expected that the more an extramarital relationship is attributed to such dissatisfaction, the more intense the jealousy will be. Furthermore, it seems likely that jealousy will become stronger when an individual interprets the behavior of the partner as reflecting aggressive intentions (cf. Jones & Davis, 1965). On the other hand, when the partner's behavior is attributed to environmental pressures or special circumstances, jealousy can be expected to be less extreme.

Some support for these predictions was found in Study 2 (the extramarital sample). In this study, six types of attributions for a partner's most important (or only) extradyadic involvement were identified. For conceptual clarity, a brief version of the earlier-mentioned Actual Sexual Jealousy Scale (Buunk, 1990c), which included only emotional reactions and excluded cognitions, was used. As shown in Table 7.2, jealousy was, as expected, correlated in both genders with the attribution of aggression ("He or she wanted to take revenge") and with the attribution of marital deprivation ("He or she missed something in our relationship"). This is in line with the findings of White (1984a). Furthermore, among males, jealousy was stronger when it was attributed to a need of variety ("He or she had a need for sexual variety"); particularly among females, jealousy was more extreme when it was seen to be caused by pressure by the third person ("The third person pressed for it"). A stepwise multiple-regression analysis showed that this last attribution was the most important among women, followed by marital deprivation; among men, the attributions of aggression and need of variety were the most important. The situational attributions of attraction to the rival and of circumstances were not correlated with jealousy, although among women lack of attraction to the rival was included in the regression analysis (Buunk, 1984).

The fact that attribution to a need for (sexual) variety seems to make men more jealous than women is in line with other findings from the same study (reported in Buunk, 1986a), and with White's (1984a) research. A separate measure consisting of two items assessed the extent to which the extramarital relationship had led to a deterioration of the sexual relationship. Among men, this sexual deterioration score correlated substantially with jealousy ($r = .40$, $p < .01$), whereas among women the correlation was not significant ($r = .13$). Other research also suggests that male jealousy, more so than female jealousy, is related to the perception that the partner is *sexually* interested in someone else, even when this interest is restricted to the fantasy level. In a cross-cultural study encompassing seven nations, men indicated significantly more often than women that they would become upset if their partners would have sexual fantasies about someone else (Buunk & Hupka, 1987). Francis (1977) employed a free association task in which people came up with as many situations as possible that could evoke jealousy. Among men, it appeared that jealousy was related to the sexual aspects of their partners' being involved with others and of comparing themselves to the rivals. Among women, the fact that their partners spent time with the rivals and talked with the rivals was more important. Even more than 50 years ago, Gottschalk (1936) found that, among men, jealousy manifested itself mainly as a feeling of shock at being sexually rejected,

**TABLE 7.2. Correlations between Jealousy and Causes Attributed to the Partner's Extradyadic Behavior**

| Partner's extradyadic behavior attributed to . . . | Males | Females |
|---|---|---|
| Aggression | .38** | .30** |
| Marital deprivation | .45** | .29** |
| Variety | .25** | .12 |
| Attraction | −.03 | −.13 |
| Circumstances | −.10 | −.03 |
| Pressure by third person | .21* | .34** |

*Note.* From "Jealousy as Related to Attributions for the Partner's Behavior" by B. Buunk, 1984, *Social Psychology Quarterly*, *47*, 107–112. Copyright 1984 by the American Sociological Association. Reprinted by permission.
*$p < .05$.
**$p < .01$.

resulting in a simultaneous and sudden release of feelings of rivalry (for an English summary of this study, see Bohm, 1960). Daly, Wilson, and Weghorst (1982) have documented that male sexual jealousy is prevalent in all cultures, and have suggested that such jealousy has the function of defending paternity confidence. Indeed, such findings seem to confirm sociobiological claims that evolution has fostered male jealousy to be specifically focused upon the sexual aspects of the partner's extramarital activities (Symons, 1979).

In making attributions for the partner's behavior, among the pieces of information that will be given attention are the characteristics of the "rival." It can be assumed that in general, individuals will feel more upset when their partners feel attracted to unattractive persons than to attractive persons (cf. Bryson, 1977), as this will lead to the attribution of negative characteristics to the partners. First, a person may conclude that the partner apparently does not have much taste and is not very selective. Second, based upon Kelley's (1967) discounting principle, the individual can make the inference that the partner apparently has a very strong desire to engage in extradyadic relationships or to leave the relationship, since the threshold needed to evoke the behavior seems so low.

To test these assumptions, in Study 1 (Buunk, 1978), each subject was given six different descriptions of individuals. For each of these descriptions, the subject was asked how upset he or she would be if his or her partner became sexually involved with that person. The six descriptions consisted, in fact, of three pairs, each pair containing the extremes on a particular dimension: "disliked" versus "liked," "physically attractive" versus "physically unattractive," and "having a lot to offer to others" versus "having little to offer to others." In all three of these cases, the person with the more negative characteristics evoked *more* negative feelings. All differences were significant for men as well as women. These findings suggest that the partner's attraction to an unattractive other is indeed interpreted more negatively than his or her interest in an attractive person. This is the more noteworthy because a "better" rival might in fact be perceived as more threatening to the relationship, but is not.

## JEALOUS CONFLICTS: SELF'S OUTCOMES VERSUS PARTNER'S OUTCOMES

Close relationships involve dynamic processes that change over time. Whereas features of the relationship such as degree of dependency and lack of trust may give rise to jealousy, a jealousy event may *affect* the relationship as well. For instance, from an exchange-theoretical perspective, McDonald and Osmond (1980) have suggested that the threat of competition for the resources provided by the partner (such as love, sexual gratification, and time) shifts the exchange relationship toward a type of exchange strategy based more on self-interest, and that this will affect the way the individual handles the conflict generated by the partner's extramarital affair.

From the perspective of Kelley's (1979) interdependency theory, conflict styles depend primarily on the degree to which someone is willing to take the outcomes of the partner into account in addition to his or her own outcomes. Conflict styles can thus be viewed to differ along two dimensions: the extent to which a given behavior serves the interests of the actor, and the degree to which the actor pays attention to the interests of the relationship and is responsive to the partner's interests. On the basis of these two loose dimensions, five conflict styles can be distinguished (Buunk, Schaap, & Prevoo, in press; Schaap, Buunk, & Kerkstra, 1988): (1) "pushing/aggression," a style that stems from seeing one's own interests as opposite of to those of the spouse, and that is characterized by minimal respect for the spouse's feelings; (2) "avoidance," which consists of physical or emotional retreat from the situation and unwillingness to discuss the situation; (3) "compromise," which is an attempt to find a fair solution, involving consensus of both partners; (4) "soothing," which involves trying to prevent an open conflict and the expression of negative feelings, and covering up the differences between both parties; and (5) "problem solving," which includes the open, direct, and cooperative expression of feelings, the exploration of causes of the conflict, the clarification of misunderstandings, and the search for a solution that is satisfying to both partners. This typology is quite compatible with other typologies for marital conflict strategies, including the work of Fitzpatrick (1984), who makes a distinction among "avoidance" (here, soothing and avoidance), "competition" (here, pushing/aggression), and "cooperation" (here, problem solving and compromise).

In a normal, satisfying relationship there will usually be a preference for problem solving and compromise, and for taking into account the interests of the other person. However, when the other shows a clear interest in someone else, the tendency to be cooperative will diminish. Given the predominance of anger in jealousy (Buunk, 1986b), the more jealousy one experiences, the more likely aggressive behavior will be. In Study 2 (the extramarital sample), scales were developed for the various conflict styles to describe the conflict experienced as a consequence of the partner's most significant extradyadic relationship; these were correlated with the Actual Sexual Jealousy Scale, which has been mentioned several times (Buunk, 1990c). As shown in Table 7.3, the more jealously people reacted to their spouses' extramarital behavior, the more they tended to exhibit *all* types of conflict resolution behavior except for problem solving, which became less prevalent as individuals became more jealous. Although jealousy was also accompanied by avoidance, soothing, and compromise seeking, pushing/aggression was particularly characteristic of jealousy. Obviously, when a spouse's affair evokes jealousy in an individual, the willingness for coordination and taking care of the relationship substantially decreases, and the individual's attitude seems to become less cooperative and more competitive and aggressive. In addition,

**TABLE 7.3. Correlations between Conflict Styles and Jealousy**

| | |
|---|---|
| Pushing/aggression | .78 |
| Avoidance | .27 |
| Compromise | .42 |
| Soothing | .40 |
| Problem solving | −.21 |

*Note.* For all correlations, $p < .01$. From "Marital Conflict Resolution" by C. Schaap, B. Buunk, and A. Kerkstra, 1988, in P. Noller & M. A. Fitzpatrick (Eds.), *Perspectives on marital interaction* (Monographs in Social Psychology of Language, Vol. 1, pp. 203–244). Philadelphia: Multilingual Matters. Copyright 1988 by Multilingual Matters. Reprinted by permission.

Study 2 showed that the more conflicts an extradyadic affair had generated, the more likely it was that an actual divorce or breakup had occurred. Other variables that were considered important from an exchange-theoretical perspective—in particular, the lack of interdependence and the positive evaluation of alternatives—did not play a role (Buunk, 1987a). Apparently, the most important factor governing a breakup is the lowered level of correspondence of outcomes in the current relationship, rather than the decreased degree of dependence upon this relationship.

## FEATURES OF INTERDEPENDENCE
## AND REACTIVE JEALOUSY

From the perspective of interdependency theory, it is apparent that jealousy is related to characteristics of the relationship. With respect to correspondence of outcomes, jealousy may decrease the degree to which the relationship is rewarding and may at the same time be an indication of problems with the coordination of behavior. Indeed, in Study 2 and Study 3, moderate negative correlations between actual sexual jealousy and relational satisfaction were documented, though they were somewhat higher among men than among women (Buunk, 1981a, 1986a). In the 5-year follow-up of Study 3 (Study 6), relational satisfaction at Time 1 was a significant predictor of a decrease in jealousy over time (Buunk, 1987b). Satisfaction has also produced moderately negative correlations with jealousy in other studies (Bringle & Evenbeck, 1979; Bringle, Evenbeck, & Schmedel, 1977), although sometimes no correlation between the two variables has been found (Hansen, 1983).

On the basis of Kelley's (1979) theory, the amount and intensity of jealousy should covary particularly with the degree of dependency on the relationship. Someone who is highly dependent has more to lose, and the fact that the partner becomes involved in an extradyadic relationship makes the individual even more relatively dependent upon the relationship. A number of studies have indeed shown relationships between dependency and jealousy. For instance, Mathes and Severa (1981) found that individuals who maintained separate identities (including having their own activities that did not include their partners), and those who did not do everything together, were less jealous than people who were highly meshed with their partners. In the present program, the importance of dependency for understanding jealousy has been examined in various ways. First, it was assumed that Rubin's (1970) Love Scale can be viewed as a measure of dependency, and that this is not the case for Rubin's Liking Scale, which merely reflects a positive attitude toward the partner (Buunk, 1981b). As expected, in Study 4 (the student sample), the Anticipated Sexual Jealousy Scale correlated more highly with Rubin's Love Scale ($r = .39$ for men, .46 for women; in both cases, $p < .001$) than with Rubin's Liking Scale ($r = .13$ and .22, respectively; n.s.). The differences between these two sets of correlations were significant. This finding has been corroborated by other research (Mathes & Severa, 1981; White, 1984b).

Furthermore, in Study 2 (the extramarital sample), it was found that individuals who said they had increased their independence over the past years had become significantly less jealous (Buunk, 1981a). Also, as described earlier, individuals who were more dependent said that they would react with more anger, and would engage more in finding reasons for their partners' behavior, if their spouses would become involved with others. However, the results have not always been consistent. For example, the Anticipated Sexual Jealousy Scale has not in all cases been found to correlate with the emotional dependency scale, whereas this last scale is the most unambiguous operationalization of Kelley's (1979) degree of dependency (Buunk, 1982a).

When the actual or potential outcomes of the partner are considered to be higher than one's own outcomes, one is (relative to the partner) more dependent upon the relationship; within social exchange theory, such relative dependency has been particularly closely connected with jealousy (Kelley, 1988). Recently, Bush, Bush, and Jennings (1988) have shown how jealousy-provoking situations increased subjects' perceptions of themselves as more involved in their relationships. In particular, White (1981a) has maintained that jealousy is more prevalent in individuals who feel relatively more dependent—that is, more involved in their relationships than their partners are. This is determined in each case by the relative availability of opposite-sex friends, the perception of the partner's relative involvement, and the relative physical attractiveness. However, the correlations between relative dependency and jealousy found by White have been rather low, and White's research typically deals with individuals who are still in a testing stage of their relationships (a minority are living together, engaged, or married), who are still assessing what they may mean to their partners, and who still may feel that their partners are monitoring their attractiveness. These findings cannot be generalized to married individuals.

As is apparent from the foregoing, the findings on the association between jealousy and the various relationship features have not been very consistent, or have not been replicated among married couples. In Study 6 it was assumed that the contradictory findings may be due to the fact that there are various types of jealousy, which bear different relationships to the various features of interdependence (Buunk, 1989). As noted before, reactive jealousy is a response to behavior that is generally disapproved, and is seen as a serious breach of trust and loyalty. A negative emotional response from the partner of an adulterer is so well understood that many individuals would not call it "jealousy," but refer to it as "anger" (Hupka, 1984). It seems that the word "jealous" is often used to refer to more "abnormal" behaviors. The question of the distinction between "normal" and "neurotic" or "abnormal" forms of jealousy has occupied many theorists and therapists, from Sigmund Freud (1922/ 1940) to Albert Ellis (1977). According to the latter author, there is a clear difference between "rational" jealousy (based upon a real threat— e.g., a high probability that one is going to lose one's partner) and "irrational" jealousy (based upon dogmatic, absolutistic, unfounded beliefs). In an article by Hoaken (1976), a useful distinction was made between "provoked" and "unprovoked" (morbid or pathological) jealousy, and within the provoked category between "normal" and "excessive" (or neurotic) jealousy.

Using this last taxonomy as a partial guide, I have distinguished two other types of jealousy in addition to reactive jealousy. Taken together, these three types probably account for the majority of experiences that people refer to as "jealousy." The taxonomy offered here seems quite compatible with the distinction among "emotional," "behavioral," and "cognitive" jealousy developed by Pfeiffer and Wong (1989), and with the more "normal" and more "neurotic" jealousy factors found by Mathes, Roter, and Joerger (1982).

"Preventive" jealousy probably constitutes what individuals usually refer to when they say "I am a very jealous person" or "My partner is so jealous." This type of jealousy stems from a fear that the partner may become sexually involved with someone else; therefore, even signs of the partner's minor interest in someone else are interpreted as threatening. This can go so far as to include the fact that the partner watches attractive women or men on TV. Typical for preventive jealousy is that the person goes to considerable efforts to prevent contact of the partner with a third person. Individuals may be very active in controlling the behavior of their partners to prevent any situation that could evoke their jealousy. Reports from abused women testify to the extreme behavior to which some husbands resort in an effort to limit the autonomy of their wives, as the result of their insecurity about the mere possibility of the wives' being unfaithful (Buunk, 1986a). In several ways, this type of jealousy differs from reactive jealousy. First, it is in general socially disapproved. Second, it is not an emotional reaction evoked by an actual event, but a behavior aimed at preventing such an event. Third, it involves by definition active attempts to control and influence the behavior of the partner.

"Self-generated" jealousy implies an active *cognitive* process of the individual. In this type of jealousy, the individual generates images of the partner's becoming involved with someone else, which leads to more or less obsessive anxiety and worrying. Sometimes this may include the more or less paranoid conviction that the partner *is* actually involved with someone else. The similarity to reactive jealousy is that negative affect is evoked by some event; however, in the case of this type of jealousy, these events are self-generated by the individual. Self-generated and preventive jealousy are not always easy to distinguish. Nevertheless, in a factor analysis all three types of jealousy were quite clearly recognizable. One difference with preventive jealousy is that this type of jealousy is more dependent and worrying instead of active and controlling.

Study 7 focused primarily on the different ways in which these forms of jealousy correlate with various aspects of interdependence (Buunk, 1989). One hypothesis explored was that *anticipated* reactive sexual jealousy is unrelated, or even positively related, to marital satisfaction. This was expected because it comes as a particular shock to someone with a satisfying marriage to perceive that the spouse is interested in someone else. The negative correlations between satisfaction and *actual* sexual jealousy can be explained by the fact that conflicts resulting from an actual extramarital affair affect the relationship negatively. The more "clinical" forms of jealousy will in general be accompanied by a low degree of marital satisfaction. Such behaviors will be instigated by dissatisfaction over the partner's affection, and will in turn affect marital satisfaction negatively. The second hypothesis was that degree of dependence is more strongly related to reactive jealousy than to the two other types, because reactive jealousy usually implies, more than the two others, the direct possibility of losing the partner as a central source of rewards. Finally, it was hypothesized that although relative dependency may increase all forms of jealousy, this variable is more strongly related to self-generated jealousy, and to a lesser extent to dominant preventive jealousy, than to reactive jealousy. There are three reasons for this. The first is saliency. For the individual with fewer outcomes outside the relationship, the partner will be a relatively very salient part of his or her life. The second is the dependent individual's higher chance of loss. When the partner is seen as leading an interesting life with a high likelihood of meeting persons of the opposite gender, one may perceive that he or she might easily be tempted to become involved with others. The third reason is resentment. The individual feels resentment because the partner is better off, which will be increased by the thought that the partner pays attention to others. All these factors foster a negative focus of the attention on the partner, which is much more characteristic of self-generated jealousy than the two other forms of jealousy.

These variables were operationalized in the following way. As in the other studies, to measure correspondence of outcomes the Relationship Interaction Satisfaction Scale (Buunk, 1990a) was used. Degree of dependency was measured with a shortened version of the emotional dependency scale. Relative dependency was operationalized by a five-item scale assessing the outcomes one obtains outside the relationship as compared to those of the partner, such as an interesting job, freedom to do what one wants, and the opportunity to meet others (alpha reliability = .71). Reactive jealousy was measured by a slightly revised version of the Anticipated Sexual Jealousy Scale. Preventive jealousy was assessed with a scale (alpha = .93) that included 11 items such as "I don't want my partner to meet people of the opposite sex too often," "I am quite possessive," and "I get upset when my partner looks at persons of the opposite sex." A scale for self-generated jealousy consisted of six items (alpha = .88), such as "I worry that my partner finds someone else more attractive than me" and "I worry that my partner is sexually interested in someone else." In addition, scales for psychosomatic complaints (eight items; alpha = .78) and insecurity over the outcomes provided by the partner (five items; alpha = .86) were included (Buunk, 1989).

Table 7.4 presents some preliminary results of Study 7, which were largely in line with the theoretical expectations. First, relational satisfaction was not associated with reactive jealousy, had a moderate negative relationship to preventive jealousy, and had a much stronger negative relationship to self-generated jealousy. Second, the correlations with degree of dependency followed the opposite pattern: This variable had higher correlations with reactive jealousy than with preventive jealousy, whereas there was no significant correlation with self-generated jealousy. Third, relative dependency was correlated significantly with all three forms of jealousy, but, as expected, most strongly with self-generated jealousy. As the results from the multiple regression showed, reactive jealousy was predicted more by degree of dependency than by both other variables; preventive jealousy was predicted to about the same extent by degree of dependency and lack of relational satisfaction; and relative dependency was more indicative of self-generated jealousy than relational satisfaction and degree of dependency were.

Some other data provide more evidence for the different backgrounds of the three jealousy types. First, psychosomatic complaints correlated somewhat more highly with self-generated jealousy ($r = .36$, $p < .001$) and preventive jealousy ($r = .33$, $p < .001$) than with reactive

**TABLE 7.4. Correlations and Beta Coefficients between Features of Interdependence and Various Types of Jealousy**

|  | Reactive r (beta) | Preventive r (beta) | Self-generated r (beta) |
|---|---|---|---|
| Relational satisfaction | .04$_a$ (.14) | −.20 (.31) | −.41 (.43) |
| Degree of dependency | .31 (.35) | .22 (.35) | .04$_a$ (.21) |
| Relative dependency | .27 (.20) | .25 (.14) | .39 (.25) |
| Multiple $R$ | .41 | .42 | .53 |

*Note.* Except when indicated with subscript *a*, for all correlations and beta coefficients, $p < .01$. From "Types and Manifestations of Jealousy: An Exchange-Theoretical Perspective" by B. Buunk, 1989, May, in G. L. White (Chair), *Themes for progress in jealousy research.* Symposium conducted at the Second Iowa Conference on Personal Relationships, Iowa City.

jealousy ($r = .23$, $p < .001$), suggesting that this last type of reaction is the most "normal" of the three. Second, insecurity correlated much more highly with self-generated jealousy ($r = .62$, $p < .001$) than with the other two (for reactive jealousy, $r = .23$, $p < .001$; for preventive jealousy, $r = .39$, $p < .001$) (Buunk, 1989).

Of course, there are overlaps among the three types of jealousy. For instance, someone who tries everything to prevent his or her partner from being unfaithful, or worries about that possibility, will be quite upset if such an event actually occurs. Nevertheless, the various findings presented here point to distinctive differences among the three jealousy types. Compared to the other types, reactive jealousy seems more characteristic of individuals in satisfying, cohesive relationships, who experience relatively little insecurity and show relatively few signs of maladjustment. On the other hand, self-generated jealousy is found particularly among individuals who feel more dependent on their relationships than their partners, are very dissatisfied with their relationships, feel very insecure about the attitude of their partners toward them, and show more signs of maladjustment than individuals with the other types of jealousy. Preventive jealousy is somewhere between these two types: It is found in relationships that show more cohesion than self-generated jealousy, but that are nevertheless still unsatisfactory.

## FINAL NOTE

For various reasons, jealousy is an interesting and promising topic for social psychologists. These reasons include the complex emotional and behavioral character of jealousy, its often extreme manifestations, and the many theoretical approaches that can be fruitfully applied to grasp its nature and determinants. In this chapter, the aim has been to show how an exchange-theoretical approach is valuable in understanding many aspects and manifestations of jealousy. In doing so, my intention has been to highlight some issues that have often been overlooked in research in this area, including the importance of norms and rules in generating jealousy, the role of considerations of reciprocity and equity, the importance of attributional activity, and the necessity of distinguishing among various types of jealousy. It has been shown that some forms of jealousy may arise from the desire to protect a valued and satisfying relationship, whereas other types of jealousy seem to be indicative of insecurity, too much dependence, and lack of trust. Social exchange theory also may offer guidelines on how to reduce jealousy—for instance, by increasing autonomy and independence, and by changing the interpretations of the partner's behavior. At the same time, however, interdependency theory makes it quite clear that to attempt to eradicate all forms of jealousy completely would mean to give up all forms of interdependence. And that would mean giving up what can be considered the core of intimate relationships.

## ACKNOWLEDGMENTS

I thank Robert G. Bringle and Harold H. Kelley for their very valuable and helpful comments on an earlier version of this chapter.

Most of the research described in this chapter was supported by the Netherlands Organization for Scientific Research (NWO).

## REFERENCES

Berscheid, E., & Peplau, L. A. (1983). The emerging science of relationships. In H. H. Kelley, E. Berscheid, A. Chirstensen, J. H. Harvey, T. L. Huston, G. Levinger, E. McClintock, L. A. Peplau, & D. Peterson (Eds.), *Close relationships* (pp. 1–19). San Francisco: W. H. Freeman.

Bohm, E. (1960). Jealousy. In A. Ellis & A. Arbarbanel (Eds.), *The encyclopedia of sexual behavior* (Vol. 1, pp. 567–574). New York: Hawthorne.

Bringle, R. G., & Buunk, B. (1985). Jealousy and social behavior: a review of personal, relationship and situational determinants. In P. Shaver (Ed.), *Review of personality and social psychology* (Vol. 6, pp. 241–264). Beverly Hills, CA: Sage.

Bringle, R. G., & Buunk, B. (1986). Examining the causes and consequences of jealousy. In R. Gilmour & S. Duck (Eds.), *The emerging field of personal relationships* (pp. 225-240). Hillsdale, NJ: Erlbaum.

Bringle, R. G., & Evenbeck, S. (1979). The study of jealousy as a dispositional characteristic. In M. Cook & G. Wilson (Eds.), *Love and attraction* (pp. 201-204). Oxford: Pergamon Press.

Bringle, R. G., Evenbeck, S. E., & Schmedel, K. (1977, Fall). *The role of jealousy in marriage.* Paper presented at the meeting of the American Psychological Association, San Francisco.

Bryson, J. B. (1977). *Situational determinants of the expression of jealousy.* Paper presented at the meeting of the American Psychological Association, San Francisco.

Burgess, R. L., & Huston, T. L. (1979). *Social exchange in developing relationships.* New York: Academic Press.

Bush, C. R., Bush, J. P., & Jennings, J. (1988). Effects of jealousy threats on relationship perceptions and emotions. *Journal of Social and Personal Relationships, 5*, 285-303.

Buunk, B. (1978). Jaloezie 2: Ervaringen van 250 Nederlanders [Jealousy: Experiences of 250 Dutch people]. *Intermediair, 14*(12), 43-51.

Buunk, B. (1980). *Intieme relaties met derden: Een sociaal psychologische studie* [Multiple intimate relationships: A social psychological study]. Alphen aan de Rijn, The Netherlands: Samsom.

Buunk, B. (1981a). Jealousy in sexually open marriages. *Alternative Lifestyles, 4*, 357-372.

Buunk, B. (1981b). Liefde, sympathie, en jaloezie [Loving, liking and jealousy]. *Gedrag, Tijdschrift voor Psychologie, 9*, 189-202.

Buunk, B. (1982a). Anticipated sexual jealousy: Its relationship to self-esteem, dependency and reciprocity. *Personality and Social Psychology Bulletin, 8*, 310-316.

Buunk, B. (1982b). Strategies of jealousy: Styles of coping with extramarital relations of the spouse. *Family Relations, 31*, 9-14.

Buunk, B. (1983). De rol van attributies en afhankelijkheid bij jaloezie [The role of dependency and attributions in jealousy]. *Nederlands Tijdschrift voor de Psychologie, 38*, 301-311.

Buunk, B. (1984). Jealousy as related to attributions for the partner's behavior. *Social Psychology Quarterly, 47*, 107-112.

Buunk, B. (1986a). Husband's jealousy. In R. A. Lewis & R. Salt (Eds.), *Men in families* (pp. 97-114). Beverly Hills, CA: Sage.

Buunk, B. (1986b, July). Developments in jealousy research: beyond exchange and cognition. In D. Perlman (Chair), *Current developments in interpersonal relations.* Symposium presented at the 21st International Congress of Applied Psychology, Jerusalem.

Buunk, B. (1987a). Conditions that promote break-ups as a consequence of extra-dyadic involvements. *Journal of Social and Clinical Psychology, 5*, 237-250.

Buunk, B. (1987b). Long-term stability and change in sexually open marriages. In L. Shamgar-Handelman & R. Palomba (Eds.), *Alternative patterns of family life in modern societies* (Collana Monografie 1, pp. 61–72). Rome: Istituto di Ricerche sulla Popolazione.

Buunk, B. (1988a). The Anticipated Sexual Jealousy Scale. In C. M. Davis, W. L. Yarber, & S. L. Davis (Eds.), *Sexuality related measures: A compendium* (pp. 192–194). Lake Mills, IA: Graphic.

Buunk, B. (1988b). The Extramarital Behavioral Intentions Scale. In C. M. Davis, W. L. Yarber, & S. L. Davis (Eds.), *Sexuality related measures: A compendium* (pp. 99–100). Lake Mills, IA; Graphic.

Buunk, B. (1989, May). Types and manifestations of jealousy: An exchange-theoretical perspective. In G. L. White (Chair), *Themes for progress in jealousy research.* Symposium conducted at the Second Iowa Conference on Personal Relationships, Iowa City.

Buunk, B. (1990a). Relationship Interaction Satisfaction Scale. In J. Touliatos, B. F. Perlmutter, & M. A. Straus (Eds.). *Handbook of family measurement techniques* (pp. 106–107). Newbury Park, CA: Sage.

Buunk, B. (1990b). Anticipated Sexual Jealousy Scale. In J. Touliatos, B. F. Perlmutter, & M. A. Straus (Eds.), *Handbook of family measurement techniques* (pp. 263–264). Newbury Park, CA: Sage.

Buunk, B. (1990c). Actual Sexual Jealousy Scale. In J. Touliatos, B. F. Perlmutter, & M. A. Straus (Eds.), *Handbook of family measurement techniques* (pp. 262–263). Newbury Park, CA: Sage.

Buunk, B., & Bosman, J. (1985). Attitude similarity and attraction in marital relationships. *Journal of Social Psychology, 126,* 133–134.

Buunk, B., & Bringle, R. G. (1987). Jealousy in love relationships. In D. Perlman & S. Duck (Eds.), *Intimate relationships: Development, dynamics and deterioration* (pp. 123–148). Beverly Hills, CA: Sage.

Buunk, B., & Bringle, R. G., & Arends, H. (1984, July). *Jealousy—a response to threatened self-concept?* Paper presented at the International Conference on Self and Identity, Cardiff, Wales.

Buunk, B., & Hupka, R. B. (1986). Autonomy in close relationships: A cross-cultural study. *Family Perspective,, 20,* 209–221.

Buunk, B., & Hupka, R. B. (1987). Cross-cultural differences in the elicitation of sexual jealousy. *Journal of Sex Research, 23,* 12–22.

Buunk, B., Schaap, C., & Prevoo, N. (in press). Gender specific styles of conflict resolution in premarital relationships. *Journal of Social Psychology.*

Buunk, B., & Van Driel, B. (1989). *Variant lifestyles and relationships.* Newbury Park, CA: Sage.

Clanton, G., & Smith, L. G. (Eds.). (1977). *Jealousy.* Englewood Cliffs, NJ: Prentice-Hall.

Daly, M., Wilson, M., & Weghorst, S. J. (1982). Male sexual jealousy. *Ethology and Sociobiology, 3,* 11–27.

Ellis, A. (1977). Rational and irrational jealousy. In G. Clanton & L. G. Smith (Eds.), *Jealousy.* Englewood Cliffs, NJ: Prentice-Hall.

Festinger, L. (1954). A theory of social comparison processes. *Human Relations, 7,* 117–140.

Fitzpatrick, M. A. (1984). A typological approach to marital interaction: Recent theory and research. In L. Berkowitz (Ed.). *Advances in experimental social psychology* (Vol. 18, pp. 1–47). Orlando, FL: Academic Press.

Francis, J. L. (1977). Towards the management of heterosexual jealousy. *Journal of Marriage and Family Counseling, 3,* 61–69.

Freud, S. (1940). Über einige Neurotische Mechanismen bei Eifersucht, Paranoia und Homoseksualität. In *Ges. Werke* (Bd. 13). London: Imago. (Original work published 1922)

Glenn, N. D., & Weaver, C. N. (1979). Attitudes toward premarital, extramarital and homosexual relations in the U.S. in the 1970's. *Journal of Sex Research, 15,* 108–118.

Gottschalk, H. (1936). *Skinsygens problemer [Problems of jealousy].* Copenhagen: Fremad.

Groves, E. R. (1934). *The American family.* Philadelphia: J. B. Lippincott.

Gurnee, H. (1936). *Elements of social psychology.* New York: Farrar & Rinehart.

Hansen, G. (1983). Marital satisfaction and jealousy among married men. *Psychological Reports, 52,* 363–366.

Heider, F. (1958). *The psychology of interpersonal relations.* New York: Wiley.

Hoaken, P. C. S. (1976). Jealousy as a symptom of psychiatric disorder. *Australian and New Zealand Journal of Psychiatry, 10,* 47–51.

Hunt, M. (1974). *Sexual behavior in the 1970's.* New York: Dell.

Hupka, R. B. (1984). Jealousy: Compound emotion or label for a particular situation? *Motivation and Emotion, 8,* 141–155.

Jones, E. E., & Davis, K. E. (1965). From acts to dispositions: The attribution process in person perception. In L. Berkowitz (Ed.). *Advances in experimental social psychology* (Vol. 2, pp. 219–266). New York: Academic Press.

Kelley, H. H. (1967). Attribution theory in social psychology. In D. Levine (Ed.), *Nebraska symposium on motivation* (Vol. 15, pp. 192–240). Lincoln: University of Nebraska Press.

Kelley, H. H. (1979). *Personal relationships: Their structures and processes.* Hillsdale, NJ: Erlbaum.

Kelley, H. H. (1986). Personal relationships: Their nature and significance. In R. Gilmour & S. Duck (Eds.), *The emerging field of personal relationships* (pp. 3–19). Hillsdale, NJ: Erlbaum.

Kelley, H. H. (1988, July 3). *What do we know about interpersonal relations? An interdependency theory perspective.* Paper presented at the Fourth International Conference on Personal Relationships, Vancouver, British Columbia.

Knapp, J. & Whitehurst, R. N. (1977). Sexually open marriage and relationships: Issues and prospects. In R. W. Libby and R. N. Whitehurst (Eds.), *Marriage and alternatives: Exploring intimate relationships* (pp. 146–161). Glenview, IL: Scott, Foresman and Company.

La Gaipa, J. J. (1977). Interpersonal attraction and social exchange. In S. Duck (Ed.), *Theory and practice in interpersonal attraction.* London: Academic Press.

Lewin, K. (1948). *Resolving social conflicts.* New York: Harper.

Mathes, E. W., Roter, P. M., & Joerger, S. M. (1982). A convergent validity study of six jealousy scales. *Psychological Reports, 51,* 123–127.

Mathes E. W., & Severa, N. (1981). Jealousy, romantic love, and liking: Theoretical considerations and preliminary scale development. *Psychological Reports, 49,* 23–31.

McDonald, G. W., & Osmond, M. W. (1980, October). *Jealousy and trust: unexplored dimensions of social exchange dynamics.* Paper presented at the NCFR Workshop on Theory Construction and Research Methodology, Portland, OR.

Milardo, R. M., & Murstein, B. I. (1979). The implications of exchange-orientation on the dyadic functioning of heterosexual cohabitors. In M. Cook & G. Wilson (Eds.), *Love and attraction: An international conference* (pp. 279–285). Oxford: Pergamon Press.

Mills, J., & Clark, M. (1982). Exchange and communal relationships. In L. Wheeler (Ed.). *Review of personality and social psychology* (Vol. 3, pp. 121–144). Beverly Hills, CA: Sage.

Peplau, L. A. (1983). Roles and gender. In H. H. Kelley, E. Berscheid, A. Christensen, J. H. Harvey, T. L. Huston, G. Levinger, E. McClintock, L. A. Peplau, & D. Peterson (Eds.), *Close relationships* (pp. 220–264). San Francisco: W. H. Freeman.

Pfeiffer, S. M., & Wong, P. T. P. (1989). Multidimensional jealousy. *Journal of Social and Personal Relationships, 6,* 181–196.

Rubin, Z. (1970). Measurement of romantic love. *Journal of Personality and Social Psychology, 16,* 265–273.

Salovey, P., & Rodin, J. (1989). Envy and jealousy in close relationships. In C. Hendrick (Ed.), *Review of personality and social psychology* (Vol. 10, pp. 221–246). Newbury Park, CA: Sage.

Scanzoni, J. (1979). Social exchange and behavioral interdependence. In Burgess, R. L., & Huston, T. L. (Eds.), *Social exchange in developing relationships* (pp. 61–98). New York: Academic Press.

Schaap, C., Buunk, B., & Kerkstra, A. (1988). Marital conflict resolution. In P. Noller & M. A. Fitzpatrick (Eds.). *Perspectives on marital interaction* (Monographs in Social Psychology of Language, Vol. 1, pp. 203–244). Philadelphia: Multilingual Matters.

Symons, D. (1979). *The evolution of human sexuality.* New York: Oxford University Press.

Thibaut, J. W., & Kelley, H. H. (1959). *The social psychology of groups.* New York: Wiley.

Thibaut, J. W., & Kelley, H. H. (1986). *The social psychology of groups* (2nd ed.). New Brunswick, NJ: Transaction Books.

Walster, E., Walster, G. W., & Berscheid, E. (1978). *Equity: Theory and research.* Boston: Allyn & Bacon.

White, G. L. (1981a). Relative involvement, inadequacy, and jealousy: A test of a causal model. *Alternative Lifestyles, 4,* 291–309.

White, G. L. (1981b). A model of romantic jealousy. *Motivation and Emotion, 5,* 295–310.

White, G. L. (1984a). Jealousy and partner's perceived motives for attraction to a rival. *Social Psychology Quarterly, 44,* 24–30.

White, G. L. (1984b). Comparison of four jealousy scales. *Journal of Research in Personality, 18,* 115–130.

White, G. L., & Mullen, P. E. (1989). *Jealousy: Theory, research, and clinical strategies.* New York: Guilford Press.

## Chapter Eight

# *Modes of Response to Jealousy-Evoking Situations*

JEFF B. BRYSON
*San Diego State University*

Theoretical constructs and measures of those constructs should be at the same level of complexity. To the extent that they are not, those measures cannot adequately represent or test the underlying theory. A failure to achieve such equivalence between theoretical and operational definitions of jealousy has been one of the principal impediments to research in this area over the past 15 years. Theoretical definitions have generally described jealousy as a complex construct, comprised of feelings, cognitions, and behaviors aroused in situations that are considered to be jealousy-evoking (e.g., Clanton & Smith, 1977; Pines & Aronson, 1983; Shettel-Neuber, Bryson & Young, 1978; White, 1981a, 1981b, 1984). Even those theorists who limit their conceptual defintion to the affective domain recognize that jealousy is not a single emotion, but a compound of several different negative emotions, any part of which may be evoked in a particular situation (e.g., Bringle, Roach, Andler, & Evenbeck, 1979; Mathes & Severa, 1981; see also Sharpsteen, Chapter 2, this volume).

Despite this acknowledgment of the complexity of jealousy, the most commonly employed measures of this construct are scales that provide a single score as a measure of jealousy, either as a disposition (e.g., Bringle, 1981; Mathes & Severa, 1981) or as a phenomenological self-description, either of chronic jealousy or jealousy within a particular relationship (e.g., White, 1981b, 1984) or in reaction to a particular situation (e.g., Bush, Bush, & Jennings, 1988). Although these approaches make quite different assumptions, and provide different perspectives on the nature of jealousy, they are both limited to describing jealousy in terms of its intensity or extremity: An individual or group can be more or less jealous than others, or an individual may be more or less jealous in certain situations or relationships than in others. Differences in the qualitative nature of these jealous responses are lost or ignored.

More recently, however, these univariate approaches to the analysis of jealousy have been criticized (e.g., Hupka, 1984). Researchers who have focused on copying styles, or on emotional and behavioral responses to jealousy-evoking situations (e.g., Buunk, 1982; Francis, 1977; Pines & Aronson, 1983), have consistently reported a wide variety of reactions and modes of expression. Bringle and Buunk (1985) have suggested that a more complex measure—one incorporating separate emotional, behavioral, and cognitive dimensions—is necessary for more detailed analyses of jealousy, and Pfeiffer and Wong (1989) have presented a compelling argument for the need to consider jealousy as a multidimensional construct.

This chapter presents some of the results of a research program that has consistently been directed toward the development of a multidimensional conception of jealousy responses. Two different paths have been taken in this endeavor. An empirical approach has been employed to define the dimensions underlying responses to jealousy-evoking situations; this allows a comparison of qualitative, rather than just quantitative, differences in jealousy. A theoretical or conceptual approach has been utilized to examine the personal, motivational, and situational factors that underlie one's choice of response mode.

## DIMENSIONS OF JEALOUSY: AN EMPIRICAL APPROACH

In my first attempt to define the range of jealousy behaviors (Bryson, 1976), I asked a group of 30 male and 32 female college students to think about times when they had felt jealous, and then to list the feelings they had experienced and the things they had done as a consequence of being jealous. The responses for all subjects were then combined, and a 48-item jealousy questionnaire was compiled by selecting the 24 emotions and the 24 actions most frequently mentioned in these listings.

The jealousy questionnaire was administered to a new sample of subjects, 66 males and 102 females, in four separate classes. Subjects were asked to indicate how well each of these feelings and actions described what they did and felt when they were jealous.

Responses to the jealousy questionnaire were examined by means of a principal components analysis and varimax rotation. Examination of the eigenvalues led to a decision to rotate the first eight factors, which accounted for 51.2% of the total variance. Subject sex was also included as a variable, to allow us to define any sex differences in the derived factors.

The obtained factors provided a first look at the topography of jealousy responses. Instead of simply describing a person as more or less jealous, these factors provide a representation of how jealousy is manifested. Differences, between groups or between individuals, are defined in terms of the nature of the jealousy response rather than simply in terms of its extremity. It is not a question of who is more jealous, but of how that jealousy is expressed—in terms of both external behaviors and internal feelings—that is the focus of attention.

The factors, and items with the highest loadings, were as follows:

*Factor I: Emotional Devastation.* This factor seemed to represent the serious negative emotional consequences of jealousy. The items with the highest loadings on this factor included: "[feel] helpless," "like I'm in a daze," "insecure," "less able to cope with other aspects of my life," "physically ill," "inadequate," "fearful," "depressed," "uncomfortable around other people," "anxious," "confused," "exploited," and "cry when I'm alone." Subject sex correlated significantly with this factor, $r$ (166) $= .21, p < .05$, indicating that females are more likely than males to report this set of primarily emotional responses to jealousy.

*Factor II: Reactive Retribution.* Items on this factor appeared to describe attempts to "get even" with the partner for his or her complicity in a jealousy-evoking situation. This factor included such items as "start going out with other people," "do something to get my partner jealous," "become more sexually aggressive with other people," "try to make my partner think I don't care," "make critical comments about my partner in front of other people," and "get a friend to go talk to my partner." This factor was also significantly correlated with subject sex ($r = -.27$, $p < .01$), indicating that males are more likely than females to respond in this manner.

*Factor III: Arousal.* The items on this factor seemed to provide a defintion of the arousal properties of jealousy, or a relationship-intensifying reaction. Items loading highly on this factor included "pay more attention to my partner than before," "become more sexually aggressive with my partner," "try to monopolize my partner's time," "[feel] more sexually aroused by my partner," and a negative loading for "resign myself to the situation." This pattern of results indicates that jealousy can serve to intensify a lover's ardor and interest in his or her partner, or that there is a rational basis for the "jealousy game" (White, 1980) of trying to make the partner jealous. However, the presence of other, less positive reaction patterns suggests that this game is a dangerous one. Although White (1980) reported that females were more likely than males to attempt to elicit this response from their partners, suggesting that males might be more likely to respond in this manner, this factor was not significantly correlated with subject sex; male and female respondents were equally likely to endorse these items.

*Factor IV: Need for Social Support.* The items on this factor included "talk to close friends about my feelings," a negative loading for "refuse to talk about my feelings with others," "cry when I'm alone," "check with others who might confirm or disconfirm my feelings," and "get away from the situation." Taken together, these items seem to represent a motivation to distance oneself from the jealousy-inducing situation—not by withdrawal from any social contact, but by more intensive interaction with friends who can provide both informational and social support. These items were endorsed more by females than by males, $(r = .27, p < .01)$.

*Factor V: Intropunitiveness.* Items loading on this factor included "feel guilty about being jealous," "get involved in other nondating activities," "feel angry at myself," and negative loadings for "feel like getting even," and "hope that my partner ends up being hurt." Taken together, these items seem to reflect a tendency to blame and punish oneself for being jealous, rather than directing any negative affect toward the partner. The correlation with subject sex indicated that males scored somewhat higher on this factor than did females $(r = -.19, p < .05)$.

*Factor VI: Confrontation.* This factor was represented by positive loadings for "ask my partner to explain the situation" and "confront the other person directly," and negative loadings for "try to make other people think I don't care," "try to make my partner think I don't care," and "feel inadequate." This cluster of items seems to represent a tendency to see this as a challenge and to confront the jealousy situation directly, rather than trying to hide one's feelings or experiencing a drop in self-esteem. There was a tendency for males to endorse these items more ($r = -.18$, $p < .05$).

*Factor VII: Anger.* The items loading high on this factor refer uniformly to feelings of anger: "feel anger toward my partner," "feel angry toward the other person," "feel that my partner has made a mistake," "feel betrayed," "feel disappointed in my partner," and "feel like getting even." It was interesting to see that there was no differentiation between the partner and the other person; either or both were likely to be the target of anger. Females were found to endorse these items more than males ($r = .24$, $p < .01$), a finding that has since been corroborated in surveys of additional college students, high school students, and both married and divorced adults.

*Factor VIII: Impression Management.* The items with high loadings on this bipolar factor seemed to represent two quite distinct methods for dealing with the problem of impression management when jealous. On the one hand there were high positive loadings for "try to make my partner think I don't care," "try to make other people think I don't care," and "feel more irritable toward other people," while at the other extreme was a high negative loading for "get drunk or high." Subject sex was most strongly related to this factor ($r = .43$, $p < .01$): Women are more likely to react in the former style, and men in the latter. This bifurcation represents clearly the sex differences in impression management orientation imposed by our culture. Women cannot overtly express their emotions for fear of threatening their relationships, and consequently must be stoic about their partners' infidelities. Men can express their emotions only under the cover of intoxication, for it provides a convenient excuse for reactions that might otherwise threaten self-esteem.

It seems clear that this analysis has demonstrated considerable support for the argument that jealousy is a multifaceted and complex emotional state. The results indicate that it is comprised of at least eight distinct response styles, encompassing a variety of cognitive, emotional, and behavioral reactions. It is important to remember that these factors are independent of one another. Thus, one may experience all of these, some subset, or only a single reaction in response to a particular jealousy-evoking situation. This is, it seems, a sufficient reason for the sense of confusion and ambivalence that one may feel when jealous, for many of these responses seem opposed or contradictory. When a person is jealous it is possible to feel both angry and sad, to want to hurt one's partner and to blame one's self, to want to get even by going out with others and to feel more aroused by one's partner, to try to hide one's feelings and to seek the advice of friends—with all of these occurring virtually simultaneously or in close succession. If one is to describe jealousy adequately it seems clear that multiple response dimensions must be examined.

## JEALOUSY STYLES: A CROSS-CULTURAL ANALYSIS

It has become almost obligatory for writers on jealousy to note that it is, in large part, a product of one's culture. However, relatively little work has been directed toward examining the role that culture plays in the determination of jealousy responses. The work that has been done has focused on the role that culture plays in determining what situations will be defined as jealousy-evoking (e.g., Buunk & Hupka, 1987; Hupka et al., 1985), or what factors make a culture more or less jealous (i.e., to define more or fewer situations as jealousy-evoking; Hupka, 1981). However, it seems reasonable to hypothesize that cultures or societies will differ not only in terms of what situations will elicit jealousy, but also in terms of how that jealousy will be expressed. To examine this hypothesis, and to better understand the generality of the jealousy response style identified earlier, we conducted a large-scale cross-cultural study of jealousy responses, comparing samples drawn from the United States and four western European countries: France, Germany, Italy, and the Netherlands (Bryson et al., 1984).

This study would not have been possible without the gracious and able assistance of a number of collaborators and colleagues who aided me in developing, cross-translating, and administering the various versions of the questionnaire: Paolo Alcini, Universita di Roma, who developed, cross-translated, and administered the Italian version; Bram Buunk, University of Groningen, the Netherlands, who did the same for the Dutch version; Marita Rosch Inglehart and Fritz Strack, formerly and presently (respectively) at the Universität Mannheim, Federal Republic of Germany, who cross-translated and helped to administer the German-language version developed by Liane Bryson; Francis Ribey, Université de Strasbourg, France, for developing and administering the French-language version; and Didier van den Hove, Université Catholique de Louvain-le-Neuve, Belgium, for the French cross-translation.[1]

The questionnaire developed for this study was considerably longer and more complex than the original 48-item jealousy reactions questionnaire. The present instrument included sections for demographic data; description of current and prior relationships; attitudes and beliefs concerning romantic relationships; a 20-item jealousy situations questionnaire similar to Bringle's (1981) Interpersonal Jealousy Scale; and 45 items comprising an amended jealousy reactions survey, similar to the original 48-item scale but with some deletions, modifications, and additions.

This questionnaire was administered to approximately 100 male and 100 female students at each of the universities listed above and at a large state university in the United States. Questionnaires completed by subjects who were not native to the country of administration were discarded, as were those with more than 10 inappropriate omissions (i.e., failure to respond to questions concerning current relationships was not considered as an inappropriate omission, as the subject may have simply considered them not personally relevant). The resulting sample sizes (for males and females, respectively) were as follows: France, 65 and 72; Germany, 58 and 68; Italy, 100 and 97; Netherlands, 95 and 112; United States, 106 and 106. (Exact numbers vary somewhat between analyses because of missing data.)

### Principal Components Analysis

As a preliminary step, separate principal components analyses of the 45 jealousy reactions items were performed for each national sample, and the resulting rotated factors were compared. Like Hupka et al. (1985), we found considerable congruence in factor structures. However, we decided to go beyond that form of analysis in the present study. In order to facilitate comparisons across national groups, we combined all groups and performed an overall principal components analysis of the jealousy reactions items. Examination of eigenvalues led to a decision to rotate nine factors, accounting for 51% of the total variance, to the varimax criterion. These factors, and items with primary loadings above .40 on each, are presented in Table 8.1.

Although the modifications of the questionnaire items from those used in the earlier study make it impossible to provide numerical estimates of congruence, an examination of the items and their loadings indicates that there is a considerable degree of similarity between these factors and those obtained earlier, despite the differences in samples and item content. Five of the factors in the present analysis (Emotional Devastation, Impression Management, Reactive Retribution, Intropunitiveness, and Social Support Seeking) are essentially equivalent to those found earlier. The Relationship Improvement factor obtained here seems to provide a fuller explanation of the Arousal factor identified earlier: The increase in attraction toward and interest in the partner is apparently related to a motivation to enhance or strengthen the relationship.

There are no similar correspondences for the Anger and Confrontation factors obtained earlier. Instead, it seems that the inclusion in the

**TABLE 8.1. Principal Components Analysis of Jealousy Reactions Items**

Factor I. Reaction to Betrayal (7.33% of variance after rotation)
.74 Feel betrayed
.68 Doubt my partner
.65 Feel angry toward my partner
.54 Give my partner the cold shoulder
.54 End the relationship
.42 Spy on my partner

Factor II. Emotional Devastation (6.30%)
.75 Feel less able to cope with other aspects of my life
.58 Feel physically ill
.57 Cry when I'm alone
.57 Feel insecure
.55 Not be able to stop thinking about the situation

Factor III. Aggression (6.20%)
.82 Threaten the other person
.79 Become physically aggressive with the other person
.48 Confront the other person
.42 Be physically aggressive with my partner
.41 Demand that my partner not see the other person

Factor IV. Impression Management (6.01%)
.62 Try to make my partner think I don't care
.60 Try to make other people think I don't care
−.60 Tell my partner that I feel jealous
.55 Try to ignore the situation
.44 Indirectly let my partner know that I know what is going on

Factor V. Reactive Retribution (5.89%)
.74 Flirt or go out with other people
.72 Do something to get even
.67 Do more than my partner has done and then tell him/her about it
.51 Do something to make my partner jealous
.41 Get drunk

Factor VI. Relationship Improvement (5.87%)
.66 Become more sexually active with my partner
.66 Try to make myself more attractive to my partner
.61 Try to improve our relationship
.57 Feel even more attracted to my partner

Factor VII. Monitoring (4.53%)
.59 Question my partner about his/her activities
.58 Ask my partner to explain his/her actions
.40 Keep an eye on my partner when the other person is around

Factor VIII. Intropunitiveness (4.24%)
.76 Feel guilty about being jealous
.71 Feel angry with myself
.48 Blame myself
.41 Resign myself to enduring the situation

Factor IX. Social Support Seeking (3.56%)
.74 Talk to close friends about my feelings
.42 Check with others who might confirm or disconfirm my feelings

cross-cultural questionnaire of items relating to monitoring the partner's behavior caused the two earlier factors to split rather differently. Some confrontation items joined with anger items to create the Aggression factor, while other items (e.g., "ask my partner to explain his/her actions") helped to define Monitoring—a new factor whose content seems comparable to Pfeiffer and Wong's (1989) "detective/protective" measures.

Items related to the overt, but not explicitly aggressive, expression of anger toward the partner (e.g., giving him or her the "cold shoulder," ending the relationship, or spying on the partner) seem to have combined to form a new factor, Reaction to Betrayal.

Overall, the correspondence in factor structures between analyses involving these quite different samples provides considerable confidence in the stability and psychological meaningfulness of the jealousy reaction styles identified to date. The underlying equivalences of analyses of the separate national samples provides further support for the use of a common set of factors to make comparisons among these groups.

### Cross-National and Sex Differences in Jealousy Reactions

Factor scores were computed for each subject, and these scores were analyzed in nine separate 2 (gender of subject) $\times$ 5 (nationality) analyses of variance, examining the separate and combined effects of these two influences on the various jealousy response styles. Cell means and sample sizes for these analyses are presented in Table 8.2.

The analysis of Factor I, Reaction to Betrayal, revealed significant main effects for both gender, $F(1, 818) = 10.35$, $p < .001$, and nationality, $F(4, 818) = 16.89$, $p < .001$. Females ($M = .10$) were more likely to endorse items describing these reactions than were males ($M = -.12$). Comparisons across nations revealed that the French ($M = .41$) obtained the highest scores, the Italian ($M = .17$) and U.S. ($M = .04$) samples were intermediate, and the German ($M = -.19$) and Dutch ($M = -.36$) samples obtained the lowest scores on this factor. The interaction was not significant ($F = 0.38$), indicating that the obtained sex differences are relatively constant across these different countries.

Emotional Devastation scores also revealed significant effects for both gender, $F(1, 818) = 11.24$, $p < .001$, and nationality, $F(4, 818) = 8.66$, $p < .001$, and a nonsignificant interaction. Again, females ($M = .10$) were more likely to report these reactions than were males ($M = -.11$). However, in this case it was the Dutch sample that was most likely to endorse these responses ($M = .21$), followed by the Italians ($M = .12$) and Ger-

**TABLE 8.2. Mean Factor Scores by Gender and Nationality**

| Factor | France | | Germany | | Italy | | Netherlands | | United States | |
|---|---|---|---|---|---|---|---|---|---|---|
| | M | F | M | F | M | F | M | F | M | F |
| I. Reaction to Betrayal | .26 | .53 | −.29 | −.10 | .11 | .24 | −.54 | −.19 | −.08 | .12 |
| II. Emotional Devastation | −.41 | −.22 | −.07 | .21 | −.06 | .30 | .20 | .21 | −.40 | −.08 |
| III. Aggression | .45 | .44 | −.32 | −.39 | .06 | −.25 | −.04 | −.26 | 1.03 | −.32 |
| IV. Impression Management | .05 | .15 | −.18 | .02 | −.20 | −.02 | −.07 | −.14 | −.05 | .49 |
| V. Reactive Retribution | .01 | −.07 | .07 | .09 | .14 | −.10 | −.22 | −.14 | .41 | .02 |
| VI. Relationship Improvement | .26 | .19 | .39 | −.14 | −.29 | −.21 | −.06 | −.20 | .17 | .23 |
| VII. Monitoring | −.21 | −.16 | .00 | .17 | −.33 | −.39 | .20 | .28 | .42 | .11 |
| VIII. Intropunitiveness | .38 | .10 | .14 | −.03 | −.38 | −.51 | .03 | .10 | .14 | .28 |
| IX. Social Support Seeking | −.36 | .09 | −.18 | .08 | −.72 | −.21 | .11 | .48 | −.05 | .61 |

187

mans ($M = .08$), with the U.S. ($M = -.21$) and French ($M = -.31$) samples obtaining the lowest scores.

Analysis of scores on the Aggression factor revealed main effects for both gender, $F (1, 818) = 36.11$, $p < .001$, and nationality, $F (4, 818) = 17.17$, $p < .001$, and the presence of a significant interaction, $F (4, 818) = 12.69$, $p < .001$. Overall, males ($M = .20$) obtained substantially higher scores on Aggression than did females ($M = -.17$). Aggression scores were highest in the French ($M = .44$) and U.S. ($M = .22$) samples, lower among the Italians ($M = -.09$) and Dutch ($M = -.16$), and lowest for the Germans ($M = -.36$). However, examination of the cell means reveals that the significant interaction was caused by variation in the magnitude of sex differences across the national samples; that is, although male and female scores were very similar within the French and German samples, they were markedly different in the United States, with males obtaining much higher scores.

Females ($M = .09$) were more likely than males ($M = -.10$) to endorse the Impression Management items, $F (1, 818) = 7.59$, $p < .01$. Examination of means relevant to the significant main effect for nationality, $F (4, 818) = 3.59$, $p < .01$, revealed that the U.S. sample ($M = .27$) was more likely to endorse these items than was any other group. A marginally significant ($p < .10$) interaction effect was caused by slightly greater sex differences in Impression Management scores in the U.S., German, and Italian samples than in the French and Dutch samples.

Reactive Retribution scores differed only marginally across genders, $F (1, 818) = 3.11$, $p < .10$; males' scores ($M = .06$) were slightly higher than females' scores ($M = -.05$). The significant nationalities effect, $F (4, 818) = 3.63$, $p < .01$, reflected the relatively greater popularity of these items among the U.S. sample ($M = .18$) and their rejection by the Dutch sample $M = -.17$), relative to the other groups. The interaction was not significant ($F = 1.51$, $p > .10$).

Analyses of Relationship Improvement scores revealed a significant effect for nationality, $F (4, 818) = 8.10$, $p < .001$, but only marginal effects for gender, either alone, $F (1, 818) = 2.95$, $p < .10$, or in interaction, $F (4, 818) = 2.21$, $p < .10$. Overall, it appears that these items were endorsed more strongly by subjects in the United States ($M = .21$), France ($M = .23$), and Germany ($M = .11$) than by those in the Netherlands ($M = -.14$) or Italy ($M = -.25$).

Monitoring behavior did not differ as a function of gender, either as a main effect, $F (1, 818) = 0.04$, or in interaction, $F (4, 818) = 1.32$, $p > .20$. However, the main effect for nationality was significant, $F (4, 818) = 14.22$, $p < .001$: Reports of these behaviors were highest in the Netherlands ($M = .24$) and the United States ($M = .23$), lower in German ($M = .09$) and France ($M = -.18$), and lowest in Italy ($M = -.36$).

Contrary to our earlier work using only U.S. samples, no sex differences were found for Intropunitiveness, $F (1, 818) = 1.15$. However, there were substantial effects due to nationality, $F (4, 818) = 14.70$, $p < .001$, with the French ($M = .24$) and U.S. ($M = .22$) samples more likely to report this reaction, the Dutch ($M = .07$) and Germans ($M = .05$) next, and the Italians ($M = -.45$) much less likely to blame themselves for their jealous feelings.

Social Support Seeking manifested large effects attributable to gender, $F (1, 818) = 74.15$, $p < .001$ and nationality, $F (4, 818) = 21.95$, $p < .001$. Females ($M = .23$) were much more likely to report these activities than were males ($M = -.26$). The U.S. ($M = .35$) and Dutch ($M = .31$) samples were the highest-ranking on this factor, followed by the Germans ($M = -.04$) and French ($M = -.13$); the Italians ($M = -.47$) were extremely low on this factor.

Overall, these analyses indicate that there are some sex differences in reactions to jealousy that are relatively stable across cultural and national boundaries. Examination of the means in Table 8.2 reveals that, in addition to the overall comparisons being statistically significant, females obtained higher scores in all five national groups on Reactions to Betrayal, Emotional Devastation, and Social Support Seeking, and were higher in four of the five national groups on Impression Management. Men, in contrast, were significantly and consistently higher across all five national groups on Aggression and Intropunitiveness. Comparisons of scores on Reactive Retribution, Relationship Improvement, and Monitoring revealed no consistent or significant sex differences. It is interesting to note a pattern that seems to underlie these differences: Females consistently obtained higher scores on measures of emotional responses (Reactions to Betrayal and Emotional Devastation) and those concerning the display of emotions (Social Support Seeking and Impression Management), males were higher on measures of aggression and self-blame (Aggression and Intropunitiveness). The latter findings seem consistent with Clanton and Smith's (1977) suggestion that men are more likely to respond to jealousy with violence and then to experience remorse at their actions. However, measures of reactions that serve either directly or indirectly to alter relationship status, such as Reactive Retribution, Relationship Improvement, and Monitoring, showed no strong or consistent pattern of sex differences.

One may also characterize each national group in terms of its characteristic jealousy reaction styles. Figure 8.1 provides a rather different

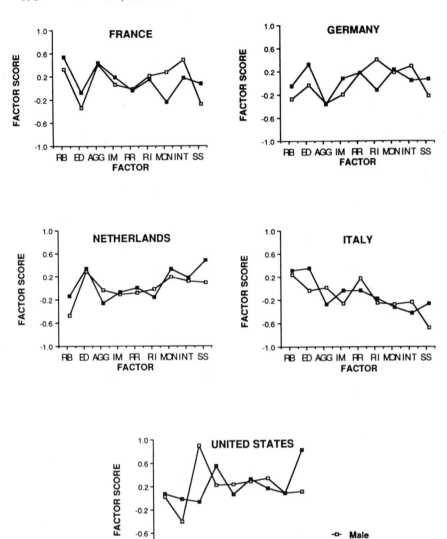

**FIGURE 8.1.** Factor score profiles by nationality and gender. RB, Reaction to Betrayal; ED, Emotional Devastation; AGG, Aggression; IM, Impression Management; RR, Reactive Retribution; RI, Relationship Improvement; MON, Monitoring; INT, Intropunitiveness; SS, Social Support Seeking.

presentation of the data in Table 8.2, providing profiles of scores across all nine factors for males and females within each of the five countries. Comparison of these graphs across countries indicates that there do seem to be national differences in jealousy responses. Each country does appear to have a distinct, characteristic profile of responses, different from the response pattern found in other cultures: The French profiles are high in Reaction to Betrayal, Aggression, and Intropunitiveness, and low in Emotional Devastation; the Germans are identified by low scores on Aggression and Reaction to Betrayal; the Italians tend primarily to be low in Social Support Seeking, Monitoring, and Intropunitiveness; the Dutch tend to be low in Reaction to Betrayal and high in Emotional Devastation; and the U.S. profiles are relatively high in Social Support Seeking, Impression Management, and Aggression. As an overall summary, one may characterize each national group in terms of its most extreme profile features: It appears that, when jealous, the French get mad, the Dutch get sad, the Germans would rather not fight about it, the Italians don't want to talk about it, and the Americans are concerned about what their friends think!

When the sexes within a given country are compared, it may be noted that in most cases the profiles of responses for males and females are quite similar. The only notable exception to this pattern is found in the U.S. samples, where the male and female profiles differ drastically.

This visual inspection is supported by the results of a cluster analysis of mean factor scores for male and female samples from each country. The dendogram for this analysis is presented in Figure 8.2. As may be seen, initial clusters for the French and Italian samples were between the two sexes. The basic similarities in the German and Dutch samples were demonstrated in their clustering sequence: The Dutch males and females combined first, and then the German females and males were added in turn to that cluster. The U.S. samples, however, showed little similarity to each other or to any other national sample. If clustering were to stop at the halfway point, when the number of groups has been reduced from 10 to 5, one would obtain a French cluster, an Italian cluster, a German–Dutch cluster, and individual profiles for the two U.S. samples. These two profiles are joined with the others only at the end of the clustering sequence. The U.S. females finally are forced into the French cluster at the shift from four to three groups, and the U.S. males, the very most different group, are forced into the sequence only on the very last step.

It appears, then, that in most cases there is considerable similarity between the sexes within countries in terms of their behavior when jealous. In addition, the clustering provides at least some evidence of international similarity (e.g., in the Dutch–German clustering sequence)

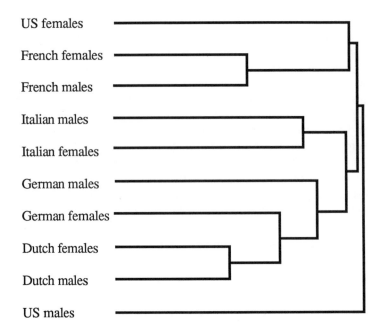

**FIGURE 8.2.** Cluster analysis of jealousy response profiles by nationality and gender.

as well. The only apparent exception to these generalizations is the U.S. sample, in which the sexes differed from each other and from the other national groups as well.

It was, admittedly, a surprise to find that the only country to display strong sex differences was the United States. My initial hypothesis had been that countries with a more overt tradition of male chauvinism or sexual inequality, such as Italy or France, would manifest the greatest sex differences in jealousy reactions, while a country such as the United States, with a more established (or at least more vigorously promoted) ethic of sexual equality, would show the fewest sex differences. The results, in fact, were opposite to those expectations.

The failure of such an "obvious" hypothesis requires some additional examination. First of all, of course, it may indeed be that sex differences in jealousy behaviors are greater in the United States than they are in these European countries. Sommers (1984) found that Americans see jealousy as something to be suppressed or disguised from others. Such attempts to hide rather than express jealousy, which are consistent with our finding that the U.S. sample was highest on the Impression Management factor, could result in less awareness of others' (and particularly romantic partners') jealous feelings, and hence in less pressure for convergence of response styles. However, the hypothesis that sex differences in jealousy responses should be less in these European countries does not agree with the judgments of my collaborators and other natives of those countries who are also familiar with American culture. Their uniform expectation has been that sex differences should be less, or at least no greater, in the U.S. sample than in the other countries. Consequently, while this is a possible explanation for these results, other factors should be considered.

A second possibility is that the instrument itself is somehow biased toward the measurement of sex differences as expressed in American jealousy reaction styles. That is, in constructing the questionnaire I may have been judging items from an American perspective, and thus may have been unconsciously predisposed to consider behaviors on which American men and women differ to be more interesting; as a consequence, I may have overlooked or not asked about behaviors on which the sexes are more likely to differ in the European countries. However, I do not think that this is the primary cause of the present results. A number of European colleagues who have looked at these data have assured me that the items selected for the questionnaire are an appropriate and representative sample of jealousy reactions for their cultures (in fact, some of the items had been suggested by my collaborators). Also, there are sex differences on some of these factors that are consistently represented across these national samples—they are simply larger in the U.S. data.

Another possibility is that students in the United States have adopted a public posture of sexual equality that is not reflected in more private behaviors. There is considerable pressure on American college students not to manifest behaviors or beliefs that could be construed as nonegalitarian, or even as implying differences between the sexes. In such a climate it may be that individuals who feel they must publicly express a belief in sexual equality without privately accepting that position must seek more subtle and socially acceptable methods for establishing a sense of gender identity and uniqueness. In romantic relationships such individuals may maintain a façade of equality yet express their different sex-role orientations through divergent jealousy reactions. In other countries, where a rhetoric of equality is not so strongly promoted, such methods for maintaining sex-role differences would not be as necessary, for there would be less conflict between public expression and private belief.

A fourth possibility, and perhaps the most likely, is that the obtained sex differences reflect a difference in the nature of the college student populations in Europe and the United States. Students in an American state university such as that used in this study are drawn from a wide range of backgrounds, ability levels, interests, and attitudes. European universities, in contrast, represent a much more highly selected and homogeneous group within a country. It may be that, as one becomes increasingly selective in terms of educational background and ability level, sex differences in social attitudes and interpersonal behaviors diminish. Overall, then, gender differences should be less in these more selective populations. In fact, there may be a paradoxical enhancement of the appearance of equality in those societies that discriminate most against women. As a general rule, it seems likely that pre-existing differences between two groups in the general population may be expected to be reduced in selected samples to the extent that the selection process is biased toward the dominant group. In a case such as the present one, when both males and females are obtained from a setting in which women have been screened more stringently than men, then only the most able, assertive, and motivated women will have survived the selection process, and they may be acceptable in large part because they resemble the masculine standard.

## Relationships of Jealousy Response Styles to Other Jealousy Measures

There is one concern that remains in assessing the utility of these jealousy response styles: Are they, in fact, measures of jealousy? One approach to answering this question is to examine correlations between scores on these factors and scores on other measures of jealousy, such as self-descriptions (e.g., White, 1981b) or measures of how "upset" one would get summed across a set of jealousy-evoking situations, similar to Bringle's (1981) Interpersonal Jealousy Scale. To the degree that these different measures converge they may be considered to measure a common construct (e.g., White, 1984).

However, one might approach this question somewhat differently on behavioral or deterministic grounds. That is, one could argue that any behavior that regularly or consistently occurs after exposure to a particular stimulus is a response to that stimulus. Thus, if we agree that certain situations are jealousy-evoking, then any behavior that becomes more likely in those situations is by definition a jealousy response. This approach has considerable theoretical merit, for it allows us a measure of jealousy that is independent of subjects' personal definitions of what constitutes jealousy, which are fraught with semantic confusion (e.g., Salovey & Rodin, 1986; Smith, Kim, & Parrott, 1988), social desirability bias (e.g., White, 1981b), and problems of denial (Clanton & Smith, 1977).

Two alternative measures of jealousy were computed for each subject. One score, here termed Self-Description Jealousy, was equivalent to White's (1981b) phenomenological measure: Subjects' responses to five items reflecting a tendency to describe oneself as jealous were summed. A second score, Situational Jealousy, was obtained by summing subjects' reports of how "upset" they would be in each of 20 potentially jealousy-evoking situations, a method similar to that used by Bringle (1981) in his Interpersonal Jealousy Scale.

Correlations of Self-Description (SD) and Situational Jealousy (SIT) with each other and with scores for the nine factors were computed separately within each national sample. These values are presented in Table 8.3. As may be seen, the two self-report measures were significantly correlated in all five national samples, indicating that, across cultures, people who consider themselves to be jealous also tend to report that they would be more upset in a variety of jealousy-evoking situations. These two jealousy measures were also significantly correlated with Reaction to Betrayal, Emotional Devastation, and Reactive Retribution in all five countries. Aggression and Monitoring were significantly correlated with Situational Jealousy in all five countries, but with Self-Description Jealousy in only three countries each (France, the Netherlands, and Italy for Aggression; France, the Netherlands, and the United States for Monitoring). Relationship Improvement was the only remaining factor with at least half of the correlations attaining significance (with both measures in the Netherlands and the United States, and with Situational Jealousy in France). The remaining factors were not consistently correlated with either of these self-report jealousy measures, having three or fewer significant correlations across groups.

In essence, then, people who describe themselves as jealous or who report that they would be more upset across a variety of jealousy-evoking situations also tend to describe themselves as reacting to jealousy by feeling anger at the betrayal, by being emotionally devastated, by getting even, by aggressively confronting the partner and/or the other person or by monitoring the partner's activities, and, in some cultures, by trying to improve the relationship. However, people who react to jealousy situations by trying to hide their feelings, by blaming themselves, or by seeking the support of their friends are not necessarily likely to see themselves as jealous. One may view this as a shortcoming of these latter measures, in that they fail to manifest evidence of convergent validity.

**TABLE 8.3. Correlations of Self-Description (SD) and Situational (SIT) Jealousy Measures and Factor Scores**

| Response mode | France | | Germany | | Italy | | Netherlands | | United States | |
|---|---|---|---|---|---|---|---|---|---|---|
| | SD | SIT | SD | SIT | SD | SIT | SD | SIT | SD | SIT |
| Reaction to Betrayal | .20** | .40** | .28** | .37** | .32** | .54** | .36** | .53** | .21** | .35** |
| Emotional Devastation | .36** | .32** | .43** | .38** | .31** | .38** | .35** | .52** | .44** | .38** |
| Aggression | .28** | .42** | .11 | .25** | .19** | .34** | .33** | .48** | .05 | .41** |
| Impression Management | .02 | −.03 | .23** | .24** | .06 | −.02 | .15* | .21* | .05 | .00 |
| Reactive Retribution | .19* | .21* | .33** | .31** | .20** | .23** | .40** | .33** | .17* | .23** |
| Relationship Improvement | .16 | .20* | .07 | .13 | −.00 | .08 | .17* | .23** | .25** | .26** |
| Monitoring | .26** | .40** | .14 | .32** | .05 | .28** | .17* | .32** | .20** | .35** |
| Intropunitiveness | .03 | .02 | .00 | −.18* | .18* | −.09 | .18** | .06 | .10 | .04 |
| Social Support Seeking | .16 | .21* | .12 | .00 | .23** | .18* | .15* | .10 | .16* | .07 |
| Correlation of SD and SIT | | .52** | | .50** | | .36** | | .48** | | .47** |
| N = | 143 | | 127 | | 197 | | 208 | | 212 | |

*p < .05.
**p < .01.

196

Alternatively and more accurately, however, this may be considered as a shortcoming of the self-report measures, for they fail to provide an adequate representation of the variety of jealousy response styles defined by the empirical approach.

## DIMENSIONS OF JEALOUSY:
## A CONCEPTUAL ANALYSIS

The empirical approach to defining the dimensions of jealousy behaviors has provided important information regarding the range of responses available to the jealous individual. This approach has served to demonstrate and emphasize that jealousy cannot be adequately described by a single score on some scale. Instead, it is a complex of feelings and actions, of multiple modes of response, any part of which can be an expression or manifestation of jealousy, and which can be adequately described only by the use of multiple response indicators. The definition of these multiple response modes has allowed us an opportunity to define gender and nationality differences in their use. At the same time, the presence of eight or nine different types of jealousy reactions is theoretically unwieldy and hardly satisfying to a desire to simplify and organize these behaviors within a more general, theoretically derived conceptual structure that explains the mechanisms underlying the selection among responses.

However, one study (Shettel-Neuber et al., 1978) that employed multiple response scales to measure separate jealousy reaction styles provided some important insights into these underlying motivations. Subjects viewed a videotape of a presumably jealousy-evoking situation, in which the apparent return of a former boyfriend or girlfriend of one member of a couple constituted the jealousy threat. One of the interesting findings was that there was an interaction between sex of subject and the experimentally varied attractiveness of the interloper: Males became more likely, and females less likely, to seek retribution (e.g., go out with others) when the interloper was attractive. If we assume that an attractive interloper is seen as more threatening to the relationship, then as the threat increased males were more likely to seek solace or to bolster their self-esteem by pursuing alternative relationships. Under those conditions, however, females were less likely to engage in behaviors that would threaten the relationship.

This suggested that many, if not all, jealousy responses might be characterized in terms of two distinct, independent motivational goals: a desire to maintain the relationship, and a desire to maintain self-esteem

(Bryson, 1977). The relative influence or importance of these two motivations may be assumed to underlie one's choice of response to a jealousy-evoking situation. Some actions represent attempts to achieve both goals; others to achieve one goal, but at the expense of the second; and still others reflect a failure to strive for either goal. A representation of this structure is presented in Figure 8.3.

A desire to achieve both goals may be considered to be represented by some jealousy responses, such as communication, certain forms of confrontation, or relationship improvement. Other actions, such as emotional withdrawal from the relationship or intropunitiveness, do not seem to be directed toward achieving either goal. One may attempt to maintain self-esteem, but at the possible expense of losing or endangering the relationship, through such reactions as retribution or terminating the relationship. Conversely, one may attempt to maintain the relationship, but at the expense of self-esteem, by clinging, by emphasizing dependency on the partner, or by trying to act as if nothing has happened. It should be emphasized that the principal concern in classifying responses is not the likelihood that they will be successful in achieving their goals, but rather the motivations, however rational or irrational, that underlie the choice of that action.

White (1981b) incorporated these two motivations in his model of jealousy responses. In this model the primary appraisal of a jealousy-evoking situation is seen as involving the division of threat into two components: threat of loss of relationship rewards and threat of loss of self-esteem. Each of these components then contributes to determining the emotional and behavioral responses to the jealousy-evoking situation. Mathes, Adams, and Davies (1985) have extended this, demonstrating that these two threats do have different emotional consequences: Threats to the relationship cause depression, and threats to self-esteem cause anger.

My original thinking was that this dual-motivation model provided a reasonable framework for conceptualizing and explaining some of the sex differences in jealousy responses. Females, who for a variety of reasons have been socialized to be the relationship maintainers in our society (e.g., O'Leary, 1977), should be more likely to respond to jealousy with actions that attempt to maintain the relationship, even at the expense of self-esteem. Males, on the other hand, should be more inclined to respond with behaviors intended to preserve self-esteem, even at the expense of the relationship. White (1981b), in a somewhat different context, has reported effects consistent with these hypotheses: Self-reported male jealousy was found to be related to self-esteem but not to dependence on the relationship, while female self-reports of jealousy

RELATIONSHIP MAINTENANCE

|  | | *Yes* | *No* |
|---|---|---|---|
| **SELF-ESTEEM MAINTENANCE** | *Yes* | Communication<br><br>Relationship improvement | Retribution<br><br>Termination |
| | *No* | Emphasizing dependency<br><br>Impression management | Emotional withdrawal<br><br>Intropunitiveness |

**FIGURE 8.3.** Dual-motivation analysis of jealousy responses.

were correlated with dependence on the relationship but not with self-esteem.

Unfortunately, an initial empirical test failed to confirm these hypotheses (Rodgers & Bryson, 1978). Instead, females rather than males were more likely to report behaviors that maintained only self-esteem, and no gender effects were found for behaviors that attempted to maintain the relationship without regard to self-esteem. Because of these confusing results, and the lack of a satisfactory explanation for them, this model was put aside while work proceeded in other directions.

Recently, however, my interest in this model was revived upon learning of work by Rusbult (1987), in which she analyzed and classified different techniques that people use to respond to broadly defined "declines in relationship quality." Although the focus, theoretical basis, and methodology of her work differed substantially from that employed in my work on jealousy responses, there are remarkable similarities between her classification scheme and the dual-motivation model.

Rusbult defined two dimensions, constructive–destructive and active–passive, presumed to underlie responses to declines in relationship quality. The poles of these two dimensions combine to describe four distinct response classes: exit, voice, loyalty, and neglect (EVLN). A schematic representation of the EVLN model is presented in Figure 8.4. The destructive–constructive dimension seems virtually identical to the relationship maintenance dimension of the dual-motivation model. Although the active–passive dimension differs in intent from the self-esteem maintenance desire, the impact is similar: Active responses seem to be

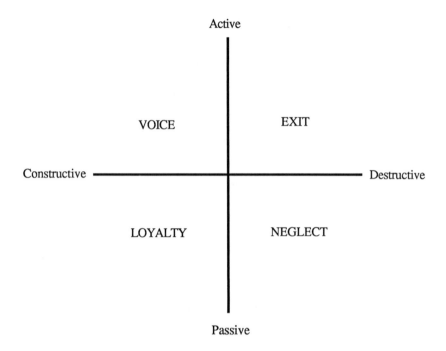

**FIGURE 8.4.** Dimensions and response modes in Rusbult's EVLN model.

self-esteem-enhancing, while passive responses fail to serve self-esteem needs.

The resultant modes of response defined by the two models also share a considerable conceptual overlap. Rusbult's descriptions of the four response modes serve to illustrate these similarities:

1. Exit (active/destructive): ending or threatening to end the relationship (i.e., actions that seek to maintain self-esteem, possibly at the expense of the relationship).
2. Voice (active/constructive): expressing one's dissatisfaction, with the intent of improving conditions (i.e., actions that seek to maintain both self-esteem and the relationship).
3. Loyalty (passive/constructive): waiting and hoping that conditions will improve (i.e., attempting to maintain the relationship, possibly at the expense of self-esteem).

4. Neglect (passive/destructive): allowing, but not actually causing, the relationship to atrophy (i.e., actions that are not directed toward either goal).

Rusbult (1987) has examined the adequacy of this model in describing responses to declines in relationship quality, and found support for predictions derived from the investment model for ongoing relationships (Rusbult, 1980). Prior satisfaction with and greater investment in a relationship increase the likelihood of constructive (voice and loyalty) responses and decrease the likelihood of destructive (exit and neglect) responses; higher alternative quality serves to increase the likelihood of active (voice and exit) responses, while lower alternative quality increases passive (loyalty and neglect) responses. In addition, Rusbult (1987) advanced some predictions regarding the role of gender in the likelihood of these responses: Females, because of their greater orientation toward relationship maintenance, should favor constructive responses (voice and loyalty), while males should be more likely to select destructive responses (exit and neglect). Although some support was found for these predictions (which are essentially equivalent to those made earlier for the dual-motivation model), the effects were not as large or consistent as those for the relationship quality variables.

Armed with this conceptual framework, we attempted to re-examine sex differences in responses to a particular kind of decline in relationship quality, that caused by jealousy-evoking situations (Bryson & Wehmeyer, 1988). Item analysis procedures were employed to develop separate four-item scales to measure each of the four response modes. Items comprising each of these scales are presented in Table 8.4. Subjects were instructed to indicate how likely they would be to perform each of these actions in a jealousy-evoking situation, and responses within each scale were summed for analyses. Sixteen separate versions of the jealousy scenario were constructed in a $2 \times 2 \times 2 \times 2$ design, varying level of investment in the relationship, prior satisfaction, alternative quality, and ambiguity of the jealousy-evoking situation. A fifth factor was defined by the sex of the subject, and different versions were written for each sex. Sixteen male and 16 female subjects responded to each of the situations in a complete factorial design; 13 subjects were subsequently eliminated for failure to follow directions, leaving a total $n$ of 499 subjects ($df = 1, 467$ for all analyses reported below). Separate analyses were conducted for each of the four response scales. Results of these analyses were remarkably straightforward: Across all four analyses, only 4 of 104 possible interaction terms achieved conventional significance levels. Likelihood of

## TABLE 8.4. EVLN Response Scale Items

*Exit*
   I would end the relationship.
   I would tell my boyfriend that I couldn't take it any more and our relationship
   was over.
   I would tell my boyfriend that he was not worth the trouble and heartache and
   I did not want to see him ever again.
   I would tell my boyfriend that I had had enough and did not want to put up
   with any more of his selfishness, and then leave.

*Voice*
   We would talk about why things had come to this point, what we needed to do
   to make things better, and proceed from there.
   I would sit down and talk things out with my boyfriend.
   I would ask my boyfriend what was wrong with our relationship.
   I would confront my boyfriend with my feelings.

*Loyalty*
   I would feel that I had invested too much of myself in this relationship to break
   it off, and would hope that he would come back to me.
   I would love my boyfriend enough that I would try to overlook what he had
   done.
   What would be important to me would be how I feel, not what others feel or
   say about my boyfriend, so I would stick by him.
   I would try to ignore what my boyfriend was doing and hope that he would .
   see how foolish it was and would come back to me.

*Neglect*
   I would feel that it really didn't matter if our relationship ended or got worse.
   I would emotionally withdraw to avoid getting hurt any more.
   I would probably just kind of quit; I wouldn't try to salvage the relationship.
   I would back off and let the relationship drift.

*Note.* This table presents the female version; appropriate modifications in sex-referenced
words were made for the male version.

each of these four types of responses does seem to be an additive function
of the independent variables employed here. Means associated with the
main effects for each independent variable are presented in Table 8.5.

Consistent with Rusbult's predictions, higher levels of investment in
the relationship made people more likely to use the constructive responses of voice ($F = 16.17$, $p < .001$) and loyalty ($F = 8.83$, $p < .01$),
and less likely to use neglect ($F = 23.56$, $p < .001$). Results for exit were
not significant, but were in the appropriate direction.

Results for prior satisfaction were also consistent with predictions in
three of four cases: Greater prior satisfaction resulted in less use of the
destructive responses of exit ($F = 11.27$, $p < .001$) and neglect ($F =$

8.16, $p < .01$), and increased use of loyalty ($F = 6.38$, $p < .05$). Greater prior satisfaction also led to somewhat more use of voice, as predicted, but this effect did not reach conventional significance levels.

In the present research, alternative quality did not have any significant influence on any of the response scales. However, it seems likely that our manipulation of this variable (i.e., an old boyfriend/girlfriend was either available or not) was too specific, and not sufficient to create the effects predicted by Rusbult.

Increased ambiguity of the jealousy situation resulted, as expected, in greater use of the constructive responses, voice ($F = 11.45$, $p < .001$) and loyalty ($F = 5.91$, $p < .05$); less ambiguity resulted in more destructive responses, exit ($F = 4.30$, $p < .05$) and Neglect ($F = 6.00$, $p < .05$).

Effects of subject gender, however, had some effects quite different from those predicted by Rusbult. Although females were, as predicted, more likely to report voice responses ($F = 3.97$, $p < .05$), the male subjects were more likely to endorse the other constructive response, loyalty ($F = 20.43$, $p < .001$). Also contrary to expectation, females

**TABLE 8.5. Determinants of Exit, Voice, Loyalty, and Neglect Responses**

| Variable | Level | Exit | Voice | Loyalty | Neglect |
|---|---|---|---|---|---|
| Investment in relationship | High | 22.38 | 21.77 | 14.79 | 18.68 |
|  | Low | 23.46 | 18.83 | 12.66 | 22.85 |
| $F (1, 467) =$ |  | 1.89 | 16.17*** | 8.83** | 23.56*** |
| Prior satisfaction | High | 21.47 | 20.97 | 12.80 | 21.76 |
|  | Low | 24.38 | 19.64 | 13.67 | 20.95 |
| $F (1, 467) =$ |  | 11.27*** | 2.07 | 6.38* | 8.16** |
| Alternative quality | High | 23.11 | 20.29 | 13.67 | 20.95 |
|  | Low | 22.74 | 20.32 | 13.78 | 20.58 |
| $F (1, 467) =$ |  | 0.15 | 0.41 | 0.01 | 0.34 |
| Situation ambiguity | High | 21.95 | 21.29 | 14.51 | 19.75 |
|  | Low | 23.90 | 19.32 | 12.94 | 21.78 |
| $F (1, 467) =$ |  | 4.30* | 11.45*** | 5.91* | 6.00* |
| Sex of subject | Male | 22.00 | 19.73 | 14.98 | 20.92 |
|  | Female | 23.85 | 20.88 | 12.47 | 20.60 |
| $F (1, 467) =$ |  | 4.84* | 3.97* | 20.43*** | 0.00 |

*$p < .05$.
**$p < .01$.
***$p < .001$.

were more likely than males to report the destructive exit responses ($F = 4.84$, $p < .05$). The sexes did not differ in endorsement of neglect items.

Although these gender effects are not consistent with the idea that women are socialized to be the relationship maintainers in our society, they are consistent with another line of research (e.g., Hagestad & Smyer, 1982; Hill, Rubin, & Peplau, 1976), which has found that women are more likely to end relationships, and men are more likely to have difficulty in dealing with termination. It may be that females are more likely to engage in relationship maintenance activities such as voice or loyalty in response to less severe or more chronic sources of dissatisfaction in relationships, but not in response to more acute or intense "crisis" events such as the jealousy situations employed here. Alternatively, it seems possible that males and females differ in attributions concerning the origins of these jealousy threats: If males are, in general, presumed to be the initiators of relationships (including those that are jealousy-evoking), then our female subjects are more likely to presume that their partners have initiated the situation, while our male subjects are more likely to blame this on the interlopers. What seems clear is that further research should be conducted to determine why these unexpected sex differences occur in response to jealousy situations, and to define the circumstances, if any, under which the opposite effects are obtained.

## CONCLUSION

This chapter has examined the variety of reactions that may occur when jealousy is evoked, and has described two distinct approaches that have been taken in the conduct of this research. Each approach, taken separately, provides a valuable perspective on the issue of responses to jealousy. However, the real strength of this research lies in the interaction between these two approaches—one focused on determining the different dimensions or varieties of modes of response to jealousy, and the other focused on the factors that underlie the selection of a particular mode.

The use of factor-analytic procedures to define dimensions of responses to jealousy-evoking situations represents the empirical approach to this topic. Subjects' responses are themselves employed to define the dimensions along which they vary, and different techniques may then be employed to compare groups on these dimensions. This approach has been useful in that it has served to demonstrate and emphasize that jealousy cannot be adequately described by a single score on some scale. Instead, it is a complex of feelings and actions, of multiple modes of response, any part of which can be an expression or manifestation of jealousy, and which can be adequately described only by the use of multiple response indicators.

The approach using multiple modes of response has also allowed a much more useful characterization of cultural influences on jealousy in terms of qualitative differences in the way that jealousy is expressed, rather than simply attempting to determine which group is the "most jealous." Further work in this area should focus on understanding the personal, relational, and situational factors that influence the likelihood of each response mode, or perhaps of sequences of these responses.

The conceptual or theoretical approach begins with the postulation of underlying structures or processes that influence the availability or desirability of various modes of response, and then examines situational or personal variables that moderate these influences. The correspondence between the modes of response described by combinations of attempts to maintain self-esteem and/or the relationship, and those postulated in Rusbult's (1987) analysis of responses to declines in relationship satisfaction, provides a measure of confidence in the direction of this research. However, considerably more work needs to be done to clarify the relationship between gender and response mode and to understand the personal and situational factors that influence one's choice of response mode. Finally, we should begin to turn our efforts toward examining outcomes, or understanding the effectiveness of each of these modes of response in preserving the integrity of the relationship and/or the psychological well-being of each of the individuals involved in a jealousy-evoking situation.

## NOTE

1. I would also like to express my gratitude to Gianvittorio Caprara, Universita di Roma; Martin Irle, Universität Mannheim; and Abraham Moles, Université de Strasbourg, for their assistance in making it possible for me to meet and collaborate with these colleagues.

## REFERENCES

Bringle, R. G. (1981). Conceptualizing jealousy as a disposition. *Alternative Lifestyles, 4,* 274–290.
Bringle, R. G., & Buunk, B. (1985). Jealousy and social behavior. *Review of Personality and Social Psychology, 6,* 241–265.

Bringle, R. G., Roach, S., Andler, C., & Evenbeck, S. (1979). *Correlates of jealousy.* Paper presented at the meeting of the Midwestern Psychological Association, Chicago.

Bryson, J. B. (1976). *The natures of sexual jealousy: An exploratory study.* Paper presented at the meeting of the American Psychological Association, Washington, DC.

Bryson, J. B. (1977). Situational determinants of the expression of jealousy. In H. Sigall (Chair), *Sexual jealousy.* Symposium presented at the meeting of the American Psychological Association, San Francisco.

Bryson, J. B., Alcini, P., Buunk, B., Marquez, L., Ribey, F., Rosch, M., Strack, F., & van den Hove, D. (1984). *A cross-cultural survey of jealousy behaviors in France, Germany, Italy, the Netherlands, and the United States.* Paper presented at the International Congress of Psychology, Acapulco, Mexico.

Bryson, J. B., & Wehmeyer, N. (1988). *The exit-voice-loyalty-neglect model and responses to jealousy.* Paper presented at the meeting of the Western Psychological Association, Reno, NV.

Bush, C. R., Bush, J. P., & Jennings, J. (1988). Effects of jealousy threats on relationship perceptions and emotions. *Journal of Social and Personal Relationships, 5,* 285–303.

Buunk, B. (1982). Strategies of jealousy: Styles of coping with extramarital involvement of the spouse. *Family Relations, 31,* 13–18.

Buunk, B., & Hupka, R. B. (1987). Cross-cultural differences in the elicitation of sexual jealousy. *Journal of Sex Research, 23,* 12–22.

Clanton, G., & Smith, L. G. (Eds.). (1977). *Jealousy.* Englewood Cliffs, NJ: Prentice-Hall.

Francis, J. (1977). Toward the management of sexual jealousy. *Journal of Marriage and the Family, 39,* 61–69.

Hagestad, G. O., & Smyer, M. A. (1982). Dissolving long-term relationships: Patterns of divorcing in middle age. In S. W. Duck (Ed.), *Personal relationships: Vol. 4. Dissolving relationships* (pp. 155–188). New York: Academic Press.

Hill, C. T., Rubin, Z., & Peplau, L. A. (1976). Breakups before marriage: The end of 103 affairs. *Journal of Social Issues, 32,* 147–168.

Hupka, R. B. (1981). Cultural determinants of jealousy. *Alternative Lifestyles, 4,* 310–356.

Hupka, R. B. (1984). Jealousy: Compound emotion or label for a particular situation? *Motivation and Emotion, 8,* 141–155.

Hupka, R. B., Buunk, B., Falus, G., Fulgosi, A., Ortega, E., Swain, R., & Tarabrina, N. V. (1985). Romantic jealousy and romantic envy: A seven nation study. *Journal of Cross-Cultural Psychology, 16,* 423–446.

Mathes, E. W., Adams, H. E., & Davies, R. M. (1985). Jealousy: Loss of relationship rewards, loss of self-esteem, depression, anxiety, and anger. *Journal of Personality and Social Psychology, 48,* 1552–1561.

Mathes, E. W., & Severa, N. (1981). Jealousy, romantic love, and liking: Theoretical considerations and preliminary scale development. *Psychological Reports, 49,* 23–31.

O'Leary, V. E. (1977). *Toward understanding women.* Monterey, CA: Brooks/ Cole.

Pfeiffer, S. M., & Wong, P. T. P. (1989). Multidimensional jealousy. *Journal of Social and Personal Relationships, 6,* 181–196.

Pines, A. M., & Aronson, E. (1983). Antecedents, correlates, and consequences of sexual jealousy. *Journal of Personality, 51,* 108–136.

Rodgers, M. A., & Bryson, J. B. (1978). *Self-esateem and relationship maintenance as responses to jealousy.* Paper presented at the meeting of the Western Psychological Association, San Francisco.

Rusbult, C. E. (1980). Commitment and satisfaction in romantic associations: A test of the investment model. *Journal of Experimental Social Psychology, 16,* 172–186.

Rusbult, C. E. (1987). Responses to dissatisfaction in close relationships: The exit–voice–loyalty–neglect model. In D. Perlman & S. W. Duck (Eds.), *Intimate relationships: Development, dynamics, and deterioration* (pp. 209–237). Beverly Hills, CA: Sage.

Salovey, P., & Rodin, J. (1986). The differentiation of social-comparison jealousy and romantic jealousy. *Journal of Personality and Social Psychology, 50,* 1100–1112.

Shettel-Neuber, J., Bryson, J. B., & Young, L. E. (1978). Physical attractiveness of the "other person" and jealousy. *Personality and Social Psychology Bulletin, 4,* 612–615.

Smith, R. H., Kim, S. H., & Parrott, W. G. (1988). Envy and jealousy: Semantic problems and experiential distinctions. *Personality and Social Psychology Bulletin, 14,* 401–409.

Sommers, S. (1984). Adults evaluating their emotions: A cross-cultural perspective. In C. Malatesta & C. Izard (Eds.), *Emotion in adult development* (pp. 319–338). Beverly Hills, CA: Sage.

White, G. L. (1980). Inducing jealousy: A power perspective. *Personality and Social Psychology Bulletin, 6,* 222–227.

White, G. L. (1981a). A model of romantic jealousy. *Motivation and Emotion, 5,* 295–310.

White, G. L. (1981b). Some correlates of romantic jealousy. *Journal of Personality, 49,* 129–147.

White, G. L. (1984). Comparison of four jealousy scales. *Journal of Research in Personality, 18,* 115–130.

# PART III

# FAMILY, SYSTEMS, AND CULTURE IN JEALOUSY AND ENVY

Jealousy and envy are experienced in the context of larger sociocultural structures, such as the family, ethnicity, and nationality. Gary Hansen believes that to understand jealousy, the focus of research should be on couples rather than individuals, because jealousy is likely when relationship loss is threatened and individuals perceive themselves as having few relationship alternatives. Hansen argues that jealousy should be considered from the standpoint of family stress theory. Like many stresses in families—divorce, death, relocation—jealousy creates ambiguity in family boundaries. In turn, jealousy can serve as a boundary-setting mechanism that demarcates important relationships like marriage.

Gregory White develops some of these themes further in his chapter. White advances a systems view of jealousy that emphasizes the importance of studying all three relationships in the jealousy triangle, as well as the manner in which these relationships are embedded in larger friendship and kinship systems. Jealousy can be viewed as a stabilizer of distressed systems, but also as an outside force that can rock systems that were previously stable.

Ralph Hupka discusses the importance of cultural variables in determining how and when jealousy is experienced. Although he acknowledges the importance of evolutionary factors in understanding jealousy, he argues that culture carries much more weight in determining the jealousy experience. Hupka argues that the capacity to experience jealousy is part of our human neuroanatomical and physiological "hardware" inherited through evolution, but that culture provides the "software" that determines which situations provoke jealousy and how it is manifested.

In the final chapter, Alexander Rothman and I argue that what is especially important to the self is what determines the situations in which one is vulnerable both to envy and to jealousy. People become envious when someone else has advantages that are seen as threatening to their self-definition—that "hit them where they live." Jealousy is instigated when relationships are threatened by rivals who have these self-defining qualities. A question, though, is this: What determines this sense of self? Rothman and I argue that both social-psychological variables and cultural pressures are important in determining what is self-relevant, and hence the experience of envy and jealousy.

## Chapter Nine

# Jealousy: Its Conceptualization, Measurement, and Integration with Family Stress Theory

GARY L. HANSEN
*University of Kentucky*

The past decade has seen unprecedented advances in the study of jealousy. There have been both efforts at theoretical development (e.g., McDonald, 1982; Reiss, 1986) and a proliferation of empirical studies of jealousy (e.g., Buunk, 1981, 1982a, 1982b, 1984; Buunk & Hupka, 1987; Hansen, 1982, 1983, 1985a, 1985b; White, 1980, 1981a, 1981b, 1981c). This emerging body of literature is characterized by a variety of theoretical and methodological approaches. The purpose of this chapter is to describe the particular conceptualization of jealousy I have employed in my research, the resulting measurement technique and research findings, and a proposal for integrating family stress and jealousy theory. Before doing so, however, I briefly review the nature of jealousy so that the consistency between my conceptualization of jealousy and what we know about its nature can be assessed.

## THE NATURE OF JEALOUSY

Bringle and Buunk (1985) point out that most contemporary conceptualizations of jealousy focus on situational antecedents to define it. This makes it possible to distinguish jealousy-evoking situations from envy situations. Jealousy is viewed as being precipitated by a threat from an agent to a person's relationship with someone, whereas envy is a negative reaction that is precipitated when someone else has a relationship to a person or object. Distinguishing between jealousy and envy does not mean that they cannot occur in the same situation; they can. The overlapping occurrence of the two phenomena does not suggest that one can be reduced to the other, however (Titelman, 1981).

I believe that jealousy is best viewed as a compound emotion (Hupka, 1984). It results from the situational labeling of one or more of the primary emotions such as fear or anger. Society teaches us to label the primary emotions we experience in specific situations that threaten our significant relationships as jealousy. In other words, the primary emotion words such as "anger" and "fear" *describe* the emotional state, whereas the compound emotion word ("jealousy") *explains* the emotional state (Hupka, 1984). Since individuals learn "explanations" during the process of socialization, this conceptualization of jealousy assumes that jealousy is a social phenomenon. It is at least partially learned, and it is manifested in response to symbolic stimuli that have meaning to the individual. The social aspects of jealousy have been noted by a number of writers. Among the most prominent is Davis (1936), who argues that a comprehensive conceptualization of jealousy must include the public or community element. Indeed, evidence indicates cross-cultural differences in the elicitation of jealousy in both preindustrial (Hupka, 1981; Reiss, 1986) and industrial (Buunk & Hupka, 1987) societies.

An example of sexual jealousy illustrates the distinction between primary emotions and the compound emotion of jealousy. A husband confesses to his wife that he recently had a one-time sexual relationship with another woman while away from home on a trip. Depending upon a variety of cultural, personal, and relational factors, the wife may experience either anger, fear, disgust, sadness, or a combination of such primary emotions. Assuming that the woman is typical of most individuals in Western society, she will interpret her husband's extramarital relationship as a threat to their marriage and will have learned that people experience jealousy in such situations. Therefore, she will explain her anger, fear, and other primary emotions in terms of jealousy.

A variety of specific definitions of "jealousy" are found in the literature. Clanton (1981) defines it as a protective reaction to a perceived threat to a valued relationship. McDonald (1982), taking a structural exchange perspective, views marital jealousy as the perceived threat of diminution or loss of the valued resources of the spouse. Bringle and Buunk (1985) define it as an aversive emotional reaction that occurs as the result of a partner's extradyadic relationship that is real, imagined, or considered likely to occur. Reiss (1986) presents a sociological or group perspective by defining jealousy as a boundary-setting mechanism for what the group feels are important relationships. For the purposes of the present discussion, an expanded version of Clanton's (1981) definition is used. Jealousy is a protective reaction to a perceived threat to a valued relationship, arising from a situation in which the partner's involvement with an activity and/or another person is contrary to the jealous person's definition of their relationship.[1]

## DUAL-FACTOR CONCEPTUALIZATION OF JEALOUSY

The definition presented above implies that two factors are necessary for a person to be jealous. The person must both (1) perceive his or her partner's actual or imagined involvement with an activity and/or another person as contrary to his or her definition of the relationship, and (2) perceive the relationship as valuable.[2] (See Figure 9.1.) Factor 1 acknowledges that how one subjectively defines a relationship is of fundamental importance in understanding jealousy. Others have noted the same thing. For example, Ellis and Weinstein (1986, p. 343) state, "Jealousy occurs when a third party threatens the arena of identification that *specifically defines the relationship* [emphasis in original]." The partner's behavior referred to in Factor 1 need not be sexual. Jealousy can arise from one's partner's being involved with children, professional colleagues, or solitary activities if such behavior is contrary to the jealous person's definition of their relationship and the relationship is valued. The importance of Factor 2 (viewing the relationship as valuable) in explaining jealousy is demonstrated by cross-cultural work, which finds that the importance of marriage or the value placed on it in a society is related to jealousy (Hupka, 1981; Reiss, 1986).

The following situation, which may or may not elicit jealousy, illustrates this dual-factor conceptualization of jealousy. A man's wife has become good friends with a coworker of the opposite sex whom the man does not know very well. His wife and her friend enjoy having lunch together, discussing their respective lives, and providing each other emotional support. Their relationship does not have a sexual component. If the man defines marriage as involving emotional exclusiveness, he may

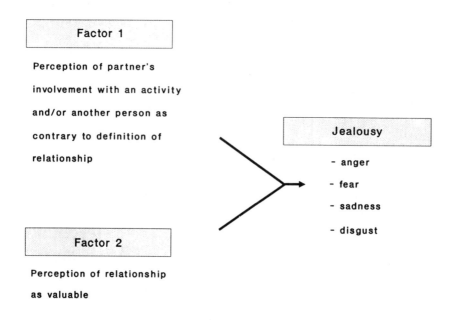

**FIGURE 9.1.** Dual-factor conceptualization of jealousy.

interpret his wife's behavior in this situation as contrary to marriage (Factor 1). If he also values the relationship with his wife (Factor 2), he will experience anger, fear, and so on, which will be explained as jealousy. On the other hand, he may not define his wife's behavior as conflicting with marriage. He may not view cross-sex friendships that provide emotional support outside of marriage as being inappropriate. In this case, he will not experience jealousy even if he values the marital relationship.

## *MEASUREMENT*

My technique for measuring jealousy (Hansen, 1982) is based on this dual-factor conceptualization. A series of hypothetical jealousy-producing events is used. The events, which are included in Table 9.1, describe the behavior of the research subject's partner in eight situations similar to the examples discussed above.[3] Subjects indicate how they would feel about their partner's behavior in each situation on a scale ranging from 1 ("extremely pleased") to 11 ("extremely disturbed or bothered").

## TABLE 9.1. Hypothetical Jealousy-Producing Events

1. Your mate has a job that requires him or her to work a normal 40 hours per week. In addition to working these 40 hours per week, your mate feels very committed to his or her job and devotes, on the average, an additional 10 hours per week to work-related activities that require him or her to go back to the office in the evenings and on weekends. Your mate does not receive extra pay for these activities.

2. Your mate enjoys a personal hobby (e.g., painting, photography, etc.) and devotes a large proportion of his or her leisure time (approximately 15 hours per week) to its pursuit. This hobby is one you do not share with your mate, so he or she engages in it alone. (The hobby does not impose a financial burden on your family.)

3. You and your mate have just had a baby. Your mate is very devoted to the child and concerned about its welfare. As a result of this devotion and concern, your mate devotes nearly all of his or her free time to playing with and taking care of the child, which has drastically reduced the amount of time you and your mate have for doing things alone with each other.

4. Your mate regularly enjoys playing cards or other types of games with his or her same-sex friends. Your mate's "night with the boys/girls" occurs about once a week.

5. Your mate has become good friends with a coworker of the opposite sex whom you do not know very well. Your mate and his or her friend enjoy having lunch together, discussing their respective lives, and providing each other emotional support. (Their relationship does not have a sexual component.)

6. You and your mate live in the same town as his or her parents and siblings. Your mate has set aside Sunday afternoons for doing things (e.g., going fishing, playing golf, visiting) with his or her family members. You do not participate with your mate in these activities with his or her family.

7. Your mate returns from a business trip to a different city and informs you that he or she met a member of the opposite sex that he or she found very physically attractive. They ended up engaging in sexual relations. Your mate informs you that their relationship was purely physical (not emotional) and that they will never be seeing each other again.

8. Your mate has developed an ongoing emotional and sexual relationship with a member of the opposite sex. Your mate receives a high degree of satisfaction from this relationship and plans to continue it. Both you and your mate have been happy and pleased with your own relationship. Your mate views his or her outside relationship as a supplment to, not a substitute for, the relationship between the two of you.

General words such as "pleased," "disturbed," and "bothered" are used because, as pointed out above, jealousy is a combination of emotions, and each situation is described so that the subject's partner is freely choosing to engage in the behavior described, enjoying it, and not directly affecting the welfare of the subject. If a subject reports that he or she would be disturbed by an event, the assumption can be made that he or she views the partner's behavior (involvement with an activity and/or another person) as contrary to his or her definition of their relationship (threatening to the relationship), rather than as a case of being angry over the partner's being forced to do something against his or her will or the like. Since the eight events represent a wide variety of behaviors by the partner, subject reaction to each one can be treated as a separate variable or summed to form a total jealousy score.

Hypothetical events are used, since research indicates that the use of hypothetical situations produces results similar to asking about the actual behavior of a subject's partner (White, 1981a) and that it is a better measure than asking people how jealous they are (Mathes, Roter, & Joerger, 1982). This is the case because jealousy measures that ask how jealous a subject is are associated with neuroticism and insecurity measures, and are probably contaminated by the social desirability response set (see Clanton & Kosins, Chapter 6, this volume, for more on this issue).

## RESEARCH FINDINGS

Research utilizing these jealousy-producing events indicates a wide range of subject reactions to them (Hansen, 1982, 1983, 1985a, 1985b, 1986). Involvement with a hobby (Event 2) and spending an evening a week with same-sex friends (Event 4) consistently elicit the least jealous responses, whereas, not surprisingly, the two events (7 and 8) involving extramarital sex evoke the most jealous responses. Jealous reactions to the partner's devoting extra time to work (Event 1) are relatively high, with mean values ranging from 7.52 (Hansen, 1986) to 8.25 (Hansen, 1985b). Similarly, mean values for the development of a cross-sex friendship (Event 5) range from 6.39 (Hansen, 1985b) to 8.92 (Hansen, 1983). Considering the degree of commitment required for success in many professions and the myriad opportunities for the development of cross-sex friendships, these findings indicate that jealousy is likely to arise and be a major issue in many marriages.

The events that elicit significantly different reactions from males and females are those in which the partner is involved with a hobby

(Event 2), same-sex friends (Event 4), or family members (Event 6) (Hansen, 1985a, 1985b, 1986). These events all involve time commitments, with females reacting in a more jealous manner than males. Even though the sex differences are relatively small, they are consistent with the findings in other work (Teismann & Mosher, 1978) that females seem to feel that the loss of time and attention is more threatening than do males.

My research has consistently found a positive association between a traditional gender-role orientation and jealousy (Hansen, 1982, 1985a, 1985b, 1986). Traditional gender-role attitudes, particularly the "division of labor" associated with such gender roles, seem to foster dependency and a sense of personal inadequacy. The resulting fear of facing the world alone increases the probability of an individual's perceiving his or her partner's involvement in jealousy-producing events as personally threatening.

A related finding involves self-esteem. In my research, low self-esteem is associated with jealousy for women, but not for men (Hansen, 1985b). This sex difference may be due to women's traditionally greater ego involvement in marriage and family life. If a woman's self-esteem is significantly tied up with her marriage, a woman with low self-esteem is more likely to perceive her husband's involvements with hobbies, other people, and so on as personally threatening than is a woman with high self-esteem.

There appears to be a complex relationship between marital adjustment and jealousy. Studies that have examined the relationship between adjustment and total jealousy (total responses to all eight events) find no relationship between the two (Hansen, 1985b, 1986). Neither is the level of rewards received from the relationship related to jealousy (Hansen, 1985b). "Marital alternatives," which refer to a person's perceptions of how much better or worse off he or she would be without the present spouse and how easily that spouse could be replaced with one of comparable quality, are negatively related to jealousy, however. It appears that regardless of the actual quality of marriage, individuals who view themselves as having few alternatives to their present marriages are more likely to experience jealousy. Therefore, it appears that the importance of marital adjustment and reward level lies in how they affect an individual's perception of his or her alternatives to the present relationship, rather than how they directly affect jealousy.

Other findings are significant both for what they do and for what they do not show. There is a strong positive relationship between religiosity and jealousy (Hansen, 1986), whereas both romanticism (Hansen, 1982) and trust (Hansen, 1985b) are not related to it. These results raise questions about two common assumptions concerning jealousy: They fail to support the belief that jealousy and romantic love are intimately linked, as well as the assumption that trust decreases the probability of jealousy.

## INTEGRATING FAMILY STRESS THEORY AND JEALOUSY THEORY

In many respects, the study of jealousy and seemingly related aspects of interpersonal relationships have developed independently, with very little (if any) overlap. This is particularly noticeable for the area of family stress, which can be thought of as an upset in the steady state of the family. According to Boss (1987, p. 695), "It may be as mild as a bat flying around the house or as severe as a holocaust; it includes anything that may disturb the family, cause uneasiness, or exert pressure on the family system." If a flying bat can upset the steady state of a family, surely the proverbial rearing of the "green-eyed monster's" ugly head can too. When a partner becomes jealous, both partners experience stress, and they must cope with it if they are to function effectively as a couple. Despite the obvious link between jealousy and stress, and despite the fact that the two bodies of literature use similar concepts and terminology, jealousy is seldom mentioned within the family stress literature, and jealousy work (while sometimes discussing coping) rarely cites the family stress literature. Utilizing the dual-factor conceptualization discussed above, the rest of this chapter makes a preliminary attempt to integrate family stress and jealousy theory by viewing jealousy as a special case of stress. More specifically, jealousy is viewed as an individual's emotional response to a specific type of boundary ambiguity.[4]

The concept of "boundary ambiguity" was outlined and developed in a series of studies and publications by Boss (Boss & Greenberg, 1984). Boss (1987) argues that family boundary ambiguity is one of the more encompassing stress variables that explains and predicts the effect of a variety of family stressor events. The term refers to a situation in which family members are uncertain in their perception of who is in or out of the family or who is performing what roles and tasks within the family system (Boss & Greenberg, 1984). High boundary ambiguity occurs in one of two types of situations. First, it occurs when a family member is physically absent and psychologically present. Cases of this kind of ambiguity studied by Boss and her associates include families in which a parent has died, families of men missing in action in Vietnam, divorced families, and families of adolescents who have left home (Boss, Pearce-

McCall, & Greenwood, 1986). Boundary ambiguity also occurs when a family member is physically present and psychologically absent. A case of this type of ambiguity is a family in which a member has Alzheimer's disease and is being cared for at home.

A family's perception of a stressor event and the meaning members give it are critical in determining family membership. Therefore, Boss (1987) argues that the C factor (perception of the stressor event) of Hill's (1958) ABCX model of family stress is the crucial factor in determining both the existence and degree of boundary ambiguity.[5] In other words, it is the congruence between the members' psychological perception of who is in and who is out with the physical reality of who is in and who is out of the system that determines the extent of ambiguity.

I believe that a person experiences boundary ambiguity whenever he or she defines a partner's involvement with an activity and/or another person as conflicting with their relationship. In other words, if Factor 1 of the dual-factor conceptualization of jealousy is present, the person experiences boundary ambiguity. Using the previous example of a man whose wife has developed a cross-sex friendship, we can think of the situation as follows: If the wife's behavior (development of a close friendship with a coworker of the opposite sex) conflicts with the husband's definition of marriage, the husband begins to view the wife as psychologically absent. Simply stated, the husband reasons that "you just don't do that" when you are married. The fact that his wife has done it (become good friends with another man) calls her commitment to the marriage into question. Her "psychological presence" is questionable, even though the relationship (physical presence of the wife) continues. His emotional response, if he also values the relationship (Factor 2 of the dual-factor conceptualization), is jealousy, and we can think of him as having experienced jealousy-producing boundary ambiguity.

Viewing jealousy as the emotional response one experiences in a particular type or situation of boundary ambiguity is not a radical or dramatic departure from previous work on either jealousy or family stress. Although jealousy theorists and researchers have not explicitly addressed the issue of boundary ambiguity, a number have included, either explicitly or implicitly, the idea of a boundary in their conceptualizations of jealousy. Reiss's (1986) definition, which defines jealousy as a boundary-setting mechanism, has already been presented. He contends that jealousy performs the function of defining the legitimate boundaries of important relationships such as marriage. Jealousy occurs when those normative boundaries are violated. Two types of jealousy were described by Davis (1936): "Jealousy of rivalry" arises from a legitimate competition for desired property, whereas "jealousy of trespass" is a reaction to the perceived threat of illegitimate loss of a partner. Obviously, jealousy of rivalry would occur in the early stages of dating, but jealousy of trespass most likely would occur in marriage. The idea of trespass itself implies the crossing of a boundary.

Just as some jealousy work has included the idea of a boundary, other work has at least hinted at the idea of ambiguity. For example, McDonald (1982) views jealous behavior in marriage as an attempt to restore the spouse's commitment by increasing *certainty* through reassurance, ultimatums, negotiation, removing available alternatives, and so on. This view is consistent with the idea of jealousy's arising in specific types of situations characterized by boundary ambiguity.

Boss (1987) does not specifically mention jealousy in her discussion of boundary ambiguity, but her description of physical presence with psychological absence outlines a situation that most would agree is likely to produce it. The situation occurs when a family is technically intact but a member is psychologically absent (e.g., preoccupied with work, alcohol or drugs, or another person). The word "preoccupied" may be too strong for the situation that produces the type of jealousy-producing boundary ambiguity under consideration here. A married individual does not have to be preoccupied with another person for his or her spouse to define the individual's behavior with that other person as inconsistent with marriage, and to question the individual's commitment to their relationship. However, just as it is not a major departure from previous jealousy work, the view presented here is not a major departure from Boss's (1987) conceptualization of boundary ambiguity.

## COPING WITH JEALOUSY-PRODUCING BOUNDARY AMBIGUITY

If, as argued above, "jealousy" refers to the emotional responses people have to a specific type of family stress arising from boundary ambiguity, it should be possible to interpret jealous behavior (ways of coping) in terms of general conceptualizations of coping within the stress literature. For the present discussion, "coping" is defined as any response to external life strains that serves to prevent, avoid, or control emotional distress (Pearlin & Schooler, 1982).

Lazarus (1977) conceives of the coping process as being the result of the interaction of three factors (cognitive appraisal, emotional reaction, and coping behavior) as diagrammed across the top of Figure 9.2. As we work backwards from right to left, coping responses or behaviors can be either direct action behaviors or intrapsychic forms of coping (Lazarus,

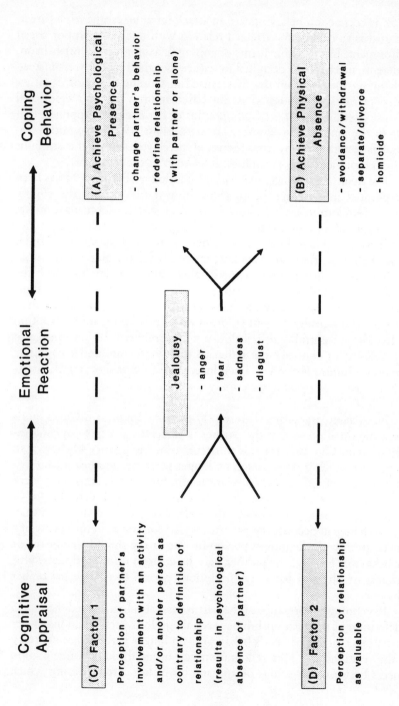

**FIGURE 9.2.** Process of coping with jealousy-producing boundary ambiguity.

1976). Direct action behaviors are an attack on or an escape from threat. The goal is to change the stressed relation with one's physical or social environment. Intrapsychic forms of coping behavior, on the other hand, are defense mechanisms designed to reduce the emotional distress instead of changing the situation that has caused it. Coping behavior of either variety (actions or thoughts) is not based upon a person's emotional response itself; rather, it is based upon his or her cognitive appraisal that leads to the emotional response (Lazarus, 1966, 1977). Cognitive appraisal is determined by the degree of perceived threat, the stimulus configuration, and the psychological makeup of the individual.

The dual-factor conceptualization of jealousy (Figure 9.1) has been incorporated into Figure 9.2 to show how it fits in with the coping process. Obviously, both Factors 1 and 2 of that conceptualization are components of an individual's cognitive appraisal of a jealousy-producing situation, while jealousy is his or her emotional reaction to it. Under coping behavior, there are two alternatives. Since the ambiguous situation that results in a person's experiencing jealousy is one in which the partner is physically present but psychologically absent, the jealous person can cope by modifying the situation so that the partner becomes either psychologically present (Option A) or physically absent (Option B). In either case, ambiguity/jealousy will be reduced. Jealousy can also be prevented or controlled at either of the two factors under cognitive appraisal (Options C and D). Therefore, there are a total of four theoretical alternatives or options for coping with jealousy.

A. *Achieve psychological presence of partner.* Option A involves modifying the situation so that the partner is perceived as being psychologically present. One way for this to occur is for the partner's behavior to change so that the jealous person no longer perceives it as being contrary to his or her definition of their relationship. Presumably, this may occur for a number of reasons. First, the partner may simply discern that his or her behavior disturbs or bothers the jealous person, and therefore may stop or change it. Second, the partner may be convinced in the course of a conversation with the jealous person that he or she should change his or her behavior. Finally, the partner may be coerced through threats, ultimatums, or physical force by the jealous person to change his or her behavior.

Psychological presence of the partner can also be achieved through a redefinition of the relationship between the jealous person and his or her partner, so that the partner's behavior is no longer perceived as contrary to the relationship. This redefinition can occur through a negotiation process between the jealous person and his or her partner during which the boundaries of their relationship are redrawn, so that the partner's behavior no longer falls outside of them. On the other hand, the redefinition process may be a solitary activity on the part of the jealous person. As the person thinks about the situation, he or she may decide that the partner's behavior is really acceptable in a relationship such as theirs after all.

The broken arrow from "Achieve Psychological Presence" in Figure 9.2 back to Factor 1 of the jealousy conceptualization indicates that Option A reduces jealousy by creating a situation in which Factor 1 is no longer present.

B. *Achieve physical absence of partner.* Option B involves reducing jealousy by creating a situation in which the jealous person's partner becomes physically, as well as psychologically, absent. One way this can be done is through avoidance of or withdrawal from the partner. In this case, the jealous person begins to act as if his or her partner is not present, even if the relationship actually continues. At best, the jealous person "goes through the motions" of interacting with the partner, while their relationship is devitalized, if not dead. Other methods of creating physical absence are more straightforward: The jealous person can simply end the relationship. Examples include divorce and homicide.

The broken arrow from "Achieve Physical Absence" in the figure back to Factor 2 indicates that Option B reduces jealousy by creating a situation in which Factor 2 is greatly, if not totally, diminished. In other words, the jealous person creates a situation in which he or she no longer perceives the relationship as very valuable.

C. *Change perception of partner's behavior.* A third way of coping with jealousy, Option C, is for the jealous person to alter his or her perception of the partner's involvement with the activity and/or other person so that it is no longer contrary to his or her definition of the relationship. In this case, the jealous person does not redefine the relationship; neither does the partner change his or her behavior. The jealous person's perception of the partner's behavior simply changes. Examples include denial that the partner's behavior actually occurred, altered perceptions of the circumstances surrounding the partner's behavior, and changes in the motives attributed to the partner by the jealous person. As in the case of redefining the relationship, changed perceptions of the partner's behavior may be the product either of interaction between the jealous person and his or her partner or of a solitary cognitive process on the part of the jealous individual.

This coping option can be illustrated with the previous example of the man whose wife develops a cross-sex friendship with a coworker. If the husband initially assumes that his wife has developed the friendship because she finds her coworker physically attractive, he may define her behavior as being contrary to his definition of marriage and experience jealousy. If after discussing the situation with his wife, however, he believes that she has developed the friendship because her coworker understands the personalities involved in office politics and is supportive of her efforts to deal with a tense work environment, he may no longer perceive her behavior as contrary to his definition of marriage, and he will have coped with the jealousy.

D. *Change perception of relationship value.* A final method of coping, Option D, is to devalue the relationship. In this case, the jealous person does not feel that the relationship is worth very much any more. He or she becomes indifferent. He or she does not really care what happens to it. Therefore, the person does not experience an emotional reaction when the partner's behavior is contrary to his or her definition of the relationship.

Family stress theorists acknowledge that coping techniques can be either functional or dysfunctional for the overall family system. With one important exception, Options A (achieve psychological presence) and C (change perception of partner's behavior) are generally functional from the viewpoint of "the family," whereas Options B (achieve physical absence) and D (change perception of relationship value) are generally dysfunctional. The exception is the use of threats, ultimatums, or physical force to coerce the partner to change his or her behavior. Although this is included under Option A, it should not be considered a functional method of coping with jealousy.[6]

It is beyond the scope of this chapter to provide a comprehensive review of the coping literature; however, it is possible to review some of the jealousy work to see whether the theoretical coping options outlined above actually have been observed. Buunk (1982b) examined the ways in which people cope with extramarital relationships of their spouses. Based upon a factor analysis of questionnaire items assessing coping styles, he identified three strategies: Avoidance (of the spouse), Reappraisal (of the situation), and Communication. The Avoidance factor included such things as considering the possibility of leaving the spouse, avoidance, and retreating, most of which would fall under what I have here called Option B (achieve physical absence). Reappraisal is another individual strategy, which refers to cognitive attempts to reduce one's jealousy. Buunk's Reappraisal factor included a critical attitude toward one's own jealousy, as well as direct attempts to get the jealousy under control by relativizing the whole situation. Generally, the techniques included in this strategy are examples of a solitary redefinition of the relationship with the partner and would be included under the present Option A (achieve psychological presence). Finally, the most common strategy, Communication, would reduce jealousy through either Option A or Option C, depending upon whether it results in a redefinition of the relationship or a changed perception of the partner's behavior.

Consistent with the present view that the coping options are either functional (Options A and C) or dysfunctional (Options B and D), Buunk (1982b) found that the Communication factor was positively related with marital satisfaction, whereas the Avoidance factor was negatively related to it. Francis (1977) reached a similar conclusion when she identified the development of communication skills as the appropriate treatment mode for sexual jealousy.

Although Buunk's study did not identify a coping strategy that fits the present Option D (change perception of relationship value), support for its inclusion as a viable alternative for coping with jealousy comes from preliminary results of a survey reported by Salovey and Rodin (1985), which indicated that "selective ignoring," defined as simply deciding that the desired object is not that important, is a coping strategy used by some.

Most recent jealousy studies have not investigated the extreme techniques of coping with jealousy, such as the use of physical force and homicide. Studies of family violence leave little doubt that they occur frequently, however. For example, Daly, Wilson, and Weghorst (1982) reviewed several studies of spousal homicide (Chimbos, 1978; Guttmacher, 1955) that used data beyond those found in police files, and concluded that male sexual jealousy may be the major source of conflict in an overwhelming majority of spousal homicides in North America. Similarly, numerous studies have noted the prevalence of jealousy as a motive in nonfatal wife abuse (e.g., Dobash & Dobash, 1979; Hilberman & Munson, 1978; Rounsaville, 1978; Whitehurst, 1971) and courtship violence (e.g., Makepeace, 1981).

Finally, a number of social-psychological studies provide some insight into some of the cognitive processes that may be involved as people cope with jealousy by changing their perceptions of their partners' behavior (Option C). Studies by White (1981a) and Buunk (1984) indicate that perceived motives or attributions for the partner's behavior are related to jealousy. Therefore, changes in perceived motives or attributions can reduce jealousy. In addition, Schmitt (1988) found that jealous people derogate their rivals on attributes they perceive to be important to their partners, but not on attributes perceived as less important to their partners. He concludes that derogation of the rival may be a way of coping with threats to a valuable relationship. These studies demonstrate that there are indeed a number of ways to reduce jealousy cognitively without either redefining the relationship or changing the partner's behavior.

## IMPLICATIONS FOR FUTURE STUDY

This chapter has summarized my particular conceptualization of jealousy, measurement technique, research program, and proposal for integrating family stress and jealousy theory. I feel that these efforts have a number of implications for the study of jealousy. The most important is that future work on jealousy should not occur in isolation from work on family stress. An established body of family stress theory and research findings exists within family studies. For example, Boss et al. (1986) present a number of theoretical propositions based on over a decade of boundary ambiguity research and theory development. Such work can provide a conceptual and theoretical basis for and an interpretation of further work on jealousy.

There are also a number of implications concerning what specific issues and topics should be addressed in the future. Identifying correlates of jealousy is one area where jealousy research already has begun to produce a substantial body of findings that are relatively consistent for some variables. For example, a number of studies have found positive associations between jealousy and relationship dependency and/or lack of alternatives for one or both sexes (Bringle & Evenbeck, 1979; Buunk, 1982a; Hansen, 1985b; White, 1981b) and between jealousy and sex-role traditionalism for one or both sexes (Hansen, 1982, 1985a, 1985b; White, 1981c). For many other variables, however, findings are either inconsistent or too few in number to allow a pattern to emerge. Clearly, there is still a need for studies designed to identify which personality characteristics, attitudes, and relationship characteristics are associated with jealousy. In other words, we need to know what type of individual is likely to perceive his or her partner's behavior as contrary to the definition of their relationship in a variety of typical jealousy-producing situations.

There is also a need for more work on coping strategies. Future work could examine the factors that influence which coping option a jealous person pursues and whether or not he or she uses the same coping strategies in other stressful situations. Considering how limited our current knowledge is on what I have referred to as Option C (change perception of partner's behavior), there is a particular need for more studies along the lines of those of White (1981a) on perceived motives and Buunk (1984) on attributions. In a related area, there is a need to identify coping resources that are particularly effective in coping with jealousy. Very few resources beyond the always-mentioned "communication" have been specifically identified in the jealousy literature.

In addition to research, there is a need for further theoretical development and elaboration. For example, the model for coping with jealousy-producing boundary ambiguity outlined here does not consider two important issues. It does not consider the partner's role in coping with jealousy. It also does not consider the family's cultural context, which can influence both how individuals perceive jealousy-producing events and how they define their relationships. Consideration of these issues could prove quite fruitful.

If family stress and jealousy theory can be integrated, there are important implications for work on family stress as well as for work on jealousy. Most importantly, family stress theorists and researchers should no longer neglect or ignore jealousy. It occurs frequently in families, it exerts pressure on the family system, and family members are struggling to cope with it.

## NOTES

1. Expanding Clanton's (1981) definition by specifying the type of situation producing a threat to a valued relationship makes it possible to distinguish jealousy from other "protective reactions to a perceived threat to a valued relationship" that clearly do not constitute jealousy (e.g., a wife trying to get her reluctant husband to see a doctor about a serious medical condition).

2. Except for the fact that the wording of Factor 1 reflects the expanded version of Clanton's (1981) definition of jealousy rather than the original one, the dual-factor conceptualization of jealousy discussed here is identical to the one I have outlined in previous work (Hansen, 1982, 1985b).

3. The present versions of the events are worded to refer to a marital relationship. Minor revisions allow for the study of jealousy in other types of relationships, however. For example, "dating partner" has been substituted for "mate" in five of the events in order to study dating jealousy (Hansen, 1985a).

4. The following effort to integrate family stress and jealousy theory was first elaborated in a 1988 paper (Hansen, 1988).

5. Hill's (1958) influential ABCX model of family stress focuses on three variables: (A) the stressor event, (B) the family's crisis-meeting resources, and (C) the definition the family makes of the event. The "X" is the stress or crisis that results from the interaction of A, B, and C.

6. Any attempt to classify coping options as categorically functional or dysfunctional is highly arbitrary and should be made with great caution. In this

case, options that usually maintain the family unit without using physical force or coercion are considered functional for "the family system," whereas others are considered dysfunctional. This does not deny the fact that some options classified as dysfunctional for the family system may be quite functional for individual family members, and vice versa. For example, divorce, which is considered dysfunctional here, is less stressful for many individuals than remaining in a dysfunctional relationship is (Bloom, Asher, & White, 1978).

## REFERENCES

Bloom, B. L., Asher, S. J., & White, S. W. (1978). Marital disruption as a stressor: A review and analysis. *Psychological Bulletin, 85*, 867–894.

Boss, P. (1987). Family stress: Perceptions and context. In M. B. Sussman & S. Steinmetz (Eds.), *Handbook of marriage and the family* (pp. 695–723). New York: Plenum.

Boss, P., & Greenberg, J. (1984). Family boundary ambiguity: A new variable in family stress theory. *Family Process, 23*, 535–546.

Boss, P., Pearce-McCall, D., & Greenberg, J. (1986). *The measurement of boundary ambiguity.* Unpublished manuscript.

Bringle, R. G., & Buunk, B. (1985). Jealousy and social behavior. A review of person, relationship, and situational determinants. In P. Shaver (Ed.), *Review of personality and social psychology: Vol. 6. Self, situations, and social behavior* (pp. 241–264). Beverly Hills, CA: Sage.

Bringle, R. G., & Evenbeck, S. (1979). The study of jealousy as a dispositional characteristic. In M. Cook & G. Wilson (Eds.), *Love and attraction* (pp. 201–204). New York: Pergamon.

Buunk, B. (1981). Jealousy in sexually open marriages. *Alternative Lifestyles, 4*, 357–372.

Buunk, B. (1982a). Anticipated sexual jealousy: Its relationship to self-esteem, depenency, and reciprocity. *Personality and Social Psychology Bulletin, 8*, 310–316.

Buunk, B. (1982b). Strategies of jealousy: Styles of coping with extramarital involvement of the spouse. *Family Relations, 31*, 13–18.

Buunk, B. (1984). Jealousy as related to attributions for the partner's behavior. *Social Psychology Quarterly, 47*, 107–112.

Buunk, B., & Hupka, R. B. (1987). Cross-cultural differences in the elicitation of sexual jealousy. *Journal of Sex Research, 23*, 12–22.

Chimbos, P. D. (1978). *Marital violence: A study of interspouse homicide.* San Francisco: R & E Research Associates.

Clanton, G. (1981). Frontiers of jealousy research: Introduction to the special issue on jealousy. *Alternative Lifestyles, 4*, 259–273.

Daly, M., Wilson, M., & Weghorst, S. J. (1982). Male sexual jealousy. *Ethology and Sociobiology, 3*, 11–27.

Davis, K. (1936). Jealousy and sexual property. *Social Forces, 14,* 395-405.
Dobash, R. E., & Dobash, R. (1979). *Violence against wives: A case against the patriarchy.* New York: Free Press.
Ellis, C., & Weinstein, E. (1986). Jealousy and the social psychology of emotional experience. *Journal of Social and Personal Relationships, 3,* 337-357.
Francis, J. L. (1977). Toward the management of heterosexual jealousy. *Journal of Marriage and Family Counseling, 3,* 61-69.
Guttmacher, M. S. (1955). Criminal responsibility in certain homicide cases involving family members. In P. H. Hoch & J. Zubin (Eds.), *Psychiatry and the law.* New York: Grune & Stratton.
Hansen, G. L. (1982). Reactions to hypothetical, jealousy-producing events. *Family Relations, 31,* 513-518.
Hansen, G. L. (1983). Marital satisfaction and jealousy among men. *Psychological Reports, 52,* 363-366.
Hansen, G. L. (1985a). Dating jealousy among college students. *Sex Roles, 12,* 713-721.
Hansen, G. L. (1985b). Perceived threats and marital jealousy. *Social Psychology Quarterly, 48,* 262-268.
Hansen, G. L. (1986). *Cognitive reasoning and reactions to jealousy-producing events.* Paper presented at the annual meeting of the National Council on Family Relations, Detroit.
Hansen, G. L. (1988). *Integrating family stress and jealousy theory: Is boundary ambiguity the key?* Paper presented at the National Council on Family Relations Preconference Theory Construction and Research Methodology Workshop, Philadelphia.
Hilberman, E., & Munson, K. (1978). Sixty battered women. *Victimology: An International Journal, 2,* 460-470.
Hill, R. (1958). Generic features of families under stress. *Social Casework, 49,* 139-150.
Hupka, R. B. (1981). Cultural determinants of jealousy. *Alternative Lifestyles, 4,* 310-356.
Hupka, R. B. (1984). Jealousy: Compound emotion or label for a particular situation? *Motivation and Emotion, 8,* 141-155.
Lazarus, R. S. (1966). *Psychological stress and the coping process.* New York: McGraw-Hill.
Lazarus, R. S. (1976). *Patterns of adjustment* (3rd ed.). New York: McGraw-Hill.
Lazarus, R. S. (1977). Cognitive and coping processes in emotion. In A. Monat & R. S. Lazarus (Eds.), *Stress and coping* (pp. 145-158). New York: Columbia University Press.
Mathes, E. W., Roter, P. M., & Joerger, S. M. (1982). A convergent validity study of six jealousy scales. *Psychological Reports, 50,* 1143-1147.
Makepeace, J. M. (1981). Courtship violence among college students. *Family Relations, 30,* 97-102.
McDonald, G. W. (1982, October). *Marital jealousy: A structural exchange perspec-*

*tive*. Paper presented at the National Council on Family Relations Preconference Theory Construction and Research Methodology Workshop, Washington, DC.

Pearlin, L. I., & Schooler, C. (1982). The structure of coping. In H. I. McCubbin, A. E. Cauble, & J. M. Patterson (Eds.), *Family stress, coping, and social support* (pp. 109–135). Springfield, IL: Charles C Thomas.

Reiss, I. L. (1986). *Journey into sexuality: An exploratory voyage.* Englewood Cliffs, NJ: Prentice-Hall.

Rounsaville, B. J. (1978). Theories in marital violence: Evidence from a study of battered women. *Victimology: An International Journal, 3,* 11–31.

Salovey, P., & Rodin, J. (1985, September). The heart of jealousy. *Psychology Today,* pp. 22–29.

Schmitt, B. H. (1988). Social comparison in romantic jealousy. *Personality and Social Psychology Bulletin, 14,* 374–387.

Teismann, M. W., & Mosher, D. L. (1978). Jealous conflict in dating couples. *Psychological Reports, 42,* 1211–1216.

Titelman, P. (1981). A phenomenological comparison between envy and jealousy. *Journal of Phenomenological Psychology, 12,* 189–204.

White, G. L. (1980). Inducing jealousy: A power perspective. *Personality and Social Psychology Bulletin, 6,* 222–227.

White, G. L. (1981a). Jealousy and partner's perceived motives for attraction to a rival. *Social Psychology Quarterly, 44,* 24–30.

White, G. L. (1981b). Relative involvement, inadequacy, and jealousy. *Alternative Lifestyles, 4,* 291–309.

White, G. L. (1981c). Some correlates of romantic jealousy. *Journal of Personality, 49,* 129–147.

Whitehurst, R. N. (1971). Violence potential in extramarital sexual responses. *Journal of Marriage and the Family, 33,* 683–691.

## Chapter Ten

# Self, Relationship, Friends, and Family: Some Applications of Systems Theory to Romantic Jealousy

GREGORY L. WHITE
*Shasta Community Mental Health, Redding, California*

In our recent book on jealousy, Paul Mullen and I suggest some applications of general systems theory to romantic jealousy (White & Mullen, 1989, pp. 14–16). In this chapter, I discuss in more detail systems theory perspectives on aspects of romantic jealousy. This analysis may open up some directions for future research, and I hope that it will be helpful in planning treatment of jealous persons and relationships. Although my comments are in part guided by systems theory, the impetus toward understanding the larger relational contexts of jealousy has come from my clinical experience in counseling individuals, couples, and families troubled by jealous conflicts.

I first briefly present the definition and model of romantic jealousy that Mullen and I have developed in some detail in our work. I reiterate our distinction of normal from pathologically reactive and symptomatic jealousies. Then relevant concepts from various systems theories are presented, along with applications of these concepts to the problem of romantic jealousy. Many of these applications are hypotheses or informed guesses about the role jealousy plays in different systems, or the way in which system aspects affect the development and nature of jealousy. The chapter ends with consideration of some ways in which jealousy, particularly jealousy coping, may be involved with both maintenance and change in persons, relationships, and friendship and kin systems. Because there is no systems-oriented research on jealousy or applicable therapeutic outcome literature, this chapter does not focus on review of previous jealousy research. Such reviews can be found elsewhere (Bringle & Buunk, 1985; White & Mullen, 1989).

## DEFINITION AND MODEL OF ROMANTIC JEALOUSY

Romantic jealousy is defined as a complex of thoughts, emotions, and actions that follows loss of or threat to self-esteem and/or to the existence or quality of the romantic relationship. The perceived loss or threat is generated by the perception of a real or potential romantic attraction between one's partner and a (perhaps imaginary) rival.

This definition stipulates that jealousy can be thought of as patterns of interrelated processes located within the individual. When taking this intrapersonal perspective, Mullen and I suggest that jealousy theory and research should focus on identifying stable or quasi-stable patterns among processes, rather than focusing on discrete emotions, behaviors, or thoughts. One reason for this suggestion is that such stability is in part evidence of the operation of a system (Hoffman, 1981; Kuhn, 1974).

However, we also argue that concentrating on the intrapersonal complex could lead to ignorance of the "interpersonal jealousy system," which refers to four sets of relationships possible among actors in a jealousy triangle. These are the primary relationship between the jealous person and the beloved; the secondary relationship of the beloved and the rival; the adverse relationship between the rival and the jealous person; and the triadic relationship of the triangle itself. Finally, each actor in the triangle is embedded within larger friendship and kin systems, whose forms and processes are to a large extent culturally driven and maintained.

Borrowing on Kelley and colleagues' metatheoretical scheme for discriminating between descriptive and causal analyses of social behavior (Kelley et al., 1983), and on Lazarus's influential cognitive–transactional model of stress and coping (Lazarus & Folkman, 1984), Mullen and I have presented a model of jealousy that is illustrated in Figure 10.1. This schematic model specifically outlines what we consider to be the elements of the intrapersonal jealousy system, which we call the "jealousy complex." There are three cognitive processes of concern: the primary appraisal of threat to or loss of self-esteem (and, by implication, self-concept) or the relationship; the secondary appraisal of what can and might be done about the threat; and cognitive efforts involved in coping with the situation or with the affect generated by the situation. The two behavioral processes of concern are the enactment of coping, and information gathering used in planning coping and in monitoring its outcome. Affective processes include the sympathetically charged emotions and their paler, more cognitive counterparts of feelings and moods. In our recent book, Mullen and I further elaborate this model and discuss research and present theory relevant to all of these processes (White & Mullen, 1989).

For my purposes here, an important part of this model is that the thoughts, behavior, and affects of all actors in the triangle are interdependent or mutually causal (cf. Bandura, 1986; Hoffman, 1981; Watzlawick, Beavin, & Jackson, 1967). More stable causes of the jealousy complex include the dyadic relationships among actors (P × O) and larger cultural and network systems (E Soc). Hence, the model in this regard merely captures our view that the behaviors of all actors and their internal processes are subject to the influences of a variety of possible systems.

## Normal, Pathological, and Symptomatic Jealousy

Mullen and I differentiate three major classes of jealousy (White & Mullen, 1989). "Symptomatic" jealousy is a consequence of a major mental illness such as paranoid disorder, schizophrenia, substance abuse, or organic brain disorders. The underlying disorder may magnify premorbid jealous suspicions; may itself lead to jealousy when the person (often reasonably) infers that the partner may be less committed to him or her because of the disorder; or may appear to be completely delusional. The jealousy frequently remits with treatment of the disorder.

"Pathological" or "pathologically reactive" jealousy occurs in those people especially sensitive to self-esteem or relationship threat, usually because of personality disorder or strong sensitizing experiences. Bringle (Chapter 5, this volume) reports on research by himself and others relevant to the dispositional aspects of jealousy that may be related to personality disorder. "Normal" jealousy occurs in those who are neither sensitized nor suffering from a major mental disorder. The theoretical

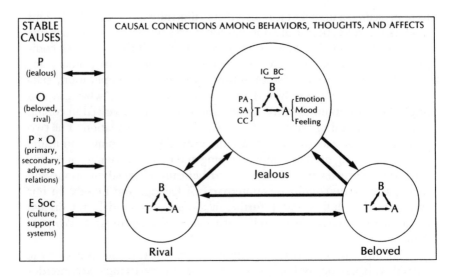

**FIGURE 10.1** A schematic model of romantic jealousy. PA, primary appraisal; SA, secondary appraisal; CC, cognitive coping efforts; IG, information gathering; BC, behavioral coping efforts; A, affects; B, behaviors; T, thoughts. From *Jealousy: Theory, Research, and Clinical Strategies* by G. L. White and P. E. Mullen, 1989, New York: Guilford Press. Copyright 1989 by The Guilford Press. Reprinted by permission.

description of the elements of normal jealousy is a major focus of our book (White & Mullen, 1989) and many of the other chapters in the present volume.

These three classes of jealousy differ in part according to the relative influences of biology, personality, and relationship on the development of the jealousy complex. There are marked differences in the capacity for reality testing, and Mullen and I suggest quite different treatment approaches. The underlying organic, affective, or thought disorder is treated for those with symptomatic jealousy, without a focus on jealousy per se except perhaps for the management of violence. For those with pathologically reactive jealousy, the primary attention of treatment is on the personality disorder or effects of unusual sensitizing experiences, while the treatment of the relationship per se is secondary. In normal jealousy, the focus is on the relationship, with a secondary emphasis on the partners as individuals.

In spite of these differences, the elements of the jealousy complex and their interrelationships may be similar across types. For example, a delusional paranoid, a person with an antisocial personality, and a normal person may all infer that a potential exists for a relationship between the beloved and a rival, and may share certain affective and behavioral reactions as a consequence. This inference may be part of a delusional system for the paranoid, may reflect early parental rejection for the antisocial, and may be based on observed flirtation for the normal. Evidence that the partner is not involved with a rival may become assimilated into the jealousy-sustaining delusional system for the paranoid, may be used by the antisocial to manipulate the beloved, and may weaken the threatening inference for the normal person. In all three cases the individuals may become angry, may be depressed, and may try to interfere with the rival relationship as a means of coping with the potential threat to self or relationship.

Although the focus of this chapter is on normal jealousy, systems processes are likely to be involved in both symptomatic and pathological jealousy as well. The extreme reactions of the symptomatic or sensitized person may reflect in part adaptation to the same system binds to which the normal person may adapt more easily.

## Three Systems of Interest

In this chapter, I focus on jealousy as an aspect of systems at three different levels: the self-system of the personality; the romantic relationship; and family/friendship networks. "Self-system" refers to the organized relationships among self-concepts and self-evaluations that transform information into self-relevant perception, inferences, moods, emotions, and behaviors. These systems are hierarchically arranged, and changes in one can lead to changes in another.

I argue that romantic jealousy can function to stabilize a system in distress as well as to create fundamental change in a system. Furthermore, jealousy may have contrary effects at different levels of systems. Jealousy may act to change a self-system while it stabilizes a romantic relationship. The often confusing oscillations of the jealous person among contradictory behaviors and conflicting emotions may be manifestations of systems that are trying to maintain themselves in the face of pressures for change. Clinical intervention to stabilize one system, such as the relationship, may destabilize other systems, such as the self-system or the family; this destabilization may lead to efforts to maintain those systems, which then in turn destabilize the relationship. Without a understanding of such dynamics, both research and intervention aimed at the intrapersonal processes of the jealous individual will be limited in theoretical scope and often unsatisfactory in clinical application.

## SOME USEFUL CONCEPTS FROM SYSTEMS THEORY

"Systems theory" is a generic term referring to a family of somewhat related descriptions of how coherent form and process are maintained and changed among seemingly discrete elements or actors of "the system." Systems theory has had a major impact in fields as diverse as engineering, computer science, ecology, anthropology, medicine, and social planning. Within psychology, its greatest impact has been on the theory and practice of community, organizational, and clinical psychology (in the last, particularly on family therapy). A comprehensive review of systems theories and their applications is not possible here, and readers are referred to such reviews elsewhere (see Bateson, 1979; Buckley, 1968; Hoffman, 1981; Katz & Kahn, 1978; Kuhn, 1974; Miller, 1978; Miller & Miller, 1980; Murrell, 1973; Segal & Bavelas, 1983; Sutherland, 1973; von Bertalanffy, 1968; Watzlawick et al., 1967). Some selected concepts from systems theory relevant to my concerns in this chapter are presented below.

### Systems as Cycles of Events

One aspect of systems is the repetitive nature of events. Cells, personalities, organizations, and relationships are all systems because they can be characterized by cycles of the input of material or information; transformation of material or information; and output of material, behavior, and information.

### Symmetrical versus Complementary Nature of Intersystem Cycles

Repetitive intrapersonal, interpersonal, or intergroup interactions tend to have two patterns. "Symmetrical" cycles are those in which each actor's (or ego state's) behavior mirrors the behavior of the other, whereas "complementary" cycles are those in which roles are quite differentiated yet require enactment of the other role (Sluzki & Beavin, 1977). Arguments and self-disclosure among equal-status friends are both examples of symmetry: Escalation of conflict or self-disclosure are both usually marked by quite similar behavior on the part of both actors. Traditional gender roles and dominance–submission patterns are examples of complementary cycles. Professors need students or research assistants in order to be professors. Traditional females need traditional males to reciprocate role behaviors. Symmetrical cycles tend to escalate until actors are exhausted or limits are externally imposed (e.g., the arms race, friendship formation), whereas complementary cycles tend to oscilate among alternating role enactments (e.g., predator–prey population cycles, parent–child conflicts). Some theorists have suggested that periods of symmetry modulate extreme swings in complementary oscillations and that complementarity acts to dampen the escalation of symmetrical cycles (Bateson, 1958, 1972; Hoffman, 1981; Maruyama, 1968; Nett, 1968; Sluzki & Beavin, 1977).

I suggest that cycles of behavior between the jealous and the beloved are quite often of a complementary or oscillating nature. The jealous and beloved may go through endless repetitions of accusation and defense, of despair and reassurance, and of disgust and heightened eroticism. The complementary roles of "jealous partner" and "accused partner" may act to stabilize the relationship by providing an exit from either escalating symmetrical conflict or escalating intimacy (which itself can provoke anxiety). However, the role complementarity that maintains the relationship may destabilize the self-system if the occupation of the complementary role threatens self-esteem or self-concept (the self-system) of the jealous person or the beloved. To put it another way, those relationships in which jealousy is marked by stable oscillations of jealousy roles may be those in which the relationship-maintaining roles are congruent with prejealousy self-systems. The function of complementarity to reduce aversive escalation of symmetry would hence be less likely to induce homeostatic processes of the self-system. (See below for a discussion of homeostasis).

## Boundaries: Repetitive Behaviors That Differentiate System Functions

External boundaries of systems are those physical and interactional features that differentiate it from its environment, including other systems. Internal boundaries of a system are patterned events that differentiate system functions, such as import and export of material or information, transformation of material or information, monitoring of transformation, and maintenance (Katz & Kahn, 1978; Miller, 1978).

Boundaries are easy to spot with many physical systems: Cells have walls, the body has skin, the school has classrooms. But boundaries of most social systems are defined by the recurring actions and interactions of their actors (Allport, 1962; Kuhn, 1974; Murrell, 1973). For example, "roles," "values," and "norms" are labels given to repetitive events (or, by some theorists, to repetitive ideas about such events; Gergen & Davis, 1985) that help differentiate one person or group from another (Katz & Kahn, 1978; von Bertalanffy, 1981).

Repetitive jealousy processes can serve as system boundaries. For example, cycles of accusation and defense often appear to provide relationship partners with a clear sense of personal identity or relationship role (differentiation of elements of the relationship system), while simultaneously differentiating the primary relationship from other types of relationships. To have a jealous conflict connotes that this relationship is of a special type distinct from more mundane relationships. (As jealousy is an element in the romanticism of many Westerners, becoming jealous implies existence of a romantic relationship.) In many cultures, friends and kin become involved in jealous conflicts; such conflicts thus act to identify and affirm friendship and kin systems (Hupka, Chapter 11, this volume; White & Mullen, 1989).

Hence, it is possible that jealousy functions to strengthen system boundaries that have become too permeable (Alderfer, 1980; Miller, 1978). Fears of intimacy, fears of relationship dissolution, and fears of family disintegration are expressions of overly permeable boundaries of the self-system, romantic relationship, and family. Repetitive intrapsychic and interpersonal jealousy cycles may stabilize and prove refractory to change because of their ability to provide coherent boundaries (cf. Alderfer, 1980; Miller, 1978).

## Hierarchical Arrangement of and Interaction among Systems

Any human system (self, romantic relationship, family) simultaneously affects and is affected by systems at three other levels. "Subsystems" carry out functions related to the overall system (e.g., import, monitoring, transformation). "Suprasystems" are larger systems in which the system is embedded, and "parallel systems" are other, discrete systems in the environment with which the system interacts. For example, the self-systems of the jealous person and the beloved are subsystems of their relationship, which itself is a subsystem of larger friendship/kinship networks. The relationship system is a parallel system to several others, including other couples, work, and school.

By extension, dysfunction in one system can affect its parallel systems, subsystems, and suprasystems. If the romantic relationship is deteriorating, partners become anxious, work quality suffers, and parents may rejoice. Likewise, if there is high job stress, if the parents interfere in the relationship, or if the self-concept of a partner changes, then the relationship may deteriorate.

## Negative Feedback Loops and System Stability

Early systems concepts emphasized the capacity of systems to maintain themselves in the face of change in subsystems, suprasystems, or parallel systems (Miller, 1978; Wiener, 1954). For example, overall family interaction patterns may remain stable if a family member leaves or if a therapist tries to change them. This capacity is called "homeostasis" or "morphostasis" (Hoffman, 1981; Maruyama, 1968; Miller, 1978).

Homeostasis is maintained by negative feedback loops. "Negative feedback" is information that change or deviation from the existing patterns of interaction is undesirable; "loops" are pathways by which information on the consequences of action is relayed back to system elements. For example, dating partners often face the dilemma of how much to disclose about themselves, particularly about their feelings for each other. Such disclosure on the part of one partner may deepen the relationship or frighten off the other partner. If the other becomes anxious or irritated upon expressions of intimacy, this is information to both that change in the relationship is not desirable, and the existing forms of interaction may remain stable (Kelley, 1979).

## System Change and Positive Feedback Loops

"Morphogenesis" refers to changes in the interactional cycles that constitute a system (Maruyama, 1968; von Bertalanffy, 1968; Watzlawick et al., 1967). Systems change when information, or "positive feedback," is received that change or deviation in interactional routines has desirable consequences. A couple whose friends and family applaud moves toward marriage are more likely to move toward redefinition of their relationship as a marriage. Systems also change as they become more differentiated in order to achieve better control over their environment, which consists mainly of other systems (Katz & Kahn, 1978; Miller, 1978). For example, marital roles may become more differentiated in order to monitor and regulate interactions with friends and neighbors, who otherwise might pose a potential threat as romantic rivals.

Whether a system changes or remains stable is presumedly the result of the preponderance of negative verses positive feedback and the timing of such feedback (Hoffman, 1981). Since information about the desirability of change can come from a number of subsystems, suprasystems, or parallel systems, the prediction of change is a complex question.

## First- and Second-Order Change

Several systems theorists have distinguished "first-order" from "second-order" change (Ashby, 1952; Nett, 1968; Watzlawick, Weakland, & Fisch, 1974). Corrective, homeostatic responses to minor perturbations in the environment are first-order changes. Second-order change involves a qualitative change in the nature of interactions among system elements as a consequence of major environmental deviations. A common example is the sequence of new parents' reactions to the birth of their first child. Many couples react at first with responses typical of the dyadic system of the lovers (e.g., trying to make the baby sleep at night so the parents can be together as adults), but eventually shift to new sets of relationships among the triadic family (Bradt, 1988). Many jealousy coping behaviors can be seen as first-order change attempts to maintain self-system or relationship homeostasis.

Second-order change is likely to be a discontinuous rather than a gradual process (Bateson, 1979; Gould & Eldredge, 1977; Hoffman, 1988; Watzlawick et al., 1974). In part, this is so because most extreme responses of first-order change have failed to coordinate the system with its environment; in part, it is so because of positive feedback loops, which rapidly enhance deviations from homeostasis (Bateson, 1979; Hoffman, 1988; Maruyama, 1968).

I suggest that jealousy coping is a first-order change process that can rapidly escalate to second-order system change under certain conditions. The attempts of the jealous person to maintain the self-system or relationship are first-order processes. However, the failure of attempts to maintain homeostasis, coupled with positive feedback for change, can propel the self-system or relationship into reorganization.

For example, in one couple I counseled, the husband was jealous of his wife's adoration of a male professor. She had just returned to college after 15 years of child raising and was thrilled by the challenges and stimulation college provided. The husband was very supportive of her return, but over the years their relationship had become rather stale and overly role-related. He became jealous when hearing his wife's descriptions of how interesting her instructor was, and he began to have somewhat obsessive fantasies about how his wife could be seduced by the instructor if the instructor so desired. He attempted to cope by trying to improve the relationship through doing more of the behaviors he had traditionally done to please her, such as taking her out for dinner more and doing more of the housework. He also derogated the professor by frequently pointing out that the professor lived in an ivory tower and could not possibly be successful in a pragmatic way. His wife realized he was jealous and tried to cope by limiting her discussion, which in turn made the husband somewhat more suspicious that his wife might be hiding her attraction for the professor. These complementary coping strategies became more extreme, with the husband becoming more disparaging of the professor and of college education in general, and engaging in stereotypically romantic actions such as presenting flowers, buying his wife gifts, and sending her love notes. She grew to be even more nonrevealing about her college life, in order to reduce his jealousy. Both were becoming increasingly dissatisfied with the marriage when they came to counseling, and both had lost confidence that their own actions could remedy the situation.

Therapy did not focus on adaptation to the wife's return to school, which would have been a first-order approach. Instead, it focused on change away from traditional sex roles, which permeated their financial, sexual, and leisure time activities. In addition, communication skills training allowed them to discuss their feelings, needs, and perceptions in a very different way from their habitual pattern. Explicit decisions about new roles and leisure activities, coupled with the new style of communicating, led to major shifts in the pattern of their relationship. The wife took more responsibility for maintenance of home and income, while the husband took more responsibility for development and expression of intimacy. These were second-order changes. The spouses became more interesting to and supportive of each other, and the husband's jealousy of the instructor ended.

## Communicational and Interpersonal Double Binds

Originally, the "double bind" was formulated as a communication process in which one person communicates to a captive receiver two contradictory messages of different types or levels (e.g., verbal vs. nonverbal or explicit vs. implicit). Both messages require the receiver to act. Furthermore, one or both messages are denied by the sender. Schizophrenia was thought to be a means of escaping the bind (Bateson, Jackson, Haley, & Weakland, 1956).

The double bind was later formulated as an interpersonal process (Haley, 1977; Weakland, 1976). In one type of interpersonal bind, the person receives messages from two senders who can each punish or reward the receiver's actions. These messages are contradictory, usually requiring the receiver to form a coalition with one message sender against the other. Furthermore, the receiver cannot easily escape from the situation, and one or both senders may deny the (often implicit) request for coalition. This bind is particularly anxiety- and anger-provoking when the two message senders are at a higher power or status level than the receiver.

Haley (1977) discusses the "perverse triangle." This type of interpersonal bind occurs when two people engage in a coalition against a third, when the two in coalition are at different levels of power, and when the coalition is denied. In organizations, this occurs when a manager and subordinate scheme against another manager; in families, this occurs when a parent and child act against the other parent. Such triangles leave the odd person out feeling angry, anxious, and depressed, and doubting his or her own sense of reality.

In the context of romantic jealousy, a communicational double bind occurs when the jealous person perceives two apparently contradictory messages from the beloved: "I love you" and "I love the rival." This second message is typically transformed into "I don't love you." The first message is often explicit, while the second is implicit in the perceived actions of the beloved toward the rival. Because of investment in and dependency upon the relationship, it may be costly for the jealous person to leave the field. If the beloved denies the perceived "I don't love you" message, then the communicational double bind is in play, with resultant confusion, anger, and helplessness exhibited by the jealous (Segal & Bavelas, 1983; Weakland, 1976).

One example of the first version of the interpersonal double bind occurs when two jealous rivals compete for the attention of the beloved, who is attracted to each. The beloved is the target of contradictory demands for coalition (relationship) and may feel powerless to escape the situation. The anxiety, vacillation, and self-doubt of the beloved is characteristic of such a double bind. Another example involves the rival of a partner in an existing romantic relationship. The beloved appears to send a message to form a relationship with the rival while the existing partner sends a message not to form a relationship. Due to strong attraction to the beloved or to situational factors, the rival may not be able to exit the field easily. Further, the beloved may deny overt messages of encouragement but appear to encourage through dress or demeanor. The rival is caught in the bind, one resolution of which is to ignore the rejection and amplify the perceived encouragement. Such amplifications may be perceived by others as grossly out of touch with reality, much in the same way that schizophrenic amplifications are seen as out of touch.

In the "perverse triangle" version of the interpersonal double bind, the jealous person may perceive the beloved and (lower-status) rival in coalition against himself or herself, but the perceived coalition is denied by the other actors. Here the lower status of the rival is either normatively prescribed within the culture (e.g., husbands have the right to control the actions of rivals) on subjectively perceived as a consequence of lack of control over the other actors. This is the position of the married person whose spouse is carrying on an affair, the impact or existence of which is denied by the errant spouse. The jealous person may seek to form a coalition with the rival against the beloved as a resolution of this bind. In my clinical experience, it is not uncommon for the jealous spouse (more likely the wife) to seek out the rival to clarify the situation or threaten retaliation, and for the jealous spouse and the rival to end up themselves in coalition against the beloved, who is causing them both so much trouble.

## JEALOUSY COPING AS A HOMEOSTATIC PROCESS

Coping efforts can help maintain the stability of the self-system, relationship, or friendship/kinship systems. Some aspects of coping as a homeostatic process are outlined below.

### Threats to or Loss of Aspects of the Self

Mullen and I (White & Mullen, 1989, pp. 19–21) discuss self-esteem and self-concept threats in jealousy. "Self-esteem" is one's valuation of aspects of oneself, whereas "self-concept" refers to beliefs about one's attributes. Together with self-efficacy beliefs, they constitute the core of the self-system, a critical subsystem of personality (Bandura, 1978; Gergen & Davis, 1985; Kohut, 1977). Such threats are abundant in jealousy situations; they stem from a variety of sources, such as the social meaning of perceived attraction of partner to a rival and outcomes of social comparison to the rival (White & Mullen, 1989).

Several behavioral and cognitive coping efforts of the jealous person function to reduce such threats and hence can be seen as maintaining homeostasis of the self-system. Examples include denial and avoidance, derogation of the rival, and development of alternative sources of esteem and affirmation. These processes have been a major focus of previous research and clinical report (Bringle & Buunk, 1985; White & Mullen, 1989).

### Threats to or Loss of Relationship Qualities

The actions of the jealous person can similarly be seen as attempts to preserve the dyadic relationship (or, at least, the perceived relationship)—in other words, to maintain or regain the status quo. Threats to or loss of certain qualities of the relationship (trust, sexual enjoyment, support) also result in negative affect, which stimulates coping efforts by one or both partners to maintain relationship homeostasis (cf. Berscheid, 1983). Such efforts have been the other major focus of previous research and clinical commentary (Bringle & Buunk, 1985; White & Mullen, 1989).

## Threats to Friendship or Kin Systems

The development of a romantic relationship between two partners may seriously disrupt existing friendship or familial systems (see Hupka, Chapter 11, this volume). Sons and daughters may leave home; previously close friends may find themselves abandoned by the mutually absorbed couple; and children may be confused and depressed if one parent has an extramarital affair discovered. It is a simple extension of our romantic jealousy model to say that friends and family members may act to maintain homeostasis of the existing sets of relationships. This may be done by various tactics of inclusion or exclusion of the new romantic partner. Friends and family can rightfully be described as (nonromantically) jealous over the new relationship.

What is not quite so obvious is that jealousy of the jealous person over real or potential attractions between the beloved and the rival can also act to maintain a larger system's homeostasis. The competing demands of friends or family and the beloved may be experienced by the jealous person as an interpersonal double bind, especially when negative feelings toward the beloved are denied by friends or family members (or vice versa). Coping efforts that move the jealous person away from the primary relationship are potentially homeostatic to the larger system and may lead to affirmation and reward by friends or family members. Hence, the perception of a rival relationship may provide the impetus to termination of the primary relationship in favor of the friendship or family system.

Mullen and I have proposed several jealousy coping strategies, but the strategies of derogation of the partner, developing alternatives to the relationship, and seeking catharsis with supportive others seem most likely to preserve or enhance existing relationships (White & Mullen, 1989, pp. 45–56). Although we discuss these three as esteem-maintaining strategies, they may at times be more uniquely related to friendship- or family-maintaining maneuvers.

More interesting is the possibility that jealousy is a route out of a bind that existed *before* the perception of a real or potential rival, and that it can actually enhance the stability of *both* the primary relationship and the family or friendship system. The jealous person may enlist the support of friends or family against the rival, and thus change their apparent antipathy toward the beloved to a coalition with the beloved. Here it is convenient to choose a rival toward whom friends or family are already ill disposed, and who can be portrayed as forcing himself or herself upon the resisting beloved. For example, a son's girlfriend may become more acceptable to parents if she is thought to be resisting the advances of a Hell's Angels biker in favor of their son.

## JEALOUSY COPING AS A MORPHOGENETIC PROCESS

Under certain conditions it is possible that jealousy functions to change the self-system, primary relationship, or friendship and kin systems. Of course, the ending of relationships is a change, but system theorists usually regard termination as an example of first-order change. That is, the possible solutions to problems in a system always include doing the opposite of being in the system, which is leaving the system. People commit suicide, couples divorce, and families separate.

My focus here is on second-order change or reorganization of the system, which is to say rearrangement in the ways in which system elements interact (Bateson, 1979; Watzlawick et al., 1974). The comments below draw on the notions of positive feedback and morphogenesis, symmetrical versus complementary relationships, and second-order change.

### Changes in Self-Esteem and Self-Concept

Mullen and I have suggested two coping strategies most likely to be involved in changes in the self-system. These strategies are "self-assessment" and "appraisal of challenge" (White & Mullen, 1989, pp. 51–54). Self-assessment is a strategy of changing one's skills, perceptions, and motivation in order to better manage affect or the situation (Lazarus & Folkman, 1984, p. 152). If these changes are successful in reducing unpleasant affects or managing the situation, or if they initiate positive feedback from others in the larger contexts of the person's life, they may become features of the reorganized self-system. For example, psychotherapy for jealousy may lead the person to be more accepting and assertive of particular needs for affection or security, with the potential of changing and reinforcing self-perception of important values and self-efficacy in obtaining those values.

In appraisal of challenge, the secondary appraisal of the jealousy situation yields a challenge to personal growth or development that leads beyond the jealousy problem per se. For example, the person may decide that his or her self-centeredness not only is a factor in the jealousy problem, but also leads to problems on the job or with family. As with self-assessment, appraisal of challenge can lead to positive feedback, which promotes further changes in the self-system.

## Changes in the Relationship

One way to cope with jealousy is to improve the primary relationship, in order to increase its attractiveness in comparison to the rival relationship (White & Mullen, 1989, p. 48). Such changes are likely to be first-order, as they do not necessarily result in fundamental changes in role relationships, in shared meanings about the nature of the relationship, or in joint maintenance activities such as problem solving (Knudson, 1985; Watzlawick et al., 1974). For example, efforts to improve the relationship by increasing one's sexual attractiveness or by complaining less may perhaps be effective, but do not require shifts in role or relationship definitions.

One way to understand second-order change in the primary relationship is to view it as a result of shifts from symmetrical to complementary patterns of relationship (Sluzki & Beavin, 1977). As mentioned earlier, complementary relationships can limit symmetrical escalations of conflict or intimacy, whereas symmetrical relationships can act to reduce extreme oscillations in complementary relationships. Jealousy can function to move a relationship from symmetrical to complementary role relationships, and vice versa, under certain conditions.

Complementary sex roles in general act to reduce relationship conflict (Ashmore & Del Boca, 1986; Ickes, 1985; Sluzki & Beavin, 1977), and these roles may serve to reduce the threat to the relationship or the self that a perceived rival poses. For example, the double standard for sexual behavior is an aspect of traditional sex roles implying that male extrarelationship sexuality is biological in impetus, rather than signaling dissatisfaction with the partner or relationship. A shift from more egalitarian and androgynous relationships to more traditional sex roles within the dyad may afford the female a less threatening attribution for the male's behavior (White & Mullen, 1989, pp. 43–44). Furthermore, this shift may engage positive feedback from others outside the jealousy situation per se and may also provide stabilizing explanations for other conflicts in the relationship, such as initiation of sexual behavior. Other complementary roles with similar outcomes are extravert versus introvert and work-oriented versus home-oriented. The partner of a beloved who is extraverted or work-oriented would have explanations for the beloved's apparent involvements with others that do not necessarily imply dissatisfaction with the partner or the primary relationship. The partner of a beloved who is introverted or home-oriented would be relatively assured that the beloved is unlikely to desire or seek a rival relationship. In all of these cases, the adoption of a complementary role may serve to de-escalate conflict over potential rival relationships.

Jealousy can also function to shift partners from oscillating role interaction to symmetrical interaction. One jealousy coping strategy is "demanding commitment" (White & Mullen, 1989, p. 50). Such demands may be accompanied by direct expression of personal needs for the relationship. More generally, attempts to resolve the jealousy problem by more direct and open communication of one's own perceived needs, goals, emotions, fantasies, and so on may be more likely to create symmetrical matching moves by the partner. The partners may be able to avoid overly rigid roles of the "jealous" and the "errant" partner if they can participate in symmetrical self-disclosure. Moreover, such moves are more likely to be perceived as directly self-expressive than routine, role-related communication. The effect may be to move the couple to new interaction patterns that had not been perceived as possible or desirable (cf. Kelley, 1979).

Jealousy can also lead to second-order change through shifts in definition of the relationship. An intense jealousy episode may signal to both partners that the relationship is no longer casual, but has assumed central importance to each partner's life. Demands for commitment may lead both partners to consider marriage. Such definitional shifts are likely to be related to normative explanations for jealousy at different stages of the relationship and to relationship scripts about the expected progression of intimacy and commitment. Persons and cultures vary in the use of jealousy as a marker of relationship shifts.

## Changes in Family or Friendship Systems

Jealousy can also lead to fundamental changes in the more extended family or friendship systems. One coping strategy is to develop alternative sources of self-esteem, identity affirmation, or relationship outcomes. Friends and family are likely sources for these needs; the development of new friendships or the alteration of former relationships to secure these goals are examples of morphogenesis. Such alterations may indirectly change the nature of relationships among other actors within the person's friendship system, as balance theories suggested long ago.

Another jealousy coping strategy Mullen and I (White & Mullen, 1989) have discussed is "support/catharsis," which functions to manage emotions through their safe expression, most usually in the company of supportive friends. Such expression is a form of intimate self-disclosure that may induce qualitative changes in existing friendships. Furthermore, friends who are mutually involved in supporting emotional expression of the jealous may themselves come to redefine their own relationship.

Jealousy episodes may affect the nature of family interaction in a variety of ways. Children who become alternative sources of esteem for a jealous parent may join cross-generational alliances against the errant spouse, with major implications for the distribution of power and love within the family. Or an intense jealousy episode of an adolescent may serve as a ritual of passage into adulthood. Jealousy is a problem with which parents may more readily identify, compared to other dilemmas of adolescence. The recognition of the adolescent as an adult may qualitatively alter relationships among many family members. As another example, a jealous spouse may try to improve the marital relationship by assuming more care of the children, and the contexts of such care may lead to different relationships among spouses and children. A husband who tries to be a better father to please an ambivalent wife may become closer to the children and more assertive of his role in their upbringing.

As these examples suggest, future research on jealousy coping will benefit from examining intended and unintended consequences of coping efforts for friendships and kin systems. I also suggest that these consequences themselves will often affect the ways in which jealousy episodes affect the self-system and the primary relationship.

## SYSTEMS, RESEARCHERS, CLINICIANS, AND JEALOUSY THEORY

To close this sketch of systems theory and its application to jealousy, I would like to suggest a dilemma for researchers and clinicians that is itself something of a systems paradox. The dilemma goes like this: In order to study jealousy, researchers may profit by considering the interactions among systems at different hierarchical levels (e.g., self-system, relationship, and family/friendship systems). However, most researchers are trained and housed within academic perspectives that take as a primary focus a system at one level (the person, interpersonal interaction, larger systems). Furthermore, academics pursuing research and clinicians pursuing change (again, usually focused on the person, relationship, or family) often have many obstacles toward effective integration of their work (e.g., different tasks, ideologies, theories, values). To arrive at a comprehensive theory of jealousy, then, researchers and clinicians not only will have to pursue each other, but will have to consider how their usual system of focus affects and is affected by others in the hierarchy. Both tasks will establish new forms of relationships among researchers and between researchers and clinicians. Hence, the study of romantic jealousy (as is true of other social phenomena) poses the challenge of second-order change to normative patterns of researchers and clinicians. It will be interesting to see whether the homeostatic forces of academic and clinical systems will vitiate jealousy research, theory, and therapy. I hope that this volume will contribute to the morphogenetic challenge posed by the comprehensive study of jealousy.

## REFERENCES

Alderfer, C. P. (1980). Consulting to underbounded systems. In C. P. Alderfer & C. L. Cooper (Eds.), *Advances in experiential social processes* (Vol. 2, pp. 267–296). New York: Wiley.

Allport, F. H. (1962). A structuronomic conception of behavior: Individual and collective. I. Structural theory and the master problem of social psychology. *Journal of Abnormal and Social Psychology, 64,* 3–30.

Ashby, W. R. (1952). *Design for a brain.* New York: Wiley.

Ashmore, R. D., & Del Boca, F. K. (1986). *The social psychology of female–male relations.* New York: Academic Press.

Bandura, A. (1978). The self-system in reciprocal determinism. *American Psychologist, 33,* 344–358.

Bandura, A. (1986). *Social foundations of thought and action.* Englewood Cliffs, NJ: Prentice-Hall.

Bateson, G. (1958). *Naven.* Stanford, CA: Stanford University Press.

Bateson, G. (1972). *Steps to an ecology of mind.* New York: Ballantine.

Bateson, G. (1979). *Mind and nature.* New York: Dutton.

Bateson, G., Jackson, D., Haley, J., & Weakland, J. (1956). Toward a theory of schizophrenia. *Behavioral Science, 2,* 251–264.

Berscheid, E. (1983). Emotion. In H. H. Kelley, E. Berscheid, A. Christensen, J. H. Harvey, T. L. Huston, G. Levinger, E. McClintock, L. A. Peplau, & D. R. Peterson (Eds.), *Close relationships* (pp. 110–168). San Francisco: W. H. Freeman.

Bradt, J. O. (1988). Becoming parents: Families with young children. In B. Carter & M. McGoldrick (Eds.), *The changing family life cycle* (2nd ed., pp. 235–254). New York: Gardner Press.

Bringle, R. G., & Buunk, B. (1985). Jealousy and social behavior. *Review of Personality and Social Psychology, 6,* 241–264.

Buckley, W. (1968). *Modern systems research for the behavioral scientist.* Chicago: Aldine.

Gergen, K. J., & Davis, K. E. (1985). *The social construction of the person.* New York: Springer.

Gould, S. J., & Eldredge, N. (1977). Punctuated equilibria: The tempo and mode of evolution reconsidered. *Paleobiology, 3,* 115–151.

Haley, J. (1977). Toward a theory of pathological systems. In P. Watzlawick & J. Weakland (Eds.), *The interactional view* (pp. 31–48). New York: Norton.

Hoffman, L. (1981). *Foundations of family therapy.* New York: Basic Books.

Hoffman, L. (1988). The family life cycle and discontinuous change. In B. Carter & M. McGoldrick (Eds.), *The changing family life cycle* (2nd ed., pp. 91–106). New York: Gardner Press.

Ickes, W. (1985). Sex-role influences on compatibility in relationships. In W. Ickes (Ed.), *Compatible and incompatible relationships* (pp. 187–208). New York: Springer.

Katz, D., & Kahn, R. L. (1978). *The social psychology of organizations.* New York: Wiley.

Kelley, H. H. (1979). *Personal relationships: Their structure and processes.* Hillsdale, NJ: Erlbaum.

Kelley, H. H., Berscheid, E., Chirstensen, A., Harvey, J. H., Huston, T. L., Levinger, G., McClintock, E., Peplau, L. A., & Peterson, D. R. (Eds.). (1983). *Close relationships.* San Francisco: W. H. Freeman.

Knudson, R. M. (1985). Marital incompatibility and mutual identity confirmation. In W. Ickes (Ed.), *Compatible and incompatible relationships* (pp. 233–252). New York: Springer.

Kohut, H. (1977). *The restoration of the self.* New York: International Universities Press.

Kuhn, A. (1974). *The logic of social systems.* San Francisco: Jossey-Bass.

Lazarus, R. S., & Folkman, S. (1984). *Stress, appraisal, and coping.* New York: Springer.

Maruyama, M. (1968). The second cybernetics: Deviation-amplifying mutual causal processes. In W. Buckley (Ed.), *Modern systems research for the behavioral scientist.* Chicago: Aldine.

Miller, J. G. (1978). *Living systems.* New York: McGraw-Hill.

Miller, J. G., & Miller, J. L. (1980). General living systems theory. In H. I. Kaplan & B. J. Sadock (Eds.), *Comprehensive textbook of psychiatry* (4th ed., pp. 13–24). Baltimore: Williams & Wilkins.

Murrell, S. A. (1973). *Community psychology and social systems.* New York: Behavioral.

Nett, R. (1968). Conformity–deviation and the social control concept. In W. Buckley (Ed.), *Modern systems research for the behavioral scientist.* Chicago: Aldine.

Segal, L., & Bavelas, J. B. (1983). Human systems and communication theory. In B. B. Wolman & G. Stricker (Eds.), *Handbook of family and marital therapy* (pp. 61–76). New York: Plenum.

Sluzki, C. E., & Beavin, J. (1977). Symmetry and complementarity: An operational definition and a typology of dyads. In P. Watzlawick & J. H. Weakland (Eds.), *The interactional view* (pp. 71–87). New York: W. W. Norton.

Sutherland, J. W. (1973). *A general systems philosophy for the social and behavioral sciences.* New York: Braziller.

von Bertalanffy, L. (1968). *General systems theory.* New York: Braziller.

von Bertalanffy, L. (1981). *A systems view of man.* Boulder, CO: Westview.

Watzlawick, P., Beavin, J., & Jackson, D. (1967). *Pragmatics of human communication.* New York: Norton.

Watzlawick, P., Weakland, J., & Fisch, R. (1974). *Change: The principles of problem formation and problem resolution.* New York: Norton.

Weakland, J. (1976). The double bind hypothesis of schizophrenia and three-party interaction. In C. Sluzki & D. Ransom (Eds.), *Double bind: The foundation of the communicational approach to the family* (pp. 173–201). New York: Grune & Stratton.

White, G. L., & Mullen, P. E. (1989). *Jealousy: Theory, research, and clinical strategies.* New York: Guilford Press.

Wiener, N. (1954). *The human use of human beings.* Garden City, NY: Doubleday/Anchor.

## Chapter Eleven

# The Motive for the Arousal of Romantic Jealousy: Its Cultural Origin

RALPH B. HUPKA
*California State University-Long Beach*

From where does romantic jealousy, the jealousy aroused in dating relationships or marriages, get its emotive power? Why is the possibility of the partner's having an affair such a devastating shock? Is the motive for the arousal of jealousy a remnant of human evolution, or is it the end product of social structures? In this chapter I comment on the unlikelihood that the motive stems from genes alone, and propose an alternative model that includes our genetic heritage but locates the motive in social structures.

## THE ANIMAL WITHIN US

A cultural perspective on jealousy cannot ignore the genetic influence on human behavior. We are social animals; the reason for that sociability lies in our long history of genetic evolution. What might have contributed to our preference for living with others? In a radical departure from the traditional view of human evolution as a consequence of brain expansion and the use of tools, Lovejoy (1981) proposed that human evolution was driven by the unique sexual and reproductive behavior of early hominids. Let us consider an adumbrated version of his behavioral model for early hominid evolution.

One of the primary causes of mortality among infant chimpanzees is "injuries caused by falling from the mother" (Van Lawick-Goodall, 1967, p. 336). Falling is more likely when the mother must both care for the infant and forage for herself. Any behavioral change that would alter such a burden would increase the rate of reproduction and survival.

Lovejoy proposed that monogamous pairbonding would increase survival and reproduction. One of the benefits of pairbonding would be that males would not compete for food with females and offspring. Instead, it would lead to direct involvement of males in the survival of offspring and the establishment of paternity. Behavior such as gathering food and returning it to the mate would increase the male's

reproductive rate by correspondingly improving the protein and calorie supply of the female who could then accommodate greater gestational and lactation loads and intensify parenting. The behavior would . . . allow a progressive increase in the number of dependent offspring because their nutritional and supervisory requirements could be met more adequately. (Lovejoy, 1981, p. 345)

Lovejoy's model provides a plausible explanation for the evolution of sociability and a genetic contribution to the preference for monogamous relationships among human beings. The need for communication in such cooperative relationships may account for the finding that the facial expressions of anger, disgust, fear, happiness, sadness, and surprise are recognized cross-culturally (e.g., Ekman et al., 1987). Most likely these emotions and the blends of their facial expressions, such as apprehensive fear, worry, contempt, sulky anger, and so on (see Ekman & Friesen, 1975), have their origin in the aeons of human evolution.

Why did the fire of jealousy evolve in human beings? Probably for the same reason that all emotions evolved, which most likely was to enhance adaptability and survival (Plutchik, 1980). Thus, disgust may prevent ingestion of life-threatening substances, and sadness-induced crying in infants may prevent separation from caregivers. The capacity to experience jealousy may consist of the affective component of the anticipation, the foreboding of impending harm, and so on. With regard to jealousy, sociobiologists do not agree with such generalized, broad-based elicitors that require the infant to learn the varied motives and dangers of the social environment into which it is born. Instead, they postulate that the arousal of male sexual jealousy is triggered by one motive whose origin has its roots in evolution. I examine the implications of that hypothesis shortly.

It appears reasonable to propose that human beings have evolved the capacity to be emotional; however, in light of their high levels of intelligence, immense investment of time in the care of offspring, and long periods of learning, it is also reasonable to propose that all other facets of emotion (e.g., their elicitation, expression, modulation, the target of the emotion, etc.) are learned. It is unlikely, given the protracted period of childhood dependency and learning, the adaptability of human beings, the variability in their cultures, and the speed at which cultures can change, that human beings come "prewired," so to speak, into the world to be emotional about anything other than the requirements for their immediate survival (e.g., Izard, Huebner, Risser, McGinnes, & Dougherty, 1980). Thus, for instance, our genetic inheritance gives us the capacity to be angry, but that which arouses our anger, whether it be an insult, a theft, or an attack on what we hold dear, is learned.

How does this apply to romantic jealousy? I define "romantic jealousy" as the cognition, physiological experience, and behavior arising when individuals are threatened by —or, in the terminology of the theories of Arnold (1960) and Lazarus (1966), make appraisals of threat in response to—the potential or imagined involvement of their loved ones or mates in relationships with interlopers. The mere sign of attraction to other individuals and undue involvement in hobbies or other activities also may trigger a sense of threat and negative physiological experiences. In sum, romantic jealousy is an anticipatory emotion. It is aroused by the threat of losing to an interloper that which is gained by establishing a relationship with someone.

As in the case of anger, our genetic heritage enables us to experience jealousy, but all else is learned. Before jealousy can be elicited, we must learn to value romantic relationships, the motive for being jealous, the target of the jealousy, the events that trigger the jealousy, who expresses it, when to express it, the manner of expressing it, who is to blame for the predicament, and so forth (Hupka, 1981). The biological heritage provides the physiological fire of jealousy, but it is ignited by a psychological spark.

Jealousy is a social construction (Averill, 1980; Harré, 1986) to the extent that it is based on learning; therefore, it may differ from culture to culture (see, e.g., Bryson, Chapter 8, this volume; Buunk & Hupka, 1987; Hupka et al., 1985). As outlined in the preceding paragraph, what

differentiates jealousy across cultures is the manner in which it is constituted or put together in each society. Although the capacity to experience jealousy is inherited, that capacity is actualized through social
structures. Jealousy requires a particular culture to give it life—the
wherefore for its expression and usefulness. There is no basis for its
elicitation without a relationship between two individuals and without
social constructs to give functional meaning to that relationship. In this
chapter, I explore a process by which the motive for the arousal of
romantic jealousy may be socially constructed. But, first, a distinction
must be made.

## JEALOUSY AS AN EMOTION AND AS A PROCESS

I differentiate between jealousy as an emotion and jealousy as a process.
The suspicion that the mate is having an affair, which arouses the
emotion of jealousy, differs from the explosion of emotional suffering in
response to, and from coping with the aftereffects of, the affair. Let us
consider this differentiation in detail.

I have defined jealousy as an emotion that is aroused by the threat of
losing one's mate to an interloper. But what is aroused when the threat
transforms into reality and the mate has an affair, or, worse yet, termi-
nates the relationship in favor of one with the interloper? Jealousy is
elicited; however, it is merely one of many emotions and, according to
our research (Barr & Hupka, 1984), is rated lower in mean likelihood of
being aroused than feeling hurt, betrayed, disappointed, angry, and
depressed. Apparently these emotions are more prominent than jealousy
in such predicaments; this suggests that jealousy contributes to the profile of reactions but is not the dominant feeling. The reactions to affairs
and to the loss of mates to interlopers are so complex that I recently
proposed that they are not captured by referring to "emotions" (which
are thought of as transitory states), but by characterizing them as comprising a "jealousy grieving process"—a process involving recurring
phases and lasting for months (Hupka, 1989).

The phases of the jealousy grieving process, adapted from a model
of grief by Averill and Nunley (1988), are as follows. To begin with,
there is (1) "shock," the initial moments of numbness of the cuckolded
individual upon discovering the liaison. This is followed by recurring
episodes of (2) "recriminations," periods of feeling hurt, angry, sad,
depressed, and so on, against a chronic background turmoil of
(3) "anguish," the ever-present feeling of betrayal, disillusionment, sense
of loss, difficulty in concentration, and preoccupation with thoughts of

the mate and the affair. As time passes, the cuckolded individual spends more and more time in (4) "accommodation," a phase marked by the search for an explanation, a desire to make sense of what happened, explorations within oneself and with the mate regarding the feasibility of repairing the relationship, and eventual adjustment to the betrayal or termination of the relationship. Finally, there is (5) "recovery," where the individual once more is able to function at the customary precrisis level.

In sum, the jealousy grieving process involves a succession of sundry emotional and cognitive reactions. It is a relearning process that requires adjusting to the crisis, possibly learning to live without the mate, and changing one's assumptions about relationships, love, trust, sexual fidelity, and so forth. Such a complex process, involving changes over months, cannot be contracted into a single emotion, whether it is jealousy, anger, depression, or feeling hurt. It is a distinct psychological process unlike the transitory states of emotions; therefore, I regard the emotion of jealousy, the experiential state in response to the threat of losing one's mate to an interloper and all the benefits that come with being in the relationship, as differing from the jealousy process, where the individual is coping not with the threat but with the grievous aftereffects of the affair.

## WHY IS ROMANTIC JEALOUSY AROUSED?

### The Motive Emanates from Evolution

Why do particular events elicit romantic jealousy? Why are they so loaded with emotional investment that they hold the power to generate jealousy and all that which is set in motion in the jealousy grieving process? Are human beings around the world born to be jealous about similar events? Or, as I elaborate upon, is it learning the benefits of having mates that, when threatened by interlopers, provokes jealousy?

Such an explanation, based on learning, is in conflict with the position of sociobiologists, who propose that the motive for elicitation of jealousy lies in our biological heritage. Before discussing the arousal of jealousy as a learned motive, let us explore the sociobiological concept of the elicitation of jealousy as an evolution-influenced desire for assurance that the children one is raising are one's own.

Daly, Wilson, and Weghorst (1982) have proposed that human males evolved defenses against wasting their efforts on raising children not sired by them. One of these defenses is the psychological propensity to be jealous. The function of male sexual jealousy is to defend paternity confidence. Males threaten violence and use violence in order to achieve sexual exclusivity and control over women, thereby satisfying their motive—their inclination (stemming from evolution) for assurance that they are passing on their own gene pool and not wasting their resources on raising the children of interlopers. Females are less concerned with sexual fidelity, because simply by giving birth they are assured of having passed their gene pool into the next generation. A woman's motive to be jealous pertains to her concern that the involvement of a man with other women does not leave sufficient resources and attention to guarantee the survival of her own offspring.

To justify tying the motive for male jealousy to remnants of human evolution, Daly et al. (1982) point to the similarity in legal restrictions on female sexual behavior in diverse societies, and note that the motive in homicide and wife beating is frequently male sexual jealousy. As an example of the cross-cultural similarity in legal restrictions on females, Daly et al. note that sexual violations are defined in accordance with the marital status of the female rather than the male. That is, it is an offense for a married woman to have sexual intercourse with someone other than her husband. But a married man does not commit adultery if he has illicit relations with a woman not his wife. Thus, the husband is the victim, "who is commonly entitled to damages, to violent revenge, or to divorce with refund of bride-price" (Daly et al., 1982, p. 12).

Yet this discriminatory attitude toward women can be accounted for more reasonably by social structures—such as the fact that economic and political power has traditionally been in the hands of the men, who then promulgate laws that are consistent with their position of power—than the hypothesis that these affronts to women stem from an evolution-selected propensity to be jealous. For verification, let us look at societies where women enjoyed some legal or economic independence.

Jacobsen (1982) reported that in medieval Iceland adultery was an affront to the woman's kin. The man had to pay a fine to her kin or, if she was married, to her husband. If she was exploited sexually, she was deemed innocent. If she consented to the affair, she lost the right to receive any inheritance to which she might have been entitled through her kin. Adultery, in contrast to Daly et al.'s (1982) generalization, was not a valid reason for divorce or violence. Thus, adultery is less likely to be defined as an affront exclusively to husbands when women have economic power (in this case, by way of inheritance).

Legal power was divided in medieval Europe between secular and ecclesiastical law systems. Canon law gave the church jurisdiction over the sacrament of marriage and, consequently, over adultery (Gold, 1982). Brundage (1982) reported that the medieval canonists considered adultery a crime against the body and not an indignity solely against the husband. It was a criminal act whether it was committed by men or women; both were punished for adulterous activities. Thus, when the legal system leans toward equitable treatment, adultery is a crime also against wives and not just against husbands.

Schlegel (1972) found in a cross-cultural sample of 66 matrilineal societies that the adultery of wives was less likely to be punished in societies where the males exerted minimal authority over the women (p. 8) than it was in societies where either the husbands or the brothers of the wives exerted power over the women (p. 67). Consistent with the hypothesis that the sexual restrictions on women are the result of the power men exert over women was Schlegel's finding that domestic power over others lay in the hands of those who controlled property, most frequently the men. In light of this association between power and control over property, it is not surprising that females were most autonomous in those matrilineal societies in which they shared with males in the control of the domestic property. The assumption that one can exercise control over other people through control over property has a long history (e.g., Hobhouse, 1906) with substantial cross-cultural empirical support (e.g., Hobhouse, 1922; Rudmin, 1988; Simmons, 1937; Sumner & Keller, 1927).

Let us turn to another issue. Daly et al. (1982) cite police investigations indicating that male jealousy is a frequent issue in spousal homicide as support for their hypothesis that the motive for the arousal of jealousy is the evolution-influenced psychological propensity for assurance of paternity confidence. Daly et al. interpret the homicide as stemming from the husband's loss of his exclusive sexual rights over his wife, his loss of control of female reproductive capacity in general, and hence his setback in the reproductive competition with other men.

What is wrong with this interpretation? It is inconsistent with Daly et al.'s definition of jealousy. They confuse prevention with revenge. These authors define jealousy as an emotion that seeks to *prevent* the loss of sexual exclusivity. Jealousy is "aroused by a perceived threat to a valued relationship or position and motivates behavior aimed at countering the threat" (Daly et al., 1982, p. 12). Yet murder in response to adultery, or the belief that adultery has been committed, is punishment for betrayal. The murder is an indication that the jealousy has failed as a prevention strategy. The cuckolded husband is seeking revenge for the putative harm done to him.

There is another problem as well. Surveys have revealed that between 37% and 50% of the respondents report having had extramarital affairs (Lampe, 1987). Yet far less than 0.01% of the U.S. male population commits murder in response to adultery. Even in a cross-cultural comparison, homicide is not the typical response (Hupka, 1981). There is even evidence to suggest that about 25% of all homicides are provoked by the victim, thereby diminishing further the homicide rate attributable to the putative jealousy of males (Wolfgang, 1959, 1968). How are we to interpret this in light of the Daly et al. (1982) hypothesis? Do more than 99% of men have a lower evolution-selected psychological propensity to defend paternity confidence than those who resort to killing of their spouses?

It is unlikely that spousal murder stems from a propensity to elevate paternity confidence. The decision to commit murder itself requires explanation. Such extreme violence is rare. There are far more reasonable explanations for spousal murder, such as socialization (Gold, 1958), lack of urban industrial discipline, ethnicity, social status, unemployment, and so on (e.g., Lane, 1979).

Even a cursory cross-cultural survey reveals many more motives for the elicitation of jealousy than Daly et al.'s focus on the desire to elevate paternity confidence. For example, among the Andalusians of Spain, jealousy maintains a man's honor in the eyes of the community (Pitt-Rivers, 1966); for the Shona of Zimbabwe, jealousy prevents the death of the couple's children (Folta & Deck, 1988); and the Yanomama husband, in response to infidelity, is less concerned about paternity confidence than about the failure of the interloper to compensate him with gifts and services (Harris, 1974).

Daly et al. (1982) also cite the prevalence of sexual jealousy as a motive in wife beating as additional support for their hypothesis that men are inclined to restrict the activities and social contacts of their mates. They believe that this inclination "is an evolved attribute that must be understood as an anticuckoldry (confidence of paternity) and sexual competition tactic" (p. 17). Again, however, more plausible explanations for wife beating are available. From a cross-cultural perspective, Schlegel (1972) found in matrilineal societies that aggression by husbands against their wives, and brothers against their sisters, was associated with the source of domestic authority. When it lay with the men, such aggression was far more likely to occur than in societies where neither husbands nor brothers were dominant in authority. Moreover, she found that a husband was more likely to have to pay substantial bridewealth (valuables given by the groom's kin group to his bride's kin group to legitimate the marriage) to the bride's family in husband-dominant matrilineal societies than in more egalitarian societies; this suggests, according to Schlegel, that substantial bridewealth buys rights over the woman.

Additional explanations for wife beating that are not based on the anticuckoldry hypothesis are available. Wife abuse has been attributed to the high need of assaultive men to exert power in relationships (Dutton & Strachan, 1987); to childhood family experiences (Goode, 1969); to a tension reduction process (Walker, 1984); and to the "legal, religious and cultural legacies which have supported a marital hierarchy, subordinated women in marriage and legalized violence against them" (Dobash & Dobash, 1977–1978, p. 426).

Perhaps the strongest challenge to the sociobiologists comes from scholars who are equally adept at reconstructing a credible evolutionary history of a particular behavior but, unlike the sociobiologists, attribute its development to the evolution of human culture rather than to natural selection. Whereas for Daly et al. (1982) the impelling force of male jealousy is the competition for females in the goal for personal offspring, Cucchiari (1981) describes a persuasive scenario in which the desire to control the sexual behavior of mates is the consequence of the social construction of the gender system. "Social construction" refers in this context to the arbitrary assignment of activities and qualities to each gender (e.g., the desire for honor, beauty, masculinity, femininity, etc.).

In pre-gender-role society, speculates Cucchiari, with its intense and unrestricted sexual expression, children are born into the horde. They are not identified as belonging to any one parent. Filiation and descent are nonissues. But with a gender-related ideology,

> Once "maleness" or "femaleness," attractiveness, sexuality, and mate getting become significant in the way men and women carve out their identities and in the way they compete among themselves, it is not difficult to understand why "cheating" or mate stealing can be threatening acts leading to severe emotional reactions. (1981, p. 59)

Thus Cucchiari places the origin of male and female jealousy in the evolution of human culture.

In sum, I have begun this section with the question of why romantic relationships have the power to provoke jealousy. The sociobiologists place the impetus, the motive, in the aeons of human evolution. Specifically, they believe that males have inherited the inclination, the psychological propensity, to want paternity confidence. Jealousy is elicited whenever it is threatened. Cited as supportive evidence for such a motive, and by inference for the idea that it must be a remnant of human evolution, are the cross-cultural restrictions on female sexuality, as well as spousal abuse in the form of husbands beating and killing wives. However, this motive and its putative basis in human evolution have been called into question with alternative explanations more closely tied to research than the narrative arguments of Daly et al. (1982).

But, then, what is the motive for the arousal of jealousy, and how is it generated? The motive, as I indicate below, is a product of the culture and can vary across cultures because it is an inescapable consequence of social structures. The term "social structures" as I use it here refers to the elements of the social organization that maintain orderly relationships among individuals, regulate the production and distribution of wealth, and provide a setting for the breeding and socialization of new members of the society. The elements include the economic and political–legal systems; the patterns of kinship, descent, and affiliation; and so on (Hunter & Whitten, 1976).

## The Motive Emanates from Social Structures

Jealousy, by definition, is elicited by the potential involvement of spouses with interlopers. But why is the possibility of losing the mate to a rival such a threat? What is the motive for getting upset? More important, whence comes the motive for the provocation of jealousy?

### The Origin of the Motive for Romantic Jealousy

The motive for jealousy is a consequence of human beings living in societies (Hupka, 1977, 1981). Such aggregate living requires the resolution of numerous issues. Among them are the selection of an economic unit (e.g., the nuclear family or the clan), provisions for the sick and elderly (e.g., the responsibility of the progeny or the government), the vesting of property (e.g., in the individual or the clan), and the regulation of sexual behavior. Whatever the manner of resolving these issues, the solutions have psychological consequences for the members of the society. They define the level of significance or value that men and women have in each other's lives.

For the sake of illustration, let us consider two societies. In Society A, one must be married in order to be recognized as an adult and hold positions of power and prestige. The nuclear family is the economic unit. This means that it has to be self-sufficient and produce its own food, clothing, shelter, utensils, and so on. In addition, many personal offspring bring prestige and provide assurance that one will be taken care of in old age. Nonmarital and extramarital sexual intercourse are forbidden. In sum, matrimony is the key to survival, recognition as an adult, personal offspring, and guilt-free recreational sex. Clearly, husbands and wives need each other—not only to enjoy that which is held dear in the society, but also to ensure survival and companionship. Understandably, interlopers are resisted fiercely because they threaten the desired lifestyle, as well as personal survival.

The converse holds for Society B, which has a clan economy. The cooperative effort of the group assures the survival of all, particularly in old age. The contribution of any one individual to the survival of the clan is not as critical as in a nuclear family. Companionship is easily satisfied in such a large group of relatives. Society B assigns the privileges of adulthood on the basis of age rather than entrance into matrimony. There are no restrictions on sexual intercourse before and after marriage; this makes it impossible to identify personal descendants and has the consequence that children are accepted and valued in their own right. In sum, matrimony, the key to so much in Society A, is not needed in Society B for survival, companionship, acceptance as an adult, recreational sex, and so forth. Men and women play less of a role in each other's lives; that is to say, they are less dependent upon each other as individuals than in Society A. Consequently, interlopers pose less of a threat.

We can now answer the question of where the motive for the arousal of jealousy comes from, or is culturally created: It is an inevitable consequence of the solutions to the problems of living as a society. The solutions, such as the selection of the nuclear family as the economic unit, have psychological consequences for the members of the society. Namely, the solutions simultaneously create goals, needs, and values—as illustrated by the comparison of Societies A and B—that the members of the society seek to attain and satisfy. By virtue of that effect, the solutions influence the level of significance that males and females have in each other's lives. When the roles of marriage partners are minimal, as in Society B, their philandering does not elicit much jealousy. Alternatively, when the roles of marriage partners are firmly linked, as in Society A, philandering causes major disruptions in the lives of the cuckolded individuals and elicits intense jealousy.

A colleague and I have provided empirical support for the cultural perspective of jealousy (Hupka & Ryan, in press). We found positive correlations in 92 preindustrial societies between the importance attached to being married, restrictions on premarital and extramarital sexual gratifications, and emphasis on private ownership of property on the one hand, and the severity of aggression of males in jealousy situations on the other. These are some of the variables that influence the degree of linkage or interdependency of individuals in pairbonding relationships.

This finding supports the proposal that the origin, the reason, or the motive for the arousal of jealousy lies in social structures. We are threatened by interlopers because of the consequences of their actions for us. And the consequences are established through the social structures. Those consequences differ across cultures, as portrayed in the present comparison of the two hypothetical societies. As the social structures vary, so does the motive for the arousal of jealousy. Consider the Kaingáng of Brazil, whose social structures do not include an ideal of love, sexual exclusivity, or the formation of a nuclear family (Henry, 1941). Therefore, because of the absence of such ideals, they cannot be a motive for the arousal of jealousy. The motive is the "flip side" of the cultural values. In the process of enculturation, the members of a society learn that which is valued in male–female relationships, thereby simultaneously acquiring the motive for jealousy.

If the motive for jealousy is indeed an inescapable outcome of social structures, then the so-called "low-jealousy" cultures may well be such in relation to one set of social structures but could be "high-jealousy" cultures in relation to different sets. The Todas of India had cultural customs similar to those of Society B when Rivers (1906) observed them at the turn of the century. Sexual intercourse with someone other than one's mate was not likely to elicit a jealousy grieving process, because they had a custom that allowed married individuals to have lovers. Hence, from the perspective of Society A, the Todas were a low-jealousy culture. However, they were threatened by events that are inconsequential in other societies. The Todas practiced tribal endogamy and primogeniture: They were upset when Toda women had sexual intercourse with non-Toda men (Peter, 1963), and when the second-born son got married before the first-born son (Rivers, 1906). With respect to those values, the Todas were a high-jealousy culture. Such responses demonstrate that the motive for jealousy is threats to learned values and customs. It is also an indication that, by virtue of the learned values and customs, jealousy is a normal response. Whatever is valued, people hate losing to rivals. Interestingly and unresolvably, whereas I interpret the cross-cultural presence of jealousy as the inevitable consequence of social structures, sociobiologists accept it as evidence that the motive for jealousy is an evolved psychological propensity (Daly et al., 1982).

## What Is the Motive for Romantic Jealousy?

What is the interloper threatening? According to Daly et al. (1982), the interloper threatens the confidence of males that they are investing their resources in the raising of their own offspring. For females, it is the concern that insufficient resources remain for the successful nurturing of their own children if their fathers are squandering them on other women.

According to the cultural perspective, whatever is gained by dating or being married is threatened by the rival. This principle applies similarly to both men and women. The interloper threatens that which is sought after or hoped to be gained in establishing the relationship in the first place, as well as preventing the successful execution of one's role as a mate or partner in a dating relationship.

As demonstrated above by the comparison of Societies A and B, however, the variety of social structures gives rise to different goals, needs, and values. Hence, the motives for the arousal of jealousy can vary across cultures. Let us acquaint ourselves with several before examining whether the different motives elicit similar experiences of jealousy.

The restriction of sexual intercourse to one's mate is an essential part of the love relationship in many industrialized nations (Buunk & Hupka, 1987; Christensen, 1973). Violation of that expectation is perceived as a betrayal of the trust and commitment of the cuckolded partner and is justifiable cause for initiating the jealousy grieving process; suspicion or anticipation of such betrayal is usually sufficient to elicit the emotion of jealousy.

However, sentimental love was not always the grounds for marriage. Poverty was a dominant condition for many pre-20th-century Europeans. To marry without consideration of the financial side of the relationship was considered imprudent (Borscheid, 1986). Merely having knowledge of someone's comfortable financial condition was sufficient reason for proposing marriage without even having met the future mate. Among the upper-class 18th- and 19th-century Nablus in Palestine, marriages were arranged as a means to broader economic and political alliances (Tucker, 1988). No doubt interlopers were as much, if not more, disliked in such marriages as in those based on love. The suspected involvement of spouses with interlopers aroused feelings of jealousy. In contrast to the motive in a love relationship, the motive or reason for the jealousy among the Nablus was the prospect of losing the economic and political power forged by the marriages.

Among the Andalusians of Spain, the husband has the responsibility of maintaining the sexual purity of his wife, daughters, mother, and sisters (Pitt-Rivers, 1966). Women are said to be incapable of doing this without his assistance. Consequently, if, say, his wife has an affair, it is the husband, not the wife or the interloper, who is the object of ridicule. He has failed in his duty. He has betrayed the values of the family and brought dishonor on its members as well as himself. Similarly, a male member of the Kabyle tribe of Algeria is socialized to defend, as a categorical imperative, the honor of the family; the good name and renown of the ancestral lineage; and his own respectability, glory, and esteem (Bourdieu, 1966). If the Kabyle's honor is impugned through, say, the illicit sexual relations of his wife, he is expected to disdain the deepest feelings for his spouse and kill the wife who has sullied the aforementioned cherished absolutes. Driven by the love of honor, he jealousy guards it against infractions with a vengeance difficult to comprehend in societies with other values.

But these different motives for the arousal of jealousy raise the question of whether the predicaments are comparable and even can be regarded as jealousy situations. Are the Andalusian husband and the Kabyle husband, when avenging the honor that has been impugned by the liaisons of their wives, propelled by the same emotions as an American husband confronting his wife's affair? The resolution of this intriguing issue lies in the distinction between the emotion of jealousy and the jealousy grieving process.

None of the individuals in the aforementioned examples wants to lose the spouse to a rival, whether for reasons of intimacy, financial security, political power, or the duty to protect honor. Each is threatened by the possibility of losing the goals, needs, and values that were satisfied through the marriage. Thus, the possibility of the spouse's having an affair elicits jealousy in each of them. That which is threatened by the interloper may differ across societies; however, the phenomenological response to the threat does not. Insofar as the capability to experience jealousy is a product of the human genetic pool, the physiological experience of jealousy most likely is similar in human beings.

But the jealousy grieving process, triggered by the discovery that the spouse did indeed have the heretofore suspected extramarital affair, probably generates a different profile of cognitions, emotions, and behavior from culture to culture, because of the differences in repercussions of the affair to the cuckolded spouse. The Kabyle husband's duty to defend his family's honor against defamation with an act of violence, even if executed with reluctance and compelled predominantly by social pressure, probably elicits a dramatically different profile of responses over time from that of an American husband who is caught in the dilemma of whether or not to continue the relationship in light of the betrayal, or who has to grapple with his wife's decision to abandon the relationship in favor of one with the interloper.

In light of such differences, is it appropriate for social scientists to do cross-cultural research on the jealousy grieving process? By doing so, do they imply that the process is comparable across cultures? To answer these questions, let us list the similarities and differences in the jealousy grieving process across cultures.

The cuckolded individual is responding to the betrayal of a norm or expectation regarding sexual behavior. In all societies, the betrayal represents the loss of something of value as a result of the interloper's interference. Moreover, the final objective of the jealousy process is either to recapture that which has been lost or to accommodate to the permanence of the loss. In addition, the reactions to the transgression can be classified according to the phases of the jealousy grieving process: shock, recriminations, anguish, accommodation, and recovery. From such a general perspective, the cultures are comparable.

The major difference across cultures lies in the repercussions of the betrayal to the cuckolded individual: loss of honor and the requirement to regain it, for the Andalusian and the Kabyle; loss of financial security, for the Nablus; or loss of an intimate relationship, feelings of being excluded, and loss of exclusivity (Buunk, 1981), and possibly self-doubt (regarding one's skills as a lover, companion, resolver of conflicts, etc.), for the typical American or other Westerner. The implication is that members of each society are driven by different goals or concerns following betrayal; therefore, the predicaments are not comparable. For example, the Kabyle's response to the betrayal is propelled by the urge to regain honor, not by aspirations for financial security or the yearning for a love relationship.

Such cultural differences are real and cannot be ignored, but they should not preclude cross-cultural comparisons. The aim of researchers should be to determine all possible repercussions of sexual betrayal across cultures, as well as within cultures; ways in which the repercussions come about and tie in with social structures; and ways in which the individuals go about recovering from the affront. Given the diversity among ethnic groups in modern nations and the multiplicity of sects, it may turn out that the repercussions are more diverse and extreme within nations than between them. More relevant to the issue of comparability is the possibility that the profile of emotions in the jealousy grieving process is due not to the nature of the repercussions, but to whatever the individual happens to be focusing on at any moment during the jealousy grieving process (Hupka, 1984). For example, the compelling force that drives an argument with the unfaithful partner may not be love (in love societies), honor (in honor societies), or greed (in alliance-forming societies), but rather the anger stemming from the unfaithful individual's disregard of the years of investment in the relationship. Thus, it remains to be determined empirically which cues—cultural factors, contextual factors, or personality traits—give rise to a particular emotion in the jealousy grieving process.

In sum, the repercussions of sexual betrayal can differ profoundly across cultures. Nevertheless, if this fact is kept in mind, there are sufficient similarities and valuable information to be gained from the cross-cultural comparisons to warrant such research.

## CONCLUSION

A computer system consists of hardware and software components. The hardware is the electronic and mechanical components of the computer, whereas the software consists of the programs that allow one to use the resources of the hardware. Although they are separate entities, each with its own history of development and principles of operation, both are required in order to have a functional computer system. One is useless without the other. I have proposed an analogous arrangement between the *capacity* to experience jealousy and the *motive* for its elicitation: The "hardware" is part of the neuroanatomical and physiological substrate that human beings have inherited through evolution, and the "software" is the diversity of cultural programs created by people regarding the elicitation and embellishment of that capacity to experience jealousy. Without culture there is no opportunity, no reason, to experience jealousy.

The social structures, the principles by which human activity is organized or programmed, have such profound ramifications for individuals that they most likely would feign jealousy and the jealousy grieving process if they were prevented from experiencing them due to spinal cord injuries (cf. Hohmann, 1962), rather than lose to rivals whatever they gain in their particular cultures by being in intimate relationships. Alternatively, if there were no social structures, there would be no motive for the arousal of jealousy. The motive is a human creation.

## REFERENCES

Arnold, M. (1960). *Emotion and personality*. New York: Columbia University Press.
Averill, J. R. (1980). A constructivist view of emotion. In R. Plutchik & H. Kellerman (Eds.), *Emotion: Theory, research, and experience. Vol. 1. Theories of emotion* (pp. 305–339). New York: Academic Press.
Averill, J. R., & Nunley, E. P. (1988). Grief as an emotion and as a disease: A social-constructionist perspective. *Journal of Social Issues, 44*(3), 79–95.
Barr, C. E., & Hupka, R. B. (1984, April). *Attribution and intention as determinants of emotions in jealousy situations*. Paper presented at the meeting of the Western Psychological Association, Los Angeles.

Borscheid, P. (1986). Romantic love or material interest: Choosing partners in nineteenth-century Germany. *Journal of Family History, 11*, 157–168.

Bourdieu, P. (1966). The sentiment of honour in Kabyle society. In J. G. Peristiany (Ed.), *Honour and shame: The values of Mediterranean society* (pp. 191–241). Chicago: University of Chicago Press.

Brundage, J. A. (1982). Adultery and fornication: A study in legal theology. In V. L. Bullough & J. Brundage (Eds.), *Sexual practices & the medieval church* (pp. 129–134). Buffalo, NY: Prometheus Books.

Buunk, B. (1981). Jealousy in sexually open marriages. *Alternative Lifestyles, 4*, 357–372.

Buunk, B., & Hupka, R. B. (1987). Cross-cultural differences in the elicitation of sexual jealousy. *Journal of Sex Research, 23*, 12–22.

Christensen, H. T. (1973). Attitudes toward marital infidelity: A nine-culture sampling of university student opinion. *Journal of Comparative Family Studies, 4*, 197–214.

Cucchiari, S. (1981). The gender revolution and the transition from bisexual horde to patrilocal band: The origins of gender hierarchy. In S. B. Ortner & H. Whitehead (Eds.), *Sexual meanings: The cultural construction of gender and sexuality* (pp. 31–79). Cambridge, England: Cambridge University Press.

Daly, M., Wilson, M., & Weghorst, S. J. (1982). Male sexual jealousy. *Ethology and Sociobiology, 3*, 11–27.

Dobash, R. E., & Dobash, R. P. (1977–1978). Wives: The "appropriate" victims of marital violence. *Victimology, 2*, 426–442.

Dutton, D. G., & Strachan, C. E. (1987). Motivational needs for power and spouse-specific assertiveness in assaultive and nonassaultive men. *Violence and Victims, 2*, 145–156.

Ekman, P., & Friesen, W. V. (1975). *Unmasking the face: A guide to recognizing emotions from facial clues.* Englewood Cliffs, NJ: Prentice-Hall.

Ekman, P., Friesen, W. V., O'Sullivan, M., Diacoyanni-Tarlatzis, I., Krause, R., Pitcairn, T., Scherer, K., Chan, A., Heider, K., LeCompte, W. A., Ricci-Bitti, P. E., Tomita, M., & Tzavaras, A. (1987). Universals and cultural differences in the judgments of facial expressions of emotion. *Journal of Personality and Social Psychology, 53*, 712–717.

Folta, J. R., & Deck, E. S. (1988). The impact of children's death on Shona mothers and families. *Journal of Comparative Family Studies, 19*, 433–451.

Gold, M. (1958). Suicide, homicide, and the socialization of aggression. *American Journal of Sociology, 62*, 651–661.

Gold, P. S. (1982). The marriage of Mary and Joseph in the twelfth-century ideology of marriage. In V. L. Bullough & J. Brundage (Eds.), *Sexual practices & the medieval church* (pp. 102–117). Buffalo, NY: Prometheus Books.

Goode, W. J. (1969). Violence among intimates. In D. J. Mulvihill & M. M. Tumin (Eds.), *Crimes of violence* (Vol. 13, Appendix 19). Washington, DC: U.S. Government Printing Office.

Harré, R. (Ed.). (1986). *The social construction of emotions.* Oxford: Basil Blackwell.

Harris, M. (1974). *Cows, pigs, wars and witches.* New York: Random House.

Henry, J. (1941). *Jungle people.* New York: J. J. Augustin.

Hobhouse, L. T. (1906). *Morals in evolution: A study in comparative ethics.* London: Chapman & Hall.

Hobhouse, L. T. (1922). The historical evolution of property, in fact and idea. In C. Gore (Ed.), *Property: Its duties and rights* (2nd ed., pp. 1–36). New York: Macmillan.

Hohmann, G. W. (1962). Some effects of spinal cord lesions on experienced emotional feelings. *Psychophysiology, 3,* 143–156.

Hunter, D. E., & Whitten, P. (Eds.). (1976). *Encyclopedia of anthropology.* New York: Harper & Row.

Hupka, R. B. (1977, August). Societal and individual roles in the expression of jealousy. In H. Sigall (Chair), *Sexual jealousy.* Symposium conducted at the meeting of the American Psychological Association, San Francisco.

Hupka, R. B. (1981). Cultural determinants of jealousy. *Alternative Lifestyles, 4,* 310–356.

Hupka, R. B. (1984). Jealousy: Compound emotion or label for a particular situation? *Motivation and Emotion, 8,* 141–155.

Hupka, R. B. (1989, May). Components of the typical response to romantic jealousy situations. In G. L. White (Chair), *Themes for progress in jealousy research.* Symposium conducted at the Second Iowa Conference on Personal Relationships, Iowa City.

Hupka, R. B., Buunk, B., Falus, A., Ortega, E., Swain, R., & Tarabrina, N. V. (1985). Romantic jealousy and romantic envy: A seven-nation study. *Journal of Cross-Cultural Psychology, 16,* 423–446.

Hupka, R. B., & Ryan, J. M. (in press). The cultural contribution to jealousy: Cross-cultural aggression in sexual jealousy situations. *Behavior Science Research.*

Izard, C. E., Huebner, R. R., Risser, D., McGinnes, G., & Dougherty, L. (1980). The young infant's ability to produce discrete emotion expressions. *Developmental Psychology, 16,* 132–140.

Jacobsen, G. (1982). Sexual irregularities in medieval Scandinavia. In V. L. Bullough & J. Brundage (Eds.), *Sexual practices & the medieval church* (pp. 72–85). Buffalo, NY: Prometheus Books.

Lampe, P. E. (1987). Adultery and the behavioral sciences. In P. E. Lampe (Ed.), *Adultery in the United States* (pp. 165–198). Buffalo, NY: Prometheus Books.

Lane, R. (1979). *Violent death in the city: Suicide, accident, and murder in nineteenth-century Philadelphia.* Cambridge, MA: Harvard University Press.

Lazarus, R. S. (1966). *Psychological stress and the coping process.* New York: McGraw-Hill.

Lovejoy, C. O. (1981). The origin of man. *Science, 211,* 341–350.

Peter, Prince of Greece and Denmark. (1963). *A study of polyandry.* The Hague: Mouton.

Pitt-Rivers, J. (1966). Honour and social status. In J. G. Peristiany (Ed.), *Honour* and shame: The values of Mediterranean society (pp. 19–77). Chicago: University of Chicago Press.

Plutchik, R. (1980). Emotion: A psychoevolutionary synthesis. New York: Harper & Row.

Rivers, W. H. R. (1906). The Todas. London: Macmillan.

Rudmin, F. W. (1988). Dominance, social control, and ownership: A history and a cross-cultural study of motivations for private property. Behavior Science Research, 22, 130–160 [corrected copy].

Schlegel, A. (1972). Male dominance and female autonomy: Domestic authority in matrilineal societies. New Haven, CT: HRAF Press.

Simmons, L. W. (1937). Statistical correlations in the science of society. In G. P. Murdock (Ed.), Studies in the science of society (pp. 493–517). New Haven, CT: Yale University Press.

Sumner, W. G., & Keller, A. G. (1927). The science of society. New Haven, CT: Yale University Press.

Tucker, J. E. (1988). Marriage and family in Nablus, 1720–1856: Toward a history of Arab marriage. Journal of Family History, 13, 165–179.

Van Lawick-Goodall, J. (1967). Mother–offspring relationships in free-ranging chimpanzees. In D. Morris (Ed.), Primate ethology (pp. 287–346). Chicago: Aldine.

Walker, L. E. (1984). The battered woman syndrome. New York: Springer.

Wolfgang, M. E. (1959). Suicide by means of victim-precipitated homicide. Journal of Clinical and Experimental Psychopathology, 20, 335–349.

Wolfgang, M. E. (1968). Patterns in criminal homicide. Philadelphia: University of Pennsylvania Press.

*Chapter Twelve*

# Envy and Jealousy: Self and Society

PETER SALOVEY
ALEXANDER J. ROTHMAN
*Yale University*

Because we are now celebrating the centennial of William James's classic and comprehensive textbook, *The Principles of Psychology*, a quote from the master seems to be an appropriate and timely way to delineate the theme of this chapter. Writing about rivalry and conflict among different selves in his seminal chapter on the consciousness of self, James provided this bit of autobiography:

> I, who for the time have staked my all on being a psychologist, am mortified if others know much more psychology than I. But I am contented to wallow in the grossest ignorance of Greek. My deficiencies there give me no sense of personal humiliation at all. Had I "pretensions" to be a linguist, it would have been just the reverse. So we have the paradox of a man shamed to death because he is only the second pugilist or the second oarsman in the world. That he is able to beat the whole population of the globe minus one is nothing; he has "pitted" himself to beat that one; and as long as he doesn't do that nothing else counts. He is to his own regard as if he were not, indeed he *is* not. (James, 1890/1983, p. 296)

This is not a chapter about social comparison processes per se, as might be suggested by the quotation (but see Salovey, 1990). Rather, it is about the circumstances under which we as human beings are most likely to experience feelings of envy or jealousy. We are not envious of just anyone's random attributes that we have not attained ourselves. Nor are we invariably jealous when our lovers flirt with random others. Rather, envy and jealousy are most likely to be felt when comparisons are made in domains that are especially important to how we define ourselves—that "hit us where we live" (Salovey & Rodin, 1983). Likewise, jealousy is most likely to be experienced when an important relationship is threatened by a rival against whom we worry that we cannot measure up in some domain that is especially important to us. Slightly more formally, these predictions, called the "domain relevance hypotheses," can be stated as follows:

Hypothesis 1: Envy is most likely to be experienced when comparisons with another person (a rival) are negative for the self, and these comparisons are in a domain that is especially important and relevant to self-definition.

Hypothesis 2: Jealousy is most likely to be experienced when the termination of an important, interdependent relationship with another person is threatened by a rival whose characteristics in especially important domains—that is, domains relevant to self-definition—appear to be better than our own.

It is the purpose of the present chapter (1) to outline the theoretical roots of these hypotheses about envy and jealousy in Tesser's self-evaluation maintenance (SEM) model of human behavior; (2) to describe a large-scale, correlational study that provided evidence supporting these hypotheses; (3) to discuss a laboratory experiment in which domain relevance was actually manipulated and whose results supported this view; and (4) to speculate about the cultural origins of domain importance. A more comprehensive review of the research on jealousy and envy conducted in our laboratory can be found in Salovey and Rodin (1989).

## A SELF-EVALUATION MAINTENANCE VIEW OF ENVY AND JEALOUSY

Tesser's SEM model begins with the premise that individuals are motivated to maintain or increase self-esteem; that is, they will behave in such a way as to promote a positive view of themselves (see Tesser, 1986, 1988, and Tesser & Campbell, 1983, for excellent overviews of this theory). The next assumption is that much of the opportunity to obtain feedback that allows individuals to maintain high self-esteem has its origins in social interactions with similar other people. Tesser has focused on two possible kinds of social interaction: one that promotes what he has labeled the "reflective process," and one that he calls the "comparison process."

In situations that instantiate the reflective process, one's self-evaluation is bolstered by the superior attributes or performances of close others. One can feel very good about oneself simply by knowing successful others—a process originally described as "basking in reflected glory" by Cialdini and his colleagues (Cialdini et al., 1976; Cialdini & Richardson, 1980). So, for example, we feel terrific about ourselves when our favorite baseball player hits a home run, when our trumpet-playing high school buddy is offered a chair in the philharmonic orchestra, when our spouse receives a deserved promotion at work, and when our children bring home report cards from school filled with A's.

In other situations, however, the superior performances and attributes of close others are quite threatening to our self-esteem. Their superior performances make us feel awful about ourselves. These are situations that Tesser (1988) described as ones invoking the comparison process. William James (1890/1983) admitted that he would feel awful in the presence of a better scholar of psychology than he. The professional golfer receives no special kicks hearing about a better-scoring competitor. And researchers in academia greet with some ambivalence the news that a colleague has won an award that they desired for themselves (cf. the discussion in Rosenhan, Salovey, & Hargis, 1981, about why professors rarely throw splashy going-away parties for colleagues leaving their university for greener pastures).

What differentiates those situations that produce reflection from those that produce comparison? Here is where the *relevance* of the performance domain becomes important. According to the SEM model, we only truly care about our performance in a limited number of life domains. When others surpass us in these domains, self-evaluation is threatened as the comparison process is invoked (Tesser & Campbell, 1982). As William James (1890/1983) claimed, he was simply not bothered by the scholarly prowess of professors of Greek. It was only the brilliance of his colleagues in psychology that could make him feel bad about himself. Jealousy and envy are more likely to be experienced under the conditions that invoke the comparison process: when we are outperformed by another person with whom we have a close relationship, and the domain of this performance is self-definitional—that is, the performance domain is important or relevant to how we see ourselves (Tesser & Collins, 1988).

How can we tell that another person is envious or jealous? Generally by observing his or her behaviors. And the behaviors in which one engages when envious or jealous usually serve the purpose of trying to restore or maintain a positive view of the self when it is threatened by comparison to others. So, for example, one can try to prevent the other person's successful performance (Tesser & Smith, 1980); one can distort one's beliefs about the other's success in a negative direction (Tesser & Campbell, 1982); one can distort one's beliefs about one's own performances and attributes in a positive direction (Salovey & Rodin, 1988; Tesser, Campbell, & Smith, 1984); one can reduce closeness with the other (Pleban & Tesser, 1981; Salovey & Rodin, 1984); and one can change one's view of what is important or relevant in order to reflect rather than compare with successful others (Tesser & Paulhus, 1983).

Each of these behaviors describes what is potentially observed when we attribute envy or jealousy to another's motives. For instance, suppose a 10-year-old boy who has played Little League baseball for several years has a friend and neighbor who always plays better than he does. If baseball is an important and relevant aspect of the boy's self-definition, he will experience the comparison process, and his self-evaluation will be threatened. This boy can prevent or terminate this threat by interfering with the other child's performance—stealing his bat, dipping his glove in a bucket of water, or socking him in the eye. Furthermore, he can distort the other child's performance—attributing his success to luck rather than skill or to colluding with opposing players. The boy may attribute his own lack of success to external forces—playing with an injury, or not having a father who hits fungos to him in the evening. More drastically, the boy may decide that he no longer desires a friendship with his rival, or, in order to maintain the friendship, may decide that baseball is simply no longer important to him (but that schoolwork is where he will now stake his reputation).

Thus, we would predict that envy and jealousy are typically instigated only in those situations where the attributes or behaviors of others threaten one's self-esteem by comparison. Envy and jealousy may reflect an eroding of one's social position (in one's own eyes and the eyes of others), and the behaviors in which one engages when envious or jealous may serve to control this diminution in status (see Sabini & Silver, 1982; Schmitt, 1988; Silver & Sabini, 1978). We now turn to work in our laboratory that more specifically investigates the role of self-definition in jealousy and envy, and that tests the domain relevance hypotheses in particular.

## CORRELATIONAL EVIDENCE SUPPORTING
## THE DOMAIN RELEVANCE HYPOTHESES

Some years ago, we (Salovey & Rodin, 1985a) came upon the opportunity to include a reader survey in *Psychology Today* on the experience of envy and jealousy. When constructing the survey, we were guided by the hypothesis that envy and jealousy would be most likely to be reported in situations that were particularly relevant to an individual's self-definition, because they involved the receipt of self-esteem-threatening feedback in a domain that was important. Thus, on the survey, respondents were asked to rate a set of four domains—wealth, fame, being liked by others (popularity), and physical attractiveness—according to how important each domain was to them. They then indicated how they ideally and actually viewed their accomplishments in each domain. Salovey and Rodin also included a measure of global self-esteem. Jealousy and envy were measured as the frequency with which respondents performed a series of behaviors associated with jealousy and envy, and the intensity of jealous and envious feelings experienced in a set of hypothetical situations. The jealous and envious behaviors and situations were grouped according to which of the four domains was made salient.

The primary hypothesis, which is illustrated schematically in Figure 12.1, was that jealousy and envy in a life domain would be predicted by the relevance of that domain for self-definition, the degree to which subjects felt they were not measuring up to their expectations in that domain, and the consequent threat to self-esteem that these cognitions should produce. Note that jealousy and envy were expected to be domain-specific: Jealousy and envy in a domain were expected to be felt most strongly in the domain rated as most relevant to self-evaluation (i.e., most important) and in the domain where self-evaluation was most threatened.

About 25,000 readers responded to the survey, and 6,482 were randomly selected for analysis (see Salovey & Rodin, 1985b, for information on the demographics of this sample). As can be seen in Table 12.1, the largest correlations were found between the importance of a particular domain and the jealousy or envy experienced in that domain. Importance of a domain was more strongly associated with jealousy or envy in that same domain than with envy or jealousy in any other domain—a pattern that had a probability of only .004 of being found by chance.

As can be seen in Table 12.2, a domain's relevance to self-definition was associated with jealousy or envy in that domain, even when threats to self-evaluation in the domain (measured as the difference between real

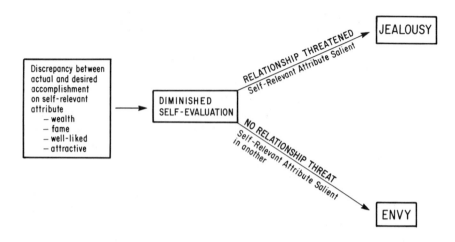

**FIGURE 12.1.** Primary hypothesis for reader survey.

and ideal ratings of accomplishment in that domain) and global self-esteem were taken into account. All three variables—relevance (importance), real–ideal discrepancies, and global self esteem—were associated with envy and jealousy.

Of course, an obvious worry in reporting data gathered through a magazine survey is that despite the large size of the sample, findings may not generalize; the sample is, after all, self-selected and nonrandom. However, Salovey and Rodin (1990) have now had the opportunity to replicate this survey on a more typical sample of 200 residents selected

**TABLE 12.1. Correlations between Domain Importance and Jealousy/Envy**

|  | Jealousy/envy | | | |
| Importance | Wealth | Fame | Popularity | Attractiveness |
| --- | --- | --- | --- | --- |
| Wealth | .20 | .12 | .04 | .10 |
| Fame | .09 | .18 | .05 | .04 |
| Popularity | .16 | .17 | .27 | .24 |
| Attractiveness | .18 | .15 | .21 | .34 |

*Note. n* = 6,472; all correlations are significant at *p* < .001. Underscored entries are those correlations predicted to be greatest in each row. The data are from Salovey and Rodin (1990).

**TABLE 12.2. Predicting Jealousy/Envy Using Multiple Regression in Reader Survey**

| Predictor | Beta | t |
|---|---|---|
| *Criterion: Jealousy/envy in wealth domain* | | |
| Wealth importance | .19 | 15.23 |
| Wealth ideal–actual discrepancy | .09 | 7.24 |
| Global self-esteem | −.19 | 15.64 |
| Model $R = .30$, $F (3, 6,168) = 205.13$, $p < .0001$ | | |
| *Criterion: Jealousy/envy in fame domain* | | |
| Fame importance | .17 | 13.79 |
| Fame ideal–actual discrepancy | .12 | 9.40 |
| Global self-esteem | −.20 | 15.61 |
| Model $R = .31$, $F (3, 6,159) = 220.41$, $p < .0001$ | | |
| *Criterion: Jealousy/envy in popularity domain* | | |
| Popularity importance | .23 | 19.02 |
| Popularity ideal–actual discrepancy | .15 | 11.84 |
| Global self-esteem | −.20 | 15.81 |
| Model $R = .39$, $F (3, 6,176) = 359.98$, $p < .0001$ | | |
| *Criterion: Jealousy/envy in attractiveness domain* | | |
| Attractiveness importance | .31 | 27.21 |
| Attractiveness ideal–actual discrepancy | .15 | 12.18 |
| Global self-esteem | −.21 | 17.23 |
| Model $R = .45$, $F (3, 6,184) = 524.64$, $p < .0001$ | | |

*Note.* All $t$ tests on the beta weights are significant at $p < .001$. The data are from Salovey and Rodin (1990).

randomly from a Northeastern urban area. As in the reader survey sample, these subjects also experienced the greatest envy and jealousy in domains that were most relevant to self-definition.

## EXPERIMENTAL EVIDENCE SUPPORTING THE DOMAIN RELEVANCE HYPOTHESES

A stronger test of the domain relevance hypotheses, however, than one offered by correlational analyses is provided by opportunities to manipulate domain relevance and then to explore the impact on jealousy and envy. Salovey and Rodin (1984) conducted such a study with a college student sample. In this study, subjects were recruited in a way that made their career choice salient: They were asked to sign up if they were interested in pursuing careers in medicine, business, or drama. Subjects were scheduled to arrive at the laboratory in pairs and assigned to two small rooms that were separated by a folding wall. Although each subject in a pair never met the other, each could overhear activity in the adjacent room through the rather thin folding wall.

The cover story for the experiment was that it explored the relationship between personality and career choice. Subjects were told that they were selected for the experiment because of their particular career orientation and that they would receive several different kinds of personality measures—one that was objective, one that was subjective, and finally a projective test. At this point, subjects were asked to begin working on the objective measure, which was in fact a bonus personality test called the Robertson–Wagner Personality Profile (RWPP), a randomized ordering of items from personality scales of interest to the investigators.

After the pair of subjects had completed the RWPP, the experimenter collected the forms and then asked the subjects to begin working on the second personality measure, the subjective one. This personality test consisted of writing a self-descriptive paragraph or two. Subjects were then left alone to work on their essays. After about 10 minutes, the experimenter returned to collect the essays. Subjects were told at this point that the experimenter had scored some of the subscales of the RWPP, and they were asked whether they would like some feedback on their performance. Naturally, every subject availed himself or herself of this opportunity. And here was where the conditions of the experiment were made salient to the subjects. On official-looking scoring grids, subjects were provided with RWPP feedback indicating that they were slightly above average in aptitude for a variety of careers and that they were either (1) well above or well below average on one of the career scales that (2) either corresponded to or did not correspond to their stated career choice (medicine, business, or drama). Furthermore, the experimenter explained that because he had run out of scoring grids, the scores of the subject in the room next door had also been plotted on this grid, but in a different color. This other subject's score was *always* depicted as well above average, and it was either in the primary subject's career area or in another area. Thus, subjects received feedback that was either (1) positive or negative, (2) relevant to their career domain or not, and (3) presented in a context in which a successful rival's performance was relevant to their career domain or not.

A measure of envy was now needed. Each subject was next given an essay to read and told it was the self-descriptive paragraphs generated by the subject next door. Subjects were told that a final measure of their personality would be indicated by this projective test: They had to read this essay and try to guess what kind of a person the other subject was. All subjects were given the same essay, which read as follows:

> I am a freshman at Yale with many interests. I enjoy backpacking and camping as well as going to movies and plays. My main interest lies in medicine [business and management/theater, music, and the performing arts in general]—I hope to be a doctor [an executive/perform professionally] some day. I'm already taking some of the required courses and doing pretty well in them—really well, actually, considering my background in this area before coming to Yale. I study a lot, and the hard work seems to be paying off.
>
> Socially, things are only O.K. I have lots of friends, but no real romantic attachments. That, however, could be changing in the near future. I certainly hope so.
>
> Academically, though, things are great. I've been one of the top in all my classes—the couple of professors that I have talked to say I have a promising future . . . I guess time will tell!!

The essay was constructed so that subjects could find both likable and annoying aspects of this person. Their judgments of him or her would then reflect how much attention they had focused on the person's assets or faults.

After reading the essay, subjects completed a number of scales on which they indicated the likely personality attributes of this other person, the degree to which they wanted to be this person's friend, and how anxious and sad they would feel upon interacting with this person at the end of the experiment. Among the measures of anxiety and sadness, we included two scales specifically measuring experienced envy and jealousy.

As hypothesized, individuals experienced the most envy (as depicted in Figure 12.2) when they received self-relevant negative feedback and subsequently thought they would associate with a similar (relevant) other person who was more successful than they were. In addition, subjects were more likely to disparage the rival (on the trait-rating task after reading the essay) in this condition than in any of the other seven, and they expected to experience more anxiety and sadness in this condition as well. Finally, subjects were least likely to desire to befriend the rival when he or she outperformed them in a relevant career domain.

In addition to the obvious importance of the relevance of the feedback domain as an antecedent of envy and jealousy, another interesting aspect of this study was that subjects reacted to envy-provoking feedback by disparaging the rival and attempting to reduce future closeness with him or her. Disparaging the rival and reducing closeness are behaviors predicted by SEM theory as ways of coping with the comparison

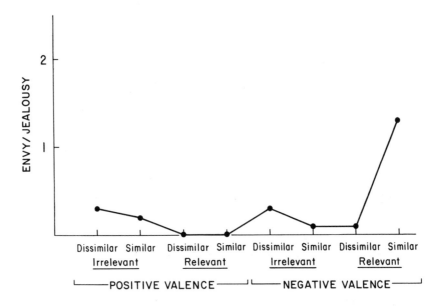

**FIGURE 12.2.** Envy and jealousy experienced in the eight conditions of the laboratory experiment. The data are from Salovey and Rodin (1984).

process, and they have been observed in other social comparison contexts as well (Cialdini & Richardson, 1980; Crocker, Thompson, McGraw, & Ingerman, 1987). Indeed, the derogation of rivals when self-evaluation is threatened is considered the defining feature of envy by some theorists (Freud, 1922/1955; Sabini & Silver, 1982).

Rival derogation is observed not just in social comparison situations that provoke envy, but in jealousy-provoking situations as well. Schmitt (1988) noted that the rival serves as an excellent target for denigration in the typical romantic triangle. First, it is the rival who most directly threatens the jealous person's self-worth. Second, the rival is an intruder who threatens to destabilize an existing relationship. Third, the jealous person often knows very little about the rival and so can easily conjure up negative visions of this person. And fourth, the jealous person would prefer to derogate the rival rather than the beloved, because continuing the relationship with the beloved is often still a desired goal. Of course, this situation presents the jealous person with an intriguing paradox: If the person loved by the jealous individual is attracted to the rival, the rival must have some redeeming characteristics. Probably they are the ones most valued by the beloved, and probably those that formed the basis of the beloved's attraction to the jealous person in the first place.

## THE CULTURAL ORIGINS OF DOMAIN RELEVANCE

Kingsley Davis (1936) was the first major sociocultural theorist to address jealousy, which he described in terms of a group's sexual property norms. Jealousy is expected to flare when sexual property rules are violated. Davis believed that norms encouraging the expression of jealousy protect societally valued relationships (e.g., sexual relationships). The delineation of valued relationships, however, in turn helps to define the behaviors considered threatening enough to provoke jealousy. For example, if sexual relationships are perceived as more valuable than work relationships, relationship-threatening behaviors would be more likely to inspire jealousy between sexual partners than between work partners.

Hupka (1981) identified several specific characteristics differentiating jealous from nonjealous cultures. Cultures low in jealousy discourage individual property rights, perceive sexual gratification and companionship as easily available, but do not consider sex a pleasurable recreational activity. In addition, these cultures place little importance on personal descendants, parental certainty, and marriage as an essential rite of passage. Cultures high in jealousy value personal property, view sexual gratification as a product only of marriage, and perceive marriage and family as important societal institutions.

Hupka's (1981) findings parallel those of Davis (1936) in suggesting that the experience of jealousy in a domain is dependent upon the value that a society ascribes to that domain. Across cultures, the same situational contexts do not always provoke jealousy. If a culture values marriage, its members may be inclined to protect such relationship jealously, and therefore the appearance of a rival may lead to jealous feelings in a married individual. However, if the culture does not place special value on marriage, it may be considered a less important domain to the individual, and so the appearance of a rival may be less threatening and consequently less jealousy-provoking.

Many sociocultural theorists (e.g., Davis, 1936; Hupka, 1981; Mead, 1936/1977; Whitehurst, 1977) have focused primarily on romantic jealousy. Their analyses, however, can be extended to other instances of social relations jealousy. Cultures can specify the importance of nonromantic relationships. For example, academic culture places a high value on relationships between graduate students and professors. Both professors and students frequently experience jealousy over threats to them, by, for example, the arrival of new first-year students (in the case of graduate students) or imperialistic colleagues (in the case of professors).

Envy, too, is also influenced by societal norms and values. It appears to exist in all cultures (Foster, 1972), although the expression of envy may vary somewhat, depending on culture. In Western society, envy is thought to inspire and motivate economic and social development (Schoeck, 1969). Envy motivates individuals to better their lot, to improve their talents and abilities, and to be more productive (Rorty, 1971). Although envy is an acknowledged motivator, admitting to it is still highly stigmatized. In a sense, society conceives of envy as a necessary evil. This somewhat more positive conception of envy emphasizes what Foster (1972) terms the "competitive axis" of envy. Competitive envy underscores wants and desires for the self, rather than those things one wants to take from others. Envy expressed in this manner motivates self-improvement. The denigration of others and their possessions that embodies the dark side of envy is not featured in this formulation. Schoeck (1969) argues that Western nations promote envy specifically in order to motivate their citizens to improve themselves. Advertising is an excellent window through which to view how societies attempt to motivate individuals to differentiate themselves from those around them. Advertisements on television and in magazines tell us to own certain cars, wear certain clothes, drink certain beers, and so on, the result of which will provoke the envy of our contemporaries. Furthermore, prestige in these societies is defined not solely as the possession of an object, but rather as the possession of something that others do not have. The elicitation of envy in others therefore can be seen as a reinforcement for the achievement of high status and prestige.

In less developed societies, envy appears to have the opposite effect on individuals. Instead of encouraging development and improvement among its members, envy in these societies inhibits deviation from the status quo (Foster, 1972; Schoeck, 1969). In these cultures, envy is aroused when a person deviates from firmly established social norms in such matters as the possession of food, the size of one's family, or the state of one's health. Because there is a fear of arousing envy in others, people try hard not to deviate from social norms. Women hide their pregnancies, farmers downplay their bumper crops, and extremely successful people may even move out of their villages to avoid arousing envy. In the Arab world, "successful people greatly fear the vicious eye and often rich people denounce the reality of their fortune to keep away the bad influence of envious eyes" (Hamady, 1960, p. 172). For example, in traditional Egyptian culture, "when a visitor comes to the house, the mother covers herself as well as the child and pretends to be feeling rather uncomfortable, either groaning or suffering from pain" (Ammar, 1954, p. 97).

The fear of arousing envy in others is so great in these societies that people believe it will result in personal misfortune. This fear of misfortune is central to the notion of the "evil eye." The evil eye is an active expression of envy that can be found across a wide range of cultures (Foster, 1972; Schoeck, 1969). The elicitation of envy in others is believed to incite the evil eye. Individuals in many cultures hold that if one is looked upon by the evil eye, one is cursed.

Envy is believed to cause crop failures, illness, even death. Consequently, children, livestock, and other possessions of great value are shielded from the evil eye. Compliments related to these valued personal possessions as well as to personal successes are discouraged or rejected by members of these cultures. For example, in Timbuctoo, there is a belief that "compliments from non-intimates bring evil upon those praised. People therefore tend to avoid direct compliments and fear those directed to them" (Miner, 1953, p. 103). Fear of the evil eye is therefore one way in which a culture's view of envy helps maintain the status quo. In these cultures, any desire to improve one's lot is mitigated by an intrinsic fear of being cursed by the evil eye.

Not only can a culture ascribe more value to certain domains, but a culture can also shape the way in which individuals experience envy and jealousy. Intrinsic to our discussion of the sociocultural influences on envy and jealousy is the manner in which people perceive situations. Whether or not a situation is jealousy-provoking is dependent upon whether or not the situation is perceived as threatening to a relationship in a valued domain.

In thinking about sociocultural influences on jealousy and envy, we have suggested that how a person interprets a behavior is dependent upon that person's cultural values. Specifically, culture can influence a person's sense of domain importance, thereby facilitating the perception of certain behaviors as jealousy- or envy-provoking. By helping to define the context in which a behavior is perceived, a culture is creating in the individual both expectancies and perceptual sets in which to interpret social behavior.

## CONCLUSION

In this chapter, we have reviewed one hypothesis that has served as an important basis for much of our laboratory's work on jealousy and envy:

Individuals are most likely to experience envy and jealousy when their self-evaluation is threatened in a domain that is especially relevant or important to their sense of self. When the rival has characteristics that one would like for oneself, envy is experienced. But when the rival threatens the stability of an established close relationship, jealousy is provoked. It should be clear that many situations in which jealousy is experienced also involve considerable envy (see Salovey & Rodin, 1986, for a more detailed discussion of this point).

The theoretical origins of these domain relevance hypotheses in Tesser's SEM model of social behavior were traced first. We then reviewed the data collected from a large-scale survey and a laboratory experiment, which support the notion that what is important to the self determines when envy and jealousy are provoked. Finally, we explored some of the sociocultural origins of jealousy and envy and noted that what is important to the self—what becomes highly valued and self-defining—is often culturally determined. Hence, the experiences of envy and jealousy offer the investigator of human emotions a unique opportunity to explore a subjective experience often generated by social interaction but with deep sociocultural roots.

## REFERENCES

Ammar, H. (1954). *Growing up in an Egyptian village: Silwa, Province of Aswan.* London: Routledge & Kegan Paul.

Cialdini, R. B., Borden, R. J., Thorne, A., Walker, M. R., Freeman, S., & Sloan, L. R. (1976). Basking in reflected glory: Three (football) field studies. *Journal of Personality and Social Psychology, 34,* 366–375.

Cialdini, R. B., & Richardson, K. D. (1980). Two indirect tactics of impression management: Basking and blasting. *Journal of Personality and Social Psychology, 39,* 406–415.

Crocker, J., Thompson, L. L., McGraw, K. M., & Ingerman, C. (1987). Downward comparison prejudice and evaluation of others: Effects of self-esteem and threat. *Journal of Personality and Social Psychology, 52,* 907–916.

Davis, K. (1936). Jealousy and sexual property. *Social Forces, 14,* 395–405.

Foster, G. (1972). The anatomy of envy: A study in symbolic behavior. *Current Anthropology, 13,* 165–202.

Freud, S. (1955). Some neurotic mechanisms in jealousy, paranoia and homosexuality. In J. Strachey (Ed. and Trans.), *The standard edition of the complete psychological works of Sigmund Freud* (Vol. 18, pp. 221–232). London: Hogarth Press. (Original work published 1922)

Hamady, S. (1960). *Temperament and character of the Arabs.* New York: Twayne.

Hupka, R. B. (1981). Cultural determinants of jealousy. *Alternative Lifestyles, 4,* 310–356.

James, W. (1983). *The principles of psychology.* Cambridge, MA: Harvard University Press. (Original work published 1890)

Mead, M. (1977). Jealousy: Primitive and civilized. In G. Clanton & L. G. Smith (Eds.), *Jealousy* (pp. 115–127). Englewood Cliffs, NJ: Prentice-Hall. (Original work published 1936)

Miner, H. (1953). *The primitive city of Timbuctoo.* Princeton, NJ: Princeton University Press.

Pleban, R., & Tesser, A. (1981). The effects of relevance and quality of another's performance on interpersonal closeness. *Social Psychology Quarterly, 44,* 278–285.

Rorty, A. O. (1971). Some social uses of the forbidden. *Psychoanalytic Review, 58,* 497–510.

Rosenhan, D. L., Salovey, P., & Hargis, K. (1981). The joys of helping: Focus of attention mediates the impact of positive affect on altruism. *Journal of Personality and Social Psychology, 40,* 899–905.

Sabini, J., & Silver, M. (1982). *Moralities of everyday life.* Oxford: Oxford University Press.

Salovey, P. (1990). Social comparison processes in envy and jealousy. In J. Suls & T. Wills (Eds.), *Social comparison: Contemporary theory and research* (pp. 261–285). Hillsdale, NJ: Erlbaum.

Salovey, P., & Rodin, J. (1983, April). *A self-esteem maintenance model of envy.* Paper presented at the annual meeting of the Eastern Psychological Association, Philadelphia.

Salovey, P., & Rodin, J. (1984). Some antecedents and consequences of social-comparison jealousy. *Journal of Personality and Social Psychology, 47,* 780–792.

Salovey, P., & Rodin, J. (1985a, February). Jealousy and envy: The dark side of emotion. *Psychology Today,* pp. 32–34.

Salovey, P., & Rodin, J. (1985b, September). The heart of jealousy. *Psychology Today,* pp. 22–25, 28–29.

Salovey, P., & Rodin, J. (1986). Differentiation of social-comparison jealousy and romantic jealousy. *Journal of Personality and Social Psychology, 50,* 1100–1112.

Salovey, P., & Rodin, J. (1988). Coping with envy and jealousy. *Journal of Social and Clinical Psychology, 7,* 15–33.

Salovey, P., & Rodin, J. (1989). Envy and jealousy in close relationships. In C. Hendrick (Ed.), *Review of personality and social psychology: Vol. 10. Close relationships* (pp. 221–246). Newbury Park, CA: Sage.

Salovey, P., & Rodin, J. (1990). *Provoking jealousy and envy: Domain relevance and self-esteem threat.* Manuscript submitted for publication.

Schmitt, B. H. (1988). Social comparison in romantic jealousy. *Personality and Social Psychology Bulletin, 14,* 374–387.

Schoeck, H. (1969). *Envy: A theory of social behavior.* New York: Harcourt, Brace & World.

Silver, M., & Sabini, J. (1978). The perception of envy. *Social Psychology, 41,* 105–117.

Tesser, A. (1986). Some effects of self-evaluation maintenance on cognition and action. In R. M. Sorrentino & E. T. Higgins (Eds.), *Handbook of motivation and cognition: Foundations of social behavior* (Vol. 1, pp. 435–464). New York: Guilford Press.

Tesser, A. (1988). Toward a self-evaluation maintenance model of social behavior. In L. Berkowitz (Ed.), *Advances in experimental social psychology* (Vol. 21, pp. 181–227). New York: Academic Press.

Tesser, A., & Campbell, J. (1982). Self-evaluation maintenance and the perception of friends and strangers. *Journal of Personality, 50,* 261–279.

Tesser, A., & Campbell, J. (1983). Self-definition and self-evaluation maintenance. In J. Suls & A. Greenwald (Eds.), *Social psychological perspectives on the self* (Vol. 2, pp. 1–31). Hillsdale, NJ: Erlbaum.

Tesser, A., Campbell, J., & Smith, M. (1984). Friendship choice and performance: Self-evaluation maintenance in children. *Journal of Personality and Social Psychology, 46,* 561–574.

Tesser, A., & Collins, J. E. (1988). Emotion in social reflection and comparison situations: Intuitive, systematic, and exploratory approaches. *Journal of Personality and Social Psychology, 55,* 695–709.

Tesser, A., & Paulhus, D. (1983). The definition of self: Private and public self-evaluation management strategies. *Journal of Personality and Social Psychology, 44,* 672–682.

Tesser, A., & Smith, J. (1980). Some effects of task relevance and friendship on helping: You don't always help the one you like. *Journal of Experimental Social Psychology, 16,* 482–590.

Whitehurst, R. N. (1977). Jealousy and American values. In G. Clanton & L. G. Smith (Eds.), *Jealousy* (pp. 136–140). Englewood Cliffs, NJ: Prentice-Hall.

# Index

## O

Open marriage, studies of, 59, 61, 71, 124, 160
Ortega y Gasset, José, 12
Osiris, myth of, 27–28
"Ought force," 83
Overgeneralization, 109
Overt behaviors, 110

## P

Pairbonding, 253
Parent–child relationship, 123, 132, 134, 135
Paternity confidence, 163, 256–257, 258–260
Personality disorder, 233, 234
Personalization, 109
Powerlessness, 41
Preventive jealousy, 168–169, 170–171
Problem solving, 164–165, 246
Projective Jealousy Scales, 63, 64
Psychological health, measuring, 63
Punishment, 66, 74, 75, 111, 153

## R

Reactive jealousy, 107, 108, 109–111, 149–168, 170–171
  coping strategies of, 110
  relationship of with suspicious jealousy, 111–112, 114
Reactive retribution, 47, 180, 185, 187, 188, 189
Reality testing, 234
Reappraisal, 53, 67–68, 75, 111, 224
Reciprocity, 156–157, 172
Relationship Interaction Satisfaction Scale, 170
Relationship Jealousy Scale, 64

Relationship rewards, 153, 155
  loss of, 55–56, 57, 72, 74, 198
  threats to, 243
Relative salience, of feelings, 26–27
Religiosity, and jealousy, 217
Rejection, 16, 21–22, 55
Resentment, 11–12, 13, 23, 81, 95, 169–170
  agent-focused vs. global, 12–15
  unsanctioned, 23, 84
Responsibility, 110
Ressentiment, 92, 96
Righteous indignation, 14, 87
Rival derogation
  in envy, 280
  in jealousy, 225, 240, 244, 280–281
Romantic Love Scale, 58, 64
Romantic relationship, studies of jealousy in, 60–65, 68–74, 114–123, 124–126, 133–143, 146–147, 151, 155–167, 169–171, 180–204, 215–218, 225
Romantic Relationship Scale (RRS), 135, 138, 143, 146–147
Rousseau, Jean-Jacques, 90–91
Rusbult, C. E., and EVLN model, 199–203

## S

Sadness
  antecedents of, 41
  prototype of, 42, 43, 44, 47
  in reactive jealousy, 111
Salieri, Antonio, 79, 80, 81–82, 84, 85–86, 95
*Schadenfreude*, 96
Scheler, M., theory of envy, 82–83, 91, 92
Schizophrenia, 241
Selective abstraction, 109
Self-assessment, 245
Self-control, 33, 36, 47